TARASCON CLINICAL REVIEW SERIES

Internal Medicine

From the publishers of the *Tarascon Pocket Pharmacopoeia*®

Joseph S. Esherick, MD, FAAFP

Associate Director of Medicine
Medical ICU Director
Ventura County Medical Center
Ventura, CA

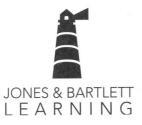

JONES & BARTLETT
LEARNING

World Headquarters
Jones & Bartlett Learning
5 Wall Street
Burlington, MA 01803
978-443-5000
info@jblearning.com
www.jblearning.com

Jones & Bartlett Learning books and products are available through most bookstores and online booksellers. To contact Jones & Bartlett Learning directly, call 800-832-0034, fax 978-443-8000, or visit our website, www.jblearning.com.

Production Credits
Senior Acquisitions Editor: Nancy Anastasi Duffy
Editorial Assistant: Marisa LaFleur
Production Assistant: Alex Schab
Manufacturing and Inventory Control Supervisor: Amy Bacus
Digital Marketing Manager: Rebecca Leitch
Composition: CAE Solutions Corp.
Cover Image: © Imagezoo/Getty Images
Cover Design: Scott Moden
Photo Research Assistant: Ashley Dos Santos
Printing and Binding: Edwards Brothers Malloy
Cover Printing: Edwards Brothers Malloy

ISBN: 978-1-4496-3642-5

6048
Printed in the United States of America
16 15 14 13 12   10 9 8 7 6 5 4 3 2 1

DEDICATION

We would like to dedicate this book to our respective families who have continued to encourage us and support us through this wonderful but long journey. I would especially like to thank my wonderful wife Gina and daughter Sophia. Without you, this project would not have been completed.

CONTENTS

Dedication.................................... iii
Contributing Authors
  and Reviewers......................... vi
Preface... vii
Abbreviations and Acronyms...... viii

**Section I Cardiovascular
  Medicine................................. 2**
1. Chest Pain 3
2. ST Elevation Myocardial
   Infarction........................... 8
3. Non-ST Elevation Acute
   Coronary Syndrome
   (NSTEMI and Unstable
   Angina)........................... 12
4. Congestive Heart Failure...... 16
5. Atrial Fibrillation................. 23
6. Bradyarrhythmias 30
7. Acute Pericarditis................. 36
8. Valvular Heart Disease......... 39
9. Perioperative Cardiovascular
   Evaluation 46
10. Hypertension 49
11. Peripheral Arterial
    Disease............................ 54
12. Shock 57
13. Syncope................................ 61

Section II Endocrinology 66
14. Inpatient Management of
    Diabetes Mellitus............. 67
15. Hyperthyroidism and
    Thyroid Storm 72
16. Hypothyroidism and
    Myxedema Coma............. 76
17. Adrenal Insufficiency........... 79
18. Calcium Disorders............... 82
19. Sodium Disorders................ 85
20. Potassium Disorders........... 88
21. Panhypopituitarism............. 91

**Section III
  Gastroenterology................. 94**
22. Evaluation of Acute
    Abdominal Pain 95
23. Upper Gastrointestinal
    Bleeding (UGIB).............. 98
24. Lower Gastrointestinal
    Bleeding (LGIB) 101
25. Diarrhea............................ 104
26. Acute Hepatitis 110
27. Cirrhosis 114
28. Acute Pancreatitis............. 120
29. Ischemic Bowel Disease..... 123
30. Esophageal Disorders 125

31. Diverticulitis 127
32. Bowel Obstruction............. 129
33. Biliary Tract Disorders....... 131

Section IV Hematology........... 136
34. Anemia.............................. 137
35. Sickle Cell Anemia 142
36. Bleeding Disorders............. 144
37. Pancytopenia..................... 146
38. Thrombocytopenia............. 147
39. Venous
    Thromboembolism 151
40. Perioperative Management
    of Anticoagulation and
    Antithrombotics............. 157

**Section V Infectious
  Disease.............................. 160**
41. Evaluation of Fever
    in the Hospitalized
    Patient............................ 161
42. Infective Endocarditis 163
43. Infections in HIV-Positive
    Patients.......................... 167
44. Meningitis 196
45. Pneumonia........................ 200
46. Management of Invasive
    Fungal Infections........... 204
47. Skin, Soft Tissue, Bone,
    and Joint Infections........ 211
48. Management of Catheter-
    Related Bloodstream
    Infections (CRBSI) 217
49. Tuberculosis...................... 219
50. Urinary Tract Infections:
    Cystitis and
    Pyelonephritis............... 222

Section VI Neurology 224
51. Acute Ischemic Stroke....... 225
52. Acute Hemorrhagic
    Stroke 230
53. Dementia 234
54. Delirium............................ 236
55. Seizures 238
56. Weakness 242

Section VII Oncology.............. 252
57. Adverse Effects of
    Chemotherapeutic
    Agents 253
58. Breast Cancer 257
59. Colorectal Cancer.............. 260
60. Chronic Leukemias............ 263
61. Lymphomas....................... 266

62. Multiple Myeloma.............. 270
63. Lung Cancer...................... 272
64. Prostate Cancer 275
65. Oncological Emergencies ... 277

**Section VIII Pulmonary
  Medicine............................ 286**
66. Evaluation of Chronic
    Cough............................. 287
67. Evaluation of Dyspnea 290
68. Evaluation of Hemoptysis... 292
69. Evaluation of Pleural
    Effusions 295
70. Asthma Exacerbation 298
71. Chronic Obstructive
    Pulmonary Disease
    Exacerbation.................. 303
72. Perioperative Pulmonary
    Evaluation and
    Management 306
73. Diffuse Interstitial Lung
    Disease........................... 308
74. Pulmonary Hypertension..... 310

Section IX Renal..................... 312
75. Evaluation of Acid-Base
    Disorders 313
76. Evaluation of Hematuria 315
77. Nephrotic Syndrome 317
78. Acute Kidney Injury............ 319
79. Chronic Kidney Disease...... 323
80. Nephrolithiasis.................. 328

Section X Rheumatology......... 330
81. Evaluation of Acute
    Monoarticular Arthritis... 331
82. Evaluation of Acute
    Back Pain 332
83. Evaluation of Polyarticular
    Arthritis......................... 336
84. Rheumatoid Arthritis.......... 341
85. Systemic Lupus
    Erythematosus............... 349
86. Systemic Vasculitis 352

**Section XI Substance
  Abuse Abstinence
  Disorders........................... 356**
87. Alcohol Withdrawal
    Syndromes..................... 357
88. Opiate Withdrawal
    Syndrome....................... 359
89. Sympathomimetic (Cocaine
    and Amphetamines)
    Withdrawal Syndrome.... 360

Section XII Appendix............... **362**
A1. ACLS Algorithms............... 363
A2. Format for Admission
Orders.......................... 370
A3. Format for History
and Physical
Exam........................... 371
A4. Format for SOAP
Progress Note.............. 372
A5. Format for Transfer
Summary..................... 373
A6. Format for Discharge
Summary..................... 374
A7. Procedure Note
Templates.................... 375
A8. ECG Interpretation........... 386
A9. How to Read a Chest
X-Ray.......................... 389
A10. How to Read an
Abdominal
X-Ray.......................... 391

A11. Empiric Antibiotics for
Common Infections in
Immunocompetent
Adults 392
A12. Antibiotic Coverage
by Class....................... 395
A13. Gram-Stain
Interpretation............... 399
A14. Common Toxidromes
and Overdoses............. 400
A15. Electrolyte Repletion......... 404
A16. Corticosteroid
Equivalency
Chart 405
A17. Acute Pain Control........... 406
A18. How to Write an
Order and a
Prescription 411
A19. Documentation of Labs
and Normal Drug
Levels 412

A20. Miscellaneous Tables
and Figures.................. 413
A21. Top Ten List for
Being a Great
Medical Student.......... 416
A22. Miscellaneous
Neurologic
Tables and
Figures........................ 417
A23. Snellen Eye
Chart 421
A24. Prophylaxis for
Hospitalized
Adults 422
A25. Equations....................... 425
A26. Urinalysis
Interpretation............... 426
A27. Peripheral Blood
Smear.......................... 427

Index 428

CONTRIBUTING AUTHORS AND REVIEWERS

Contributing Authors:

Jaehyun Byun, M.D
Family Medicine
Ventura County Medical Center
Ventura, CA

George C. Chen, D.O., M.P.H.
Family Medicine
Ventura County Medical Center
Ventura, CA

Jacob David, M.D.
Family Medicine
Ventura County Medical Center
Ventura, CA

Jeannette Kenny, M.D.
Family Medicine Resident
Ventura County Medical Center
Ventura, CA

Mish Mizrahi, M.D.
Family Medicine
Ventura County Medical Center
Ventura, CA

Suemae Ooi, M.D.
Family Medicine
Ventura County Medical Center
Ventura, CA

Mackenzie Slater, M.D.
Family Medicine Resident
Ventura County Medical Center
Ventura, CA

Reviewers: Theresa Cho, M.D., family medicine; Daniel Clark, M.D., FACC, FAHA, cardiology; Robert Dergalust, M.D., neurology; Lauren G. Ficks, M.D., endocrinology; Saumil Gandhi, M.D., nephrology; Mark Lepore, M.D., family medicine, hospitalist; Charles Menz, M.D., gastroenterology; Duane Pearson, M.D., rheumatology; Rick Rutherford, M.D., family medicine; Gail Simpson, M.D., FACP, infectious disease; Evan Slater, M.D., hematology-oncology; Ravi Bajwa, M.D., pulmonology

PREFACE

The **Tarascon Clinical Review Series: Internal Medicine** pocketbook is an evidence-based, point-of-care reference for the busy medical student or resident physician to use on your internal medicine rotation or externship. This pocket reference has all the pertinent information contained within a comprehensive internal medicine textbook consolidated into an easily navigable pocketbook. This pocketbook provides you with critical information about the evaluation and management of every common medical disorder encountered in the hospital, including the most common conditions encountered in the ICU.

This pocketbook was written in collaboration with a stellar group of resident physicians and with considerable input from medical students so that it would contain all the information that medical students and resident physicians need to answer your attending's questions (so that you shine during morning rounds)! The pocketbook includes the most important aspects of epidemiology, pathophysiology, and clinical presentation in addition to all of the key aspects of patient evaluation and management. The pocketbook is packed with tables and algorithms intended to quickly direct the busy student or resident to an evidence-based approach to manage virtually all medical disorders. It also contains templates for order writing, note writing, procedure notes, and guides to reading ECGs, X-rays, empiric antibiotics, therapeutic drug levels, interpretation of urinalyses, peripheral blood smears, and equivalency tables for corticosteroids and opioids among others.

Although the **Tarascon Clinical Review Series: Internal Medicine** pocketbook is ideal for medical students, resident physicians and midlevel providers on their internal medicine rotations, it is also a perfect reference guide for practicing hospitalists and for medical or surgical subspecialists who want a quick reference guide for internal medicine disorders.

I would like to thank all my colleagues who have passed on to me countless clinical pearls, most of which I have incorporated into this pocketbook. I would also like to thank the hospital librarian, Janet Parker, who has worked so hard to acquire virtually all of the reference articles and clinical practice guidelines that were used for the preparation of this manuscript.

The information within this pocketbook has been compiled from sources believed to be reliable. Nevertheless, the **Tarascon Clinical Review Series: Internal Medicine** pocketbook is intended to be a clinical guide only; it is not meant to be a replacement for sound clinical judgment. Although painstaking efforts have been made to find all errors and omissions, some errors may remain. If you find an error or wish to make a suggestion, please email your comments to editor@tarascon.com.

Best wishes,

Joe Esherick, MD, FAAFP

ABBREVIATIONS AND ACRONYMS

Esherick: *Tarascon Internal Medicine Pocketbook*, 2014 edition

×	for; times	AHA	American Heart Association
μL	microliter	AHCPR	Agency for Health Care Policy and Research
3TC	lamivudine		
5-FU	fluorouracil	AI	aortic or adrenal insufficiency
AA	aldosterone antagonist	AICD	automatic implantable cardioverter defibrillator
AAA	abdominal aortic aneurysm		
AAH	acute alcoholic hepatitis	AIDS	acquired immunodeficiency syndrome
Ab	antibody (antibodies)		
ABC	airway, breathing, and circulation	AIHA	autoimmune hemolytic anemia
		AIN	acute interstitial nephritis
ABCD score	**A**ge, **B**lood pressure, **C**linical findings, **D**uration of TIA	AIP	acute intermittent porphyria
		AKI	acute kidney injury
ABG	arterial blood gas	ALI	acute lung injury
ABI	ankle brachial index	ALL	acute lymphoblastic leukemia
ABLC	amphotericin B lipid complex (Abelcet)	ALT	alanine aminotransferase
		AmB	amphotericin B deoxycholate
ABPA	allergic bronchopulmonary aspergillosis	AML	acute myeloid leukemia
		AMS	acute changes in mental status
AC	anticholinergic; arterial catheter	ANA	antinuclear antibody
ACA	anterior cerebral artery	ANC	absolute neutrophil count
ACC	American College of Cardiology	ANCA	antineutrophil cytoplasmic antibodies
ACD	anemia of chronic disease		
ACE	angiotensin-converting enzyme	ANP	atrial natriuretic peptide
ACEI	angiotensin-converting enzyme inhibitor	anti-TPO	antithyroid peroxidase antibody
		AP	anteroposterior
ACLS	advanced cardiovascular life support	A/P	assessment/plan
		APACHE (score)	Acute Physiology and Chronic Health Evaluation
ACPA	anti-citrullinated protein antibody		
		APC	activated protein C; adenomatous polyposis coli (gene)
ACR	American College of Rheumatology		
		APP gene	amyloid precursor protein (coding) gene
ACS	acute coronary syndrome		
ACTH	adrenocorticotropic hormone	aPTT	activated partial thromboplastin time
ADH	antidiuretic hormone		
ADHF	acute decompensated heart failure	AR	atrial regurgitation
		ARB	angiotensin receptor blockers
ADL(s)	activities of daily living	ARDS	acute respiratory distress syndrome
ADP	adenosine diphosphate		
AED	antiepileptic drug; automated external defibrillator	ARF	acute renal failure
		ARR	aldosterone/renin ratio
AF; Afib	atrial fibrillation	ART	antiretroviral therapy
AFB	acid-fast bacillus	AS	aortic stenosis
AFP	American Family Physician	ASA	aspirin; American Society of Anesthesiologists
AG	anion gap		
AGN	acute glomerulonephritis		

ASIS	anterior superior iliac spine	CCP	cyclic citrulinated peptide (antibody)
AST	aspartate aminotransferase		
ATD	antithyroid drug(s)	CCS	Canadian Cardiovascular Society
ATN	acute tubular necrosis		
ATP	adenosine triphosphate	CD	cluster of differentiation; correction dose; Crohn's disease
ATS	American Thoracic Society		
AV	atrioventricular		
AVA	aortic valve area	CDC	Centers for Disease Control and Prevention
AVB	atrioventricular block		
AVM	arteriovenous malformation	CEA	carcinoembryonic antigen; carotid endarterectomy
AVR	aortic valve replacement		
ax	axillary	CF	complement-fixing (antibody); correction factor; cystic fibrosis,
BAE	bronchial artery embolism		
BAL	bronchoalveolar lavage		
BCG	Bacille Calmette-Guérin	CFU	colony-forming unit
BE	Barrett's esophagus	CHADS	**C**ongestive heart failure, **H**ypertension, **A**ge, **D**iabetes, prior **S**troke
bid	two times per day		
biw	two times per week		
BLS	basic life support	CHB	complete heart block
BM	bowel movement	CHF	congestive heart failure
BMI	body mass index	CI	cardiac index
BMP	basic metabolic panel	CIDP	chronic inflammatory demyelinating polyneuropathy
BMT	blood and marrow transplant		
BNP	brain natriuretic peptide		
BOOP	bronchiolitis obliterans with organizing pneumonia	CIWP-Ar	Clinical Institute Withdrawal Assessment for Alcohol
BP	blood pressure	CK	creatine kinase
BPH	benign prostatic hyperplasia	CKD	chronic kidney disease
bpm	beats per minute	CKD-EPI	Chronic Kidney Disease Epidemiology Collaboration (equation)
BRCA	breast cancer		
BSA	body surface area		
BUN	blood urea nitrogen	CK-MB	creatine kinase myocardial band
Ca	calcium		
CA	cancer	CLL	chronic lymphocytic leukemia
CABG	coronary artery bypass surgery	cm	centimeter
CAD	coronary artery disease	CML	chronic myeloid leukemia
CA-MRSA	community-acquired methicillin-resistant *Staphylococcus aureus*	CMP	comprehensive metabolic panel
		CMV	cytomegalovirus
		CNS	central nervous system
c-ANCA	cytoplasmic antineutrophil cytoplasmic antibodies	COPD	chronic obstructive pulmonary disease
CAP	community-acquired pneumonia	COX-2	cyclooxygenase type 2
cap(s)	capsule(s)	CP	chest pain
CART	classification and regression tree	CPAP	continuous positive airway pressure
		CPP	cerebral perfusion pressure
CAS	carotid artery stenosis	CPPD	calcium pyrophosphate dehydrate
cath lab	catheterization lab		
CBC	complete blood count	CPR	cardiopulmonary resuscitation
CBCD	complete blood count with differential	Cr	creatinine
		CRBSI	catheter-related bloodstream infections
CBD	common bile duct		
CC	chief complaint		
CCB	calcium channel blockers	CrCl	creatinine clearance

CREST	**c**alcinosis, **R**aynaud's phenomenon, **e**sophageal dysmotility, **s**clerodactyl and **t**elangiectasias (syndrome)	DNR	Do Not Resuscitate (order)
		DOT	directly observed therapy
		DPI	dry powder inhaler
		DS	double strength
CRH	corticotropin-releasing hormone	dsDNA	double-stranded DNA
CRP	c-reactive protein	dTMP	deoxythymidine monophosphate
crt	creatinine	DTR	deep tendon reflex(es)
CRT	cardiac resynchronization therapy (pacemaker)	dUMP	deoxyuridine monophosphate
		DUS	duplex ultrasound
CSF	cerebrospinal fluid	DVT	deep venous thrombosis
CT	computed tomography	Dx	diagnosis
CTCA	computed tomography coronary angiogram	EBL	estimated blood loss
		EBV	Epstein-Barr virus
CTPA	computed tomography pulmonary angiogram	ECG	electrocardiogram
		echo	echocardiogram
CURB score	**C**onfusion, **U**rea, **R**espiratory rate, **B**lood pressure	ECOG	Eastern Cooperative Oncology Group
CV	cardiovascular	ED	emergency department; erectile dysfunction
CVA	cerebrovascular accident (stroke)	EDTA	ethylenediaminetetraacetic acid
CVC	central venous catheter	EEG	electroencephalogram
CVD	cardiovascular disease	EG	ethylene glycol
CVP	central venous pressure	EGD	esophagogastroduodenoscopy
CXR	chest x-ray	EGFR	epidermal growth factor receptor
d5W	dextrose 5% in water		
DAS	disease activity scale	EMB	ethambutol
DBP	diastolic blood pressure	EMG	electromyogram
DC	direct current (cardioversion)	epi	epinephrine
DCC	deleted in colorectal carcinoma (gene)	EPS	electrophysiologic study
		ER	emergency room; estrogen receptor; extended release
DCIS	ductal carcinoma in situ (breast cancer)	ERCP	endoscopic retrograde cholangiopancreatography
DDAVP	desmopressin		
DDD	**D**ual mode, **D**ual chamber, **D**ual sensing (pacemaker)	ESRD	end-stage renal disease
		ESR	erythrocyte sedimentation rate
DEXA	dual-energy x-ray absorptiometry	ESWL	extracorporeal shock wave lithotripsy
		ETT	endotracheal tube
DFBCL	diffuse large B-cell lymphoma	EVL	endoscopic variceal ligation
DHEA	dehydroepiandrosterone	FAP	familial adenomatous polyposis
DI	diabetes isipidus	FAST scale	**F**unctional **A**ssessment **St**aging scale
DIC	disseminated intravascular coagulation		
		FC	flucytosine
DILD	diffuse interstitial lung disease	FDA	U.S. Food and Drug Administration
DIP	distal interphalangeal		
DIS	dissemination in space	Fe	iron
DIT	dissemination in time	FENa	fractional excretion of sodium
DKA	diabetic ketoacidosis	FEurea	fractional excretion of urea
dL	deciliter	FEV_1	forced expiratory volume in 1 second
DM	diabetes mellitus		
DMARD	disease-modifying antirheumatic drugs	FFP	fresh frozen plasma
		FISH	fluorescence in-situ hybridization
DNA	deoxyribonucleic acid		
DNI	Do Not Intubate (order)		

FN	false negative	HCAP	healthcare-associated pneumonia
FP	false positive		
FSH	follicle-stimulating hormone	HCC	hepatocellular carcinoma
fT$_4$	free levo7thyroxine	HCO$_3$	bicarbonate
FTA	fluorescent treponemal antibody	HCQ	hydroxychloroquine
FVC	forced vital capacity	Hct	hemocrit
g	gram(s)	HCTZ	hydrochlorothiazide
G6PD	glucose-6-phosphate dehydrogenase	HCV	hepatitis C virus
		HCVAb	hepatitis C surface antibody
GABA	gamma-aminobutyric acid (receptor)	HD	hemodialysis; high dose
		HDC	hemodialysis catheter
GBS	Guillain–Barré Syndrome	HDL	high-density lipoprotein
GCS	Glasgow Coma Scale; graduated compression stockings	HEENT	head, eyes, ears, nose, and throat
GD	Graves' disease	HELLP	hemolysis elevated liver enzymes and low platelets (syndrome)
GE	gastroesophageal		
GERD	gastroesophageal reflux disease		
GFR	glomerular filtration rate	HER	human epidermal growth factor receptor
GGTP test	gamma-glutamyl transpeptidase		
		HEV	hepatitis E virus
GH	growth hormone	HF	heart failure
GI	gastrointestinal	HFS	hip fracture surgery
glc	glucose	Hgb	hemoglobin
GNR	gram-negative rod	HgbA1c	glycohemoglobin
GO	Graves' ophthalmopathy	HHV	human herpesvirus
GP	glycoprotein; granulomatosis with polyangiitis	HiB	haemophilus influenzae type b (meningitis)
GS	generalized seizure	HIDA	hepatobiliary iminodiacetic acid (scan)
gtt(s)	drop(s)		
GU	genitourinary	HIT	heparin-induced thrombocytopenia
h	hour(s)		
HA	headache; heart attack	HIV	human immunodeficiency virus
HAART	**h**ighly **a**ctive **a**nti**r**etroviral therapy	HL	Hodgkin's lymphoma
		HLA	human leukocyte antigen
HACEK	**H**aemophilus aphrophilus, **A**ctinobacillus actinomycetemcomitans, **C**ardiobacterium hominis, **E**ikenella corrodens, and **K**ingella kingae	HOCM	hypertrophic obstructive cardiomyopathy
		hpf	per high power field
		HPI	history of present illness
		HR	heart rate; hormone receptor
		HS	hereditary spherocytosis
HA-MRSA	hospital-acquired methicillin-resistant Staphylococcus aureus	HSM	hepatosplenomegaly
		HSV	herpes simplex virus
		HTLV	human T-cell lymphotropic virus
HAP	hospital-acquired pneumonia	HTN	hypertension
HAV	hepatitis A virus	HUS	hemolytic-uremic syndrome
HbA	adult "normal" hemoglobin	IABP	intra-aortic balloon pump
HBeAG	hepatitis B e antigen	IBD	inflammatory bowel disease
HbF	fetal hemoglobin	IBS	irritable bowel syndrome
HBIG	hepatitis B immune globulin	IC	internal capsule
HbS	sickle-cell hemoglobin	ICD	implantable cardioverter defibrillator
HBsAb	hepatitis B surface antibody		
HBsAg	hepatitis B surface antigen	ICH	intracerebral hemorrhage
HBV	hepatitis B virus	ICP	intracranial pressure

ICS	intercostal space		LBP	lower back pain
ICSI	Institute for Clinical Systems Improvement		LCIS	lobular carcinoma in situ
ICU	intensive care unit		LDH	lactate dehydrogenase
ID	identification		LDL	low-density lipoprotein
IDA	iron deficiency anemia		LE	leukocyte esterase; lower extremity; lupus erythematosus
IDSA	Infectious Diseases Society of America			
IE	infective endocarditis		LEF	leflunamide
IFN	interferon		LFTs	liver function tests
Ig	immunoglobulin (A, E, G, M)		LGIB	lower gastrointestinal bleed
IGF-1	insulin-like growth factor 1		LH	luteinizing hormone
IGRA	Interferon Gamma Release Assay (test)		LHRH	luteinizing hormone releasing hormone
IM	intramuscular		LIMA	left internal mammary artery
INH	isoniazid		LipAmB	liposomal amphotericin B
INR	international normalized ratio		LLQ	left lower quadrant
IP	interphalangeal		LMHW	low molecular weight heparin
IPC	intermittent pneumatic compression device(s)		LMN	lower motor neuron
			LOS	length of stay
IPF	idiopathic pulmonary fibrosis		LP	lumbar puncture
iPTH	intact parathyroid hormone		LR	likelihood ratio
IRIS	immune reconstitution syndrome		LRINEC	Laboratory Risk Indicator for Necrotizing Fasciitis
IRU	immune recovery uveitis		LUQ	left upper quadrant
ITP	idiopathic thrombocytopenic purpura		LV	left ventricular
			LVAD	left ventricular assist device
IU	international units		LVEDP	left ventricular end-diastolic pressure
IV	intravenous			
IVDU	intravenous drug use		LVEF	left ventricular ejection fraction
IVIG	intravenous immunoglobulin		LVESD	left ventricular end-diastolic dimension
IVP	intravenous pyelogram			
J	joule		LVH	left ventricular hypertrophy
JAK2	JanusKinase 2		M	monoclonal
JC virus	John Cunningham virus		MAC	*Mycobacterium avium* complex
JVD	jugular venous distention		MALT	mucosa-associated lymphoid tissue (lymphoma)
K	potassium			
KCl	potassium chloride		MAOI	monoamine oxidase inhibitor
KDIGO	**K**idney **D**isease: **I**mproving **G**lobal **O**utcomes		MAP	mean arterial pressure
			MAS	macrophage activation syndrome
kg	kilogram			
KS	Kaposi's sarcoma		MAT	multifocal atrial tachycardia
KUB	kidneys, ureters, and bladder		max	maximum
L	left; liter		MCA	middle cerebral artery
LA	left atrium		MCD	multicentric Castleman's disease
LABA	long-acting β₂-agonist(s)			
LACI	lacunar infarct		mcg	microgram
LAD	left anterior descending; lymphadenopathy		MCP	metacarpophalangeal(s)
			MCTD	mixed connective tissue disease
			M-CTPA	multidetector CT pulmonary angiogram
LAM	lymphangioleiomyomatosis			
lb	pound		MCV	mean corpuscular volume
LBBB	left bundle branch block		MD	medical doctor
LBO	large bowel obstruction		MDI	metered dose inhaler

MDR	multidrug resistant		Nd-YAG	neodymium-doped yttrium aluminum garnet laser
MDRD	modification of diet in renal disease (equation)		neb	nebulized
MELD score	Model for End-State Liver Disease		NF	necrotizing fasciitis; nuclear factor
mEq	milliequivalent		ng	nanogram
METs	metabolic equivalents		NGT	nasogastric tube
mg	milligram		NHL	non-Hodgkin lymphoma
Mg	magnesium		NHLBI	National Heart, Lung, and Blood Institute
MGC	myasthenia gravis crisis			
MI	myocardial infarction		NICE	National Institute for Health and Clinical Education (UK)
MIC	minimum inhibitory concentration			
			NIH	National Institutes of Health
min	minute		NIHSS	NIH Stroke Scale
mL	milliliter		NK cell	natural killer cell
mm	millimeter		NL	normal
MM	multiple myeloma		NMDA	N-Methyl-D-aspartic acid (receptor)
mmHg	millimeter of mercury			
mmol	millimole		NNRTI	non-nucleoside reverse transcriptase inhibitor
MMSE	Mini-Mental Status Exam			
mo	months old (NOTE: this is NOT an abbreviation for "month" or "months")		NNT	numbers needed to treat
			NO	nitric oxide
			NPH insulin	neutral protamine Hagedorn insulin
mOsm	milliosmole			
MODS	multiple organ dysfunction syndrome		NPO	nothing per oral (by mouth)
			NPV	negative predictive value
MPO	myeloperoxidase		N/R	not recommended
MR	mitral regurgitation		NS	normal saline
MRA	magnetic resonance angiogram		NSAIDs	non-steroidal anti-inflammatory drugs
MRI	magnetic resonance imaging		NSCLC	non-small-cell lung carcinoma
MRSA	methicillin-resistant *Staphylococcus aureus*		NSTE-ACS	non-ST-elevation acute coronary syndrome
ms	millisecond(s)		NSTEMI	non-ST-elevation myocardial infarction
MS	mitral stenosis; multiple sclerosis			
			NSTI	necrotizing soft tissue infection(s)
MSSA	methicillin-susceptible *Staphylococcus aureus*		NT-proBNP	N-terminal prohormone of brain natriuretic peptide
MTP	metatarsophalangeal(s)			
MTX	methotrexate		NYHA	New York Heart Association
mU	milliunit		NTG	nitroglycerin
MUGA	multigated acquisition scan		NT-proBNP	N-terminal prohormone of brain natriuretic peptide
MV	mitral valve			
MVI	multivitamin		N/V	nausea/vomiting
MVR	mitral valve replacement		NVE	native valve endocarditis
Na	sodium		OA	osteoarthritis
NAC	N-acetylcysteine		OB/GYN	obstetrics/gynecology
NaCl	sodium chloride		OCD	obsessive-compulsive disorder
NaHCO₃	sodium bicarbonate (baking soda)		OCP	oral contraceptive pills
			OGTT	oral glucose tolerance test
NCCN	National Comprehensive Cancer Network		OR	operating room
			ORC mesh	oxidized regenerated cellulose mesh
NCS	nerve conduction study			

OS	opening snap		PJP	*Pneumocystis jiroveci* pneumonia
OSA	obstructive sleep apnea			
osm	osmolality		PLT	platelet
P	port; probability		PMBV	percutaneous mitral balloon valvulotomy
PA	posteroanterior; pulmonary artery		PMI	point of maximal impulse
PAC	premature atrial complex		PMN	polymorphonuclear leukocytes
PACI	partial anterior circulation infarct		PMR	polymyalgia rheumatica
PACO$_2$	partial pressure of carbon dioxide		PNA	peptide nucleic acid
			PNH	paroxysmal noctural hemoglobinuria
PAD	peripheral arterial disease; pulmonary artery diastolic (pressure)		PO	per oral (by mouth)
			PO$_4$	phosphate
			POCI	posterior circulation infarct
PAH	pulmonary arterial hypertension		POD	perfusion on demand; postoperative day
PAN	polyarteritis nodosa		PORN	progressive outer retinal necrosis
p-ANCA	peripheral/perinuclear antineutrophil cytoplasmic antibodies		PPD	purified protein derivative (test)
PAT	paroxysmal atrial tachycardia		PPI	proton pump inhibitor
PBS	peripheral blood smear		PPV	positive predictive value
PCA	patient-controlled analgesia; posterior cerebral artery		PR	per rectum; progesterone receptor
PCC	prothrombin complex concentrate		PRBC	packed red blood cell
			prn	as needed
PCI	percutaneous coronary intervention		PS	partial seizure
			PSA	prostate-specific antigen
PCP	*Pneumocystis* pneumonia		PSI	**P**neumonia **S**everity **I**ndex
PCR	polymerase chain reaction		pt	patient
PCWP	pulmonary capillary wedge pressure		PT	physical therapy; prothrombin time
PDD	Parkinson's Disease dementia		PTEN	phosphatase and tensin homolog
PE	pleural effusion; pulmonary embolism		PTH	parathyroid hormone
PEA	pulseless electrical activity		PTHC	percutaneous transhepatic cholangiography
PEDIS	**p**erfusion, **e**xtent, **d**epth, **i**nfection, and **s**ensation (assessment)		PTHrP	parathyroid hormone-related protein
PEF	peak expiratory flow		PTP	pretest probability
PEL	primary effusion lymphoma		PTSD	post-traumatic stress disorder
PET scan	positron emission tomography scan		PTT	partial thromboplastin time
			PTU	propylthiouracil
PETCO$_2$	partial pressure of end-tidal carbon dioxide		PTX	pneumothorax
			PUD	peptic ulcer disease
PF	pleural fluid		PVC	premature ventricular contraction
PFO	patent foramen ovale			
pg	picogram		PVD	peripheral vascular disease
PHTN	pulmonary hypertension		PVE	prosthetic valve endocarditis
PI	protease inhibitor(s)		PZA	pyrazinamide
PID	pelvic inflammatory disease		q	every
PIP	proximal interphalangeal		qid	four times per day
PIV	peripheral intravenous line		R	right

RA	rheumatoid arthritis; right atrium	SIADH	syndrome of inappropriate antidiuretic hormone
RAI	radioactive iodine; relative adrenal insufficiency	SIRS	systemic inflammatory response syndrome
RAS	renal artery stenosis	SL	sublingual
RBBB	right bundle branch block	SLE	systemic lupus erythematosus
RBC	red blood cell/count	SMA	superior mesenteric artery
RB-ILD	respiratory bronchiolitis-interstitial lung disease	SNF	skilled nursing facility
		SOB	shortness of breath
RCA	right coronary artery; ristocetin cofactor activity	soln	solution
		Sosm	serum osmolality
RCRI	revised cardiac risk index	sp.	species
RDW	RBC distribution width	SPECT	single photon emission computed tomography
RF	rheumatoid factor (test); risk factor(s)	SPEP	serum protein electrophoresis
RFB	rifabutin	SpO_2	saturation of peripheral oxygen
RI	reticulocyte index	SQ	subcutaneous
RIF	rifampin	SR	sustained release
RIPA	ristocetin-induced platelet aggregation	SRH	stigmata of recent hemorrhage
		SS	single strength
RLQ	right lower quadrant	SSA/SSB	Sjögren's syndrome (A, B)
RML	right middle lobe	SSD	sickle-cell anemia
RMSF	Rocky Mountain spotted fever	SSKI	potassium iodide
RNA	ribonucleic acid	SSRI	selective serotonin reuptake inhibitor
RNP	ribonucleoprotein		
ROM	range of motion	SSSS	staphylococcal scalded skin syndrome
RPGN	rapidly progressive glomerulonephritis		
		SSTI	skin and soft tissue infection
RR	relative risk; respiratory rate	ST	ST segment
RS cell	Reed–Sternberg cells	STEMI	ST-elevation myocardial infarction
RT	radiation therapy		
RTA	renal tubular acidosis	sTfR	soluble transferring receptor
rtPA	recombinant tPA	SUDEP	sudden unexplained death in epilepsy
RUQ	right upper quadrant		
RV	right ventricular	susp	suspension
Rx	prescription/therapy	SVC	superior vena cava
S_1	first heart sound	SVRI	systemic vascular resistance index
S_2	second heart sound		
S_3	third heart sound	SVT	supraventricular tachycardia
S_4	fourth heart sound	sxs	symptoms
SA node	sinoatrial node	T3 RIA	triiodothyronine radioimmunoassay
SABA	short-acting β_2-agonist(s)		
SAH	subarachnoid hemorrhage	tab	tablet
SAO_2	arterial oxygen saturation	TACI	total anterior circulation infarct
SAP	severe acute pancreatitis	TAVI	transcatheter aortic valve implantation
SBO	small bowel obstruction		
SBP	spontaneous bacterial peritonitis; systolic blood pressure	TB	tuberculosis
		Tbili	total bilirubin
		TCA(s)	tricyclic antidepressant(s)
SC	subcutaneous	TCT	thrombin clotting time
SCC	small-cell carcinoma	TD	Traveler's Diarrhea
SCD	sickle-cell disease	TDF	tenofovir
SCLC	small-cell lung cancer	TDI	total daily insulin

TE	*Toxoplasma gondii* encephalitis	UE	upper extremity
TEE	transesophageal echocardiogram	UFH	unfractionated heparin
		UGI	upper gastrointestinal
TEN	toxic epidermal necrolysis disease	UGIB	upper gastrointestinal bleed
		UIP	usual interstitial pneumonitis
TF	tissue factor	ULN	upper limit of normal
THA	total hip arthroplasty	UMN	upper motor neuron
TIA	transient ischemic attack	UNa	urine sodium
TIBC	total iron-binding capacity	UO	urine output
tid	three times per day	UPA	undifferentiated polyarthritis
TIMI	thrombolysis in myocardial infarction	UPEP	urine protein electrophoresis
		UTI	urinary tract infection
TIPSS	transjugular intrahepatic portosystemic shunt	VATS	video-assisted thoracic surgery
		VDRL	venereal disease research laboratory (test)
tiw	three times per week		
TKA	total knee arthroplasty	VF; VFib	ventricular fibrillation
TKR	total knee replacement	VIP	vasoactive intestinal polypeptide
TLC	therapeutic lifestyle change(s)		
TLS	tumor lysis syndrome	V/Q	ventricular perfusion (lung scan)
TLSO	thoracolumbosacral orthosis (brace)		
		VSD	ventricular septal defect
TMP-SMX	trimethoprim-sulfamethoxazole	VT; VTach	ventricular tachycardia
TN	true negative	VTE	venous thromboembolism
TNF	tumor necrosis factor	VVIR	**V**entricular pacing, **V**entricular sensing, **I**nhibition response and **R**ate-adaptive (pacemaker)
TnI	troponin I		
TP	true positive		
tPA	tissue plasminogen activator		
TPN	total parenteral nutrition	vWD	von Willebrand disease
TPO	thyroid peroxidase antibody	VZV	varicella zoster virus
TSH	thyroid-stimulating hormone	XDR	extremely drug resistant
TSI	thyroid-stimulating immunoglobulin	WBC	white blood cell count
		WBRT	whole brain radiation therapy
TTE	transthoracic echocardiogram	WHO	World Health Organization
TTP	thrombotic thrombocytopenic purpura	wk(s)	week(s)
		WPW	Wolff-Parkinson-White syndrome
U	unit(s); urine		
UA	unstable angina; urinalysis	wt	weight
UACS	upper airway cough syndrome	yo	years old
UC	ulcerative colitis	ZAP70	zeta-chain-associated protein kinase 70
Ucrt	urinary creatinine		

TARASCON CLINICAL REVIEW SERIES

Internal Medicine

From the publishers of the *Tarascon Pocket Pharmacopoeia*®

Section I   Cardiovascular Medicine 2
Section II   Endocrinology 66
Section III   Gastroenterology 94
Section IV   Hematology......................................136
Section V   Infectious Disease..........................160
Section VI   Neurology 224

Section VII   Oncology..252
Section VIII   Pulmonary Medicine....................286
Section IX   Renal...312
Section X   Rheumatology...................................330
Section XI   Substance Abuse
        Abstinence Disorders..................................356

SECTION 1

CARDIOVASCULAR MEDICINE

CHAPTER 1

CHEST PAIN

1. ETIOLOGIES

- See **Tables 1.1** and **1.2**.

TABLE 1.1.   Non–Life-Threatening Causes of Chest Pain

Categories	Pericarditis	Esophageal Spasm	GERD (reflux esophagitis)	Costochondritis	Pneumonia (pleurisy)	Zoster	Peptic Ulcers	Acute Cholecystitis	Panic Attack
Quality	Sharp pain, +/– pleuritic	Squeezing substernal	Burning	Localized sharp	Pleuritic chest pain	Unilateral burning	Dull pain	Sharp right lower chest	Chest tightness
Radiation	Trapezius ridges	—	—	—	—	Dermatomal pattern	+/– to back	Right scapular tip	—
Associated signs and symptoms	Pericardial rub +/– effusion	—	Acid taste in mouth	—	Cough, fever, dyspnea, pleural rub	Vesicular rash	N/V, melena	N/V, anorexia	Sweating, palpitations, SOB
Exacerbating factors	Supine position, deep breathing	Swallowing	Eating, supine position	Palpation of affected site	Deep breaths	Palpation of affected area	Meals	Fatty foods	—
Relieving factors	Leaning forward	NTG, CCB	Antacids	NSAIDs	Oxygen, NSAIDs	Antivirals, steroids	Antacids	NPO	Benzodiazepine
Diagnostic studies	ECG, 2D-echo, increased TnI = myopericarditis	UGI, esophageal manometry	EGD, pH probe, UGI	Clinical diagnosis	CXR, sputum culture, abnormal lung exam	Clinical diagnosis	EGD, H. pylori testing	RUQ, ultrasound	Diagnosis of exclusion
Therapy	NSAIDS, colchine, steroids	CCB, nitrates	Acid suppression therapy	NSAIDs	Antibiotics, thoracentesis for large effusion	Antivirals, prednisone	Acid suppression therapy	Surgery	Counseling, anxiolytics

TABLE 1.2. Life-Threatening Causes of Chest Pain

Condition	Quality	Radiation	Associated Signs and Symptoms	Exacerbating Factors	Relieving Factors	Diagnostic Studies	Therapy
Acute MI or acute coronary syndrome	Chest pressure, heaviness, tightness, poorly localized	Neck, jaw, shoulders, arms	Nausea, diaphoresis, dyspnea, Levine sign	Exertion, emotional distress	Rest, nitrates, β-blockers, calcium-channel blockers	ECG, cardiac biomarkers, myocardial perfusion studies	See pages 8–15
Pulmonary embolus	Sudden onset, pleuritic chest pain	—	Dyspnea, cough, +/- hemoptysis, +/- effusion	Deep breaths	Oxygen	CTPA, V/Q scan	Heparin or LMWH, TPA for a massive PE
Acute aortic dissection	Sudden onset, "tearing" anterior chest pain or back pain	Interscapular area	Δ SBP greater than 20 mmHg between arms, new AI murmur, CXR with widened mediastinum	Hypertension, exertion	Rest, blood pressure control	CT angiogram of aortic arch	β-blockers to keep SBP less than or equal to 110 mmHg and HR less than 60, CT surgery consultation
Tension pneumothorax	Sudden onset, unilateral pleuritic chest pain	—	Dyspnea	Exertion, deep breaths	Oxygen, rest	CXR, chest ultrasound	Needle decompression then tube thoracostomy

2. <u>**CLINICAL PRESENTATION**</u>

   Life-Threatening Causes of Chest Pain
   - MI
     - Very likely: anterior chest pressure radiating to arms, neck, or back associated with hypotension, S3 gallop [LR+ 3.2, LR− 1], diaphoresis [LR+ 2.2, LR− 0.7]
     - Unlikely: sharp or pleuritic quality [LR+ 0.2] and reproducible tenderness [LR+ 0.2]
     - Traditional hand gestures in chest pain (*none have measurable diagnostic significance*):
       - Levine sign: clenched fist against sternum
       - Palm sign: extended palm against sternum
       - Arm sign: gripping the left arm
       - Pointing sign: indicating a single location with one or two fingers
   - **Pneumonia:** fever, cough, rhonchi, dyspnea, fatigue, egophony, dullness to percussion
   - **Heart failure:** dyspnea on exertion, peripheral edema, orthopnea, rales, wheezing, paroxysmal nocturnal dyspnea, displaced apical impulse
   - **Pulmonary embolism:** dyspnea (sudden onset), pleuritic chest pain, hemoptysis, syncope, hypotension

   Non–Life-Threatening Causes of Chest Pain
   - **Chest wall pain**: palpation of tender area reproduces the same chest pain; sharp, positional pain
   - **Panic disorder**
   - **GERD/PUD**: epigastric or retrosternal burning

3. <u>**EVALUATION OF CHEST PAIN**</u>

   - **Labs**
     - ECG and cardiac enzymes q 6–8 h × 3
     - Chemistry panel, CBCD
     - Consider high-sensitivity D-Dimer test if low pretest probability of PE (98% NPV if D-Dimer is less than 500 ng/mL)
   - **Radiology**
     - Chest X-ray
     - Multi-detector CTPA if intermediate–high pretest probability for PE
     - CT angiogram of aorta to evaluate for aortic dissection
     - Doppler ultrasound of lower extremities if intermediate–high pretest probability for PE
     - Echocardiogram for acute pericarditis or congestive heart failure
   - **Additional tests**
     - 12-lead ECG q 6–8 h
   - **Microbiology**
     - Blood cultures × 2 and sputum culture with Gram stain (if pneumonia suspected)
   - See **Table 1.3**

TABLE 1.3.   Pretest Probability of Significant CAD with Different Types of Chest Pain

Pretest Likelihood of Significant Coronary Artery Disease with Chest Pain (CP)						
	Nonanginal CP (1 or less of 3 sxs)		Atypical CP (2 of 3 sxs)		Typical CP (3 of 3 sxs)	
Age (yrs)	Men	Women	Men	Women	Men	Women
30–39	4%	2%	34%	12%	76%	26%
40–49	13%	3%	51%	22%	87%	55%
50–59	20%	7%	65%	31%	93%	73%
60–69	27%	14%	72%	51%	94%	86%

-symptoms (sxs): substernal CP; CP exacerbated by exertion; CP relieved by NTG or rest
Source: Adapted from NEJM, 1979: 300; 1350 and NEJM, 1979;301:230.
Probability values are expressed as percent of patients with significant coronary artery disease (greater than 70% stenosis) by coronary angiography

Noninvasive Evaluation for Coronary Artery Disease
- See **Table 1.4**

TABLE 1.4.   Noninvasive Cardiac Testing to Assess for Significant CAD

Test	Indications	Sensitivity	Specificity
Treadmill test*	• Evaluation of CP in low-risk patients • Exercise prescription • Risk stratification post-MI/PCI/CABG • Normal baseline ECG	60–68%	75%
Exercise radionuclide[†]	• Evaluation of CP in intermediate-risk patients • Abnormal baseline ECG • Better to evaluate atypical CP in women	87%	73%
Adenosine/Persantine/ regadenoson radionuclide[†‡]	• Evaluation of CP if unable to exercise • Contraindications: asthma or 2°/3° AVB	89%	75%
Dobutamine radionuclide[†]	• Evaluation of CP if unable to exercise & adenosine/Persantine/regadenoson contraindicated	86%	80–90%
Stress echocardiography	• Evaluation of CP in intermediate-risk patients	76–92%	75–88%

* Hold β-blockers on morning of exam and hold digoxin 7 or more days (if possible)
† Thallium-201 SPECT if pt weighs less than 250 lbs; 99mTc-sestamibi SPECT preferred if weight 250–400 lbs
‡ No caffeine or theophylline prior to exam

- **CT coronary angiogram**
  - β-blocker used to titrate HR 55–65
  - Most useful for patients with atypical chest pain, equivocal ECG, negative cardiac biomarkers, and intermediate pretest probability for CAD based on Duke Clinical Score
  - Good test to rule out CAD, but not to rule in significant CAD
  - Negative CTCA results in 99% NPV for CAD

4. <u>**INDICATIONS FOR CORONARY ANGIOGRAPHY**</u>

- High-risk treadmill test (see next section) at low workload
- Large reversible defect (greater than 10–15%) during cardiac radionuclide (thallium or technetium) testing
- Very high pretest probability (even without noninvasive testing)
- Refractory angina despite optimal medical therapy
- Left ventricular systolic dysfunction of unclear etiology
- History of sudden cardiac death or sustained ventricular tachycardia
- Suspected coronary vasospasm or anomalous coronary anatomy

5. <u>**HIGH-RISK TREADMILL FEATURES**</u>

- Symptom-limited treadmill at less than 5 METs exercise by Bruce protocol
- ST segment elevation or depression more than 2 mm with exercise
- Diffuse ST segment depression with exercise
- ST segment changes last longer than 5 minutes into the recovery period
- Hypotension with exercise
- Typical angina associated with ventricular arrhythmias or exercise-induced CHF

REFERENCES

Yoon YE, Wann S. Evaluation of acute chest pain in the emergency department: "triple rule-out" computed tomography angiography. *Cardiol Rev.* 2011;19(3):115–21.

CHAPTER 2

ST ELEVATION MYOCARDIAL INFARCTION

1. ## EPIDEMIOLOGY
   - Second most frequent reason for adult ED encounters, with 8 million visits yearly; 500,000 yearly incidence
   - Every 25 seconds an American has a coronary event; every minute, an American dies from a coronary event
   - Patients present with CP; STEMI occurs 5% of the time, and NSTEMI occurs 25% of the time
   - Multicenter Chest Pain Study: 22% of patients with ACS initially present with sharp/stabbing pain (13% pleuritic and 7% reproducible on palpation)
   - Risk factor: female (1.7:1), age, black

2. ## PATHOPHYSIOLOGY OF MYOCARDIAL ISCHEMIA
   - Acute drop in coronary blood flow due to thrombus obstructing coronary artery, usually caused by plaque rupture; if totally occlusive then STEMI, if subtotally occlusive then NSTEMI
   - Chronic progressive stenosis usually not associated with NSTEMI
   - Propagation of thrombus at disrupted plaque
   - ADP, epinephrine, and serotonin release cause platelet activation
   - Thromboxane A_2 release causes coronary vasoconstriction
   - Platelet glycoprotein IIB/IIIa receptor activation leads to platelet cross-linking

3. ## CLINICAL PRESENTATION
   - Findings that support a STEMI
     - Typical angina (precipitated by exertion, improved by rest or nitroglycerin, lasts less than 10 min) [LR+ 5.8]
     - Prior MI [LR+ 3.8, LR− 0.6]
     - SBP less than 100 [LR+ 3.6, LR− 1]
     - 3rd heart sound [LR+ 3.2, LR− 1]
     - Diaphoresis [LR+ 2.2, LR− 0.7]
     - JVD [LR+ 2.4, LR− 1]
     - Crackles [LR+ 2.1, LR− 1]
   - Findings that do *not* support a STEMI
     - Duration longer than 30 minutes [LR+ 0.1]
     - Sharp, pleuritic, or positional pain [LR+ 0.3]
     - Chest wall tenderness [LR+ 0.3]

4. ## DIAGNOSIS OF ACUTE STEMI
   - Chest pain or angina equivalent
   - ECG with ST segment elevation 1 mm or more in at least 2 contiguous leads OR
     - New LBBB
   - Troponin I greater than or equal to 0.6 or elevated CK-MB
   - See **Figure 2.1**

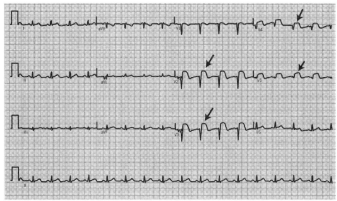

FIGURE 2.1.   ECG Demonstrating an Extensive Anterior Wall STEMI
The arrows demonstrate the concave downward ST elevations in the precordial V2-V5 leads

Source: Courtesy of Daniel Clark, M.D., Director of Medicine and Cardiology, Ventura County Medical Center, Ventura, California.

5. **DIFFERENTIAL DIAGNOSIS**
   - Aortic dissection
   - Pericarditis
   - Pulmonary embolus
   - Pulmonary edema
   - Esophageal spasm
   - Pneumothorax
   - Costochondritis
   - Panic attack

6. **WORKUP**
   - ECG within 10 minutes of arrival
   - CXR
   - Labs: cardiac enzymes q 6–8 h x 3, CBC, BMP
   - Consider echocardiogram for arrhythmias, shock, CHF, or a new regurgitant murmur

7. **TREATMENT**
   - Oxygen
   - Nitroglycerin 0.4 mg sublingual q 5 min × 3 for ongoing chest pain
   - Aspirin 325-mg tablet chewed, then 81–162 mg PO daily
   - β-blockers: metoprolol 5 mg IVP q 5 min × 3, then 25–50 mg PO q 6 h (titrate to HR 55–65)
   - Atorvastatin 80 mg PO daily, started immediately
   - Anticoagulation (one of the following):
     - Enoxaparin 30 mg IV bolus (younger than 75 yo), then 1 mg/kg SQ q 12 h (max 150 mg SQ q 12 h)
     - Heparin 60 Units/kg (max 4000 Units) IV bolus, then 12 Units/kg/h (max 1000 Units/h)
     - Fondaparinux 2.5 mg SQ daily
     - Bivalirudin 0.75 mg/kg IV bolus, then 1.75 mg/kg/h

- ADP receptor blockers (ideally given before Percutaneous coronary intervention (PCI), but withhold if high likelihood of urgent coronary artery bypass graft (CABG)):
  - Clopidogrel 300–600 mg PO load, then 75 mg PO daily
  - Prasugrel (younger than 75 yo) 60 mg PO load, then 10 mg PO daily (60 kg or higher), 5 mg/day (less than 60 kg)
- ACEI (e.g., captopril 6.25 mg PO bid), typically started on hospital day 2
- Primary PCI if symptoms within 12 hours or if more than 12 hours and ongoing/recurrent chest pain on maximal medical therapy
  - Door-to-balloon time goal is less than 90 minutes
  - If symptoms less than 12 hours and door-to-balloon time is longer than 90 minutes, thrombolysis is indicated
- Adjunctive therapy
  - Morphine 2 mg IVP q 5 min prn ongoing chest pain
  - Insulin prn fingerstick blood glucose greater than 180 mg/dL
  - Nitroglycerin infusion 5–200 mcg/min prn ongoing/recurrent chest pain
- Cardiac monitoring for arrhythmias
- 48–72 hours post-PCI or 5 days post-thrombolysis

8. **PROGNOSIS**
   - See **Table 2.1**

TABLE 2.1. TIMI Risk Score for STEMI

Historical	Points	Risk Score	30-Day Mortality in TIMI II (%)*
Age		0	0.8
• 75 yo or older	3		
• 65–74	2		
DM or HTN or Angina	1		
Exam		1	1.6
• SBP less than 100 mmHg	3	2	2.2
• HR greater than 200 bpm	2	3	4.4
• Killip II–IV	2	4	7.3
• Weight less than 67 kg (150 lbs)	1	5	12
Presentation		6	16
• Anterior ST elevation or LBBB	1	7	23
• Time to Rx more than 4 h	1	8	27
Risk Score = Total Points (0–14)		Greater than 8	38

*Entry criteria: CP longer than 30 min, elevated ST, symptom onset is less than 6 h, fibrinolytic eligible
Source: Morrow, David, et al., Clinical Investigation Reports. Circulation. 2000; 102: 2031–2037. Printed with permission by Wolters Kluwer Health.

9. **COMPLICATIONS**
   - **Left ventricular wall rupture**: incidence less than 1% and higher in first 2 weeks post-MI; larger infarct size, anterior infarct and lack of collateral flow; female; older than 70 yo; use of fibrinolytic therapy; death from hemopericardium/tamponade
   - **Interventricular septum rupture**: less frequent than free-wall rupture, typically occurs 3–5 days post-MI and as late as 2 weeks; increase in RV infarct
   - **Mitral regurgitation**: caused by ischemic papillary muscle displacement, papillary muscle or chordal rupture, and LV dilatation; 5% death from papillary muscle rupture

- **Arrhythmia:** includes SVTs, AV/intraventricular blocks, bradyarrhythmias, ventricular arrhythmias, reperfusion arrhythmias; higher incidence in STEMI vs NSTEMI; risk of ventricular fibrillation greatest within first hour of MI; risk factors include electrolyte imbalance, hypoxia, increased sympathetic activity
- **Left ventricular mural thrombus:** post anterior wall infarct; high risk of embolization
- **LV aneurysm:** incidence 3–15%; risk factors include females, complete LAD occlusion, no previous history of angina; medical therapy includes ACEIs and anticoagulation; surgical management only for severe heart failure, refractory ventricular arrhythmias, recurrent embolism
- **Pericarditis:** incidence 10%, typically within 24–96 hours of MI
- **Dressler syndrome:** autoimmune process with features of fever, chest pain; occurs 2–3 wks after MI; complications include cardiac tamponade, constrictive pericarditis, pleural effusion; treatment includes rest, NSAIDs, and steroids
- See **Figure 2.2**

FIGURE 2.2. ST Elevation Myocardial Infarction

- History of anginal-type CP or anginal equivalent
- ECG, CXR, Chem 7, CBC, PT, PTT, troponin I
- Establish IV and give oxygen

ECG with ST elevation greater than or equal to 1 mm in greater than or equal to 2 contiguous leads **or** new LBBB

Duration up to 12 h

- Primary PCI plus medical rx if door-balloon time or transfer-balloon time within 90 minutes
  OR
- TPA plus med rx if transfer or door-balloon times not achievable

Primary PCI preferred over TPA
- Cardiogenic shock
  - Adjunctive IABP
- NYHA Class III–IV CHF
- Unstable ventricular arrhythmias
- Rescue PCI if less than 50% ST segment resolution by 90 min s/p TPA
- Any contraindication for TPA

Contraindications for TPA
- Absolute
  - Prior ICH
  - Brain tumor, aneurysm, AVM
  - Ischemic stroke or closed head injury within 3 months
  - Active internal bleeding
  - Suspected aortic dissection
- Relative
  - BP greater than 180/110 mmHg
  - Ischemic stroke more than 3 months prior
  - CPR longer than 10 minutes
  - Trauma/major surgery within 3 wks
  - Internal bleed 2–4 wks ago
  - Noncompressible vessel puncture
  - Pregnancy
  - Current anticoagulation

Duration longer than 12 h

- Medical therapy
  OR
- Primary PCI plus medical rx for ongoing or recurrent chest pain

Medical Therapy for STEMI
- ASA 325 mg chewed, then 162 mg PO daily
- Metoprolol 5 mg IVP q 5 min × 3, then 25–50 mg PO q 6 h (desire HR 55–65)
- Atorvastatin 80 mg PO daily
- Anticoagulation (choose one of following to be given for entire hospitalization, up to 8 days):
  - Enoxaparin 30 mg IV bolus (younger than 75 yo), then 1 mg/kg SQ bid
    - 1 mg/kg SQ daily (CrCl 15–30 mL/min)
    - Avoid if CrCl less than 15 mL/min
  - Heparin 60 U/kg IV bolus, then 12 U/kg/h
  - Fondaparinux 2.5 mg IV, then 2.5 mg SQ daily; avoid if CrCl less than 30 mL/min
- Clopidogrel 300 mg PO × 1, then 75 mg PO daily (usually started after coronary anatomy is known)
- Nitroglycerin (SL, transdermal, or IV) for persistent chest pain
- Morphine 2 mg IV q 5 min prn severe CP
- GP IIb/IIIa inhibitor added in cath lab
- ACEI started on hospital day 2 as BP allows Earlier if needed for BP control ARB if patient is ACEI-intolerant
- Insulin titrated to chemsticks 80–150 × 48 h
- Consider eplerenone 25–50 mg PO daily if LVEF less than or equal to 0.4 post-MI *and* either DM or CHF

CHAPTER 3

NON–ST ELEVATION ACUTE CORONARY SYNDROME (NSTEMI AND UNSTABLE ANGINA)

1. <u>PATHOPHYSIOLOGY</u>
   - Mismatch between myocardial oxygen demand and supply at atherosclerotic plaque due to:
     - Plaque rupture with subtotal obstructive thrombus formation (see Chapter 2)
     - Coronary vasospasm (e.g., Prinzmetal angina)
     - Mechanical obstruction of coronary blood flow (e.g., progressive atherosclerosis)
     - Increased myocardial demand secondary to tachycardia, anemia, surgery, infection, etc.

2. <u>CLINICAL PRESENTATION</u>
   - Typical angina (50%): substernal chest pain, aggravated by exercise or mental stress and relieved by rest, lasts less than 10 minutes
   - Atypical angina (50%): shortness of breath, nausea, diaphoresis, atypical chest pain, or discomfort not located in chest

3. <u>DIAGNOSIS OF NSTE-ACS</u>
   - Chest pain or angina equivalent
   - ECG with ST segment depression 1 mm or more or localized T wave changes in at least 2 contiguous leads
   - Troponin I greater than or equal to 0.6 or elevated CK-MB indicates an NSTEMI
   - See **Figure 3.1**

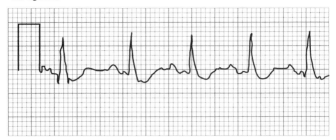

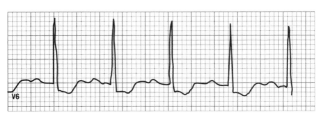

FIGURE 3.1.   Rhythm Strip Demonstrating ST Depressions Associated with an NSTEMI

Source: Courtesy of Daniel Clark, M.D., Director of Medicine and Cardiology, Ventura County Medical Center, Ventura, California.

4. **DIFFERENTIAL DIAGNOSIS**
   - Same as for STEMI
   - See **Table 3.1**

TABLE 3.1. Risk of Death or MI in Non−ST Elevation Acute Coronary Syndrome

Characteristics	High-risk ACS (Any of following)	Intermediate-risk ACS (No high risk; greater than or equal to 1 below)	Low-risk ACS (No intermediate−high risk)
History	• Accelerated tempo of ACS symptoms within 48 h	• Prior MI, PVD, CVD, CABG, or ASA use • Age older than 70 yo	• Age younger 70 yo
Pain	• Ongoing rest angina for at least 20 minutes	• Rest angina 20 min or more resolved with rest/NTG • Nocturnal angina • Severe/progressive angina within 2 weeks	• Increased frequency, severity, or duration of angina • New-onset angina
Exam	• CHF, S3, or increased rales • New/increased MR murmur • Hypotension • Age older than 75 yo	—	—
ECG	• Rest angina with ST depressed 0.5 mm or more • New LBBB • Sustained VT	• Old pathologic Q waves • Diffuse ST depressed less than 1 mm • T wave inversions	• Normal ECG or unchanged from baseline
Cardiac enzymes	• TnI greater than or equal to 0.1 ng/mL • Increased CK-MB	• TnI less than 0.1 ng/mL • Slight increase in CK-MB	• Normal after 6 h of observation

ACS = acute coronary syndrome
CABG = coronary artery bypass graft
CHF = congestive heart failure
CK-MB = MB isoenzyme of creatine kinase
TnI = Troponin I
MI = myocardial infarction
ST = ST segment
S3 = third heart sound
VT = ventricular tachycardia
Source: Adapted from 2007 ACC/AHA Guideline Update for UA/NSTEMI in JACC, 2007; 50(7): 652–726.

5. **WORKUP**
   - ECG within 10 minutes of arrival
   - CXR
   - Labs: CBC, BMP, cardiac enzymes q 6–8 h x 3
   - Consider echocardiogram for complicated ACS (arrhythmias, shock, CHF, or a new regurgitant murmur)
   - Myocardial perfusion study for low-risk ACS (TIMI Risk Score 0–2 and uncomplicated ACS) evaluating for perfusion defects

6. **TREATMENT**
   - Oxygen
   - Nitroglycerin 0.4 mg sublingual q 5 min × 3 for ongoing chest pain
   - Aspirin 325-mg tablet chewed, then 162 mg PO daily
   - β-blockers: metoprolol 5 mg IVP q 5 min × 3, then 25–50 mg PO q 6 h (titrate to HR 55–65)
   - Atorvastatin 80 mg PO daily, started immediately

- Anticoagulation (one of the following):
  - Enoxaparin 30 mg IV bolus (younger than 75 yo), then 1 mg/kg SQ q 12 h (max 150 mg SQ q 12 h)
  - Heparin 60 Units/kg (max 4000 Units) IV bolus, then 12 Units/kg/h (max 1000 Units/h)
  - Fondaparinux 2.5 mg SQ daily
  - Bivalirudin 0.75 mg/kg IV bolus, then 1.75 mg/kg/h
- ADP receptor blockers (ideally given before PCI, but withhold if high likelihood of urgent CABG)
  - Clopidogrel 300–600 mg PO load, then 75 mg PO daily
  - Prasugrel (younger than 75 yo) 60 mg PO load, then 10 mg PO daily (60 kg or more), 5 mg/day (less than 60 kg)
- GP IIb/IIIa inhibitors (consider initiating if PCI is indicated but procedure is delayed)
  - Abciximab, eptifibatide, or tirofiban
- ACEI (e.g., captopril 6.25 mg PO bid), typically started on hospital day 2 if:
  - NSTEMI, CHF, DM, HTN, or Left ventricular ejection fraction (LEVF) less than 0.4
- Cardiac catheterization with possible PCI for:
  - Intermediate–high risk ACS; persistent or recurrent angina despite optimal medical therapy; reversible ischemia more than 10–15% on myocardial perfusion study
- Adjunctive therapy
  - Morphine 2 mg IVP q 5 min prn ongoing chest pain
  - Insulin prn fingerstick blood glucose greater than 180 mg/dL
  - Nitroglycerin infusion 5–200 mcg/min prn ongoing/recurrent chest pain
- Cardiac monitoring
  - 24–48 hours post-PCI or 3–5 days post-NSTEMI treated medically

7. **PROGNOSIS**
   - See **Table 3.2**

TABLE 3.2. TIMI Risk Score for Unstable Angina/NSTEMI

TIMI Risk Score	0–1	2	3	4	5	6–7
Death/MI or urgent revascularization	4.7%	8.3%	13.2%	19.9%	26.2%	40.9%

1 point for each variable: age 65 or older; 3 or more CAD risk factors; known coronary stenosis 50% or more; ST depressed by 0.5 mm or more; greater than or equal to 2 anginal events within 24 h; ASA use within 7 days; elevated TnI or CK-MB
Source: Adapted from JAMA, 2000; 284(7): 835–42.

8. **COMPLICATIONS**
   - Mitral regurgitation
   - Arrhythmia (includes SVTs, AV/intraventricular blocks, bradyarrhythmias, ventricular arrhythmias)
   - Pericarditis
   - Dressler syndrome
   - See **Table 3.3** and **Figure 3.2**.

TABLE 3.3. When Invasive Strategy is Preferred Over Conservative Strategy for ACS

- Refractory angina
- TIMI Risk Score of 3 or more
- High-risk ACS
- Intermediate-risk NSTEMI
- CHF
- Sustained ventricular tachycardia
- PCI in last 6 months
- CABG
- LVEF less than 0.4
- New ST segment depressions by 0.5 mm or more
- High-risk findings on stress test

Source: Adapted from 2007 ACC/AHA Guideline Update for UA/NSTEMI in JACC, 2007; 50(7): 652–726.

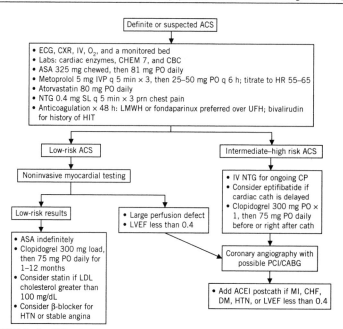

FIGURE 3.2.   Non—ST Elevation Acute Coronary Syndrome

References: JACC, 2007; 50: 652–726, Ann Emer Med, 2008; 51(5): 591–606 and NEJM, 2004; 350(15): 1495–504.

CHAPTER 4

CONGESTIVE HEART FAILURE

1. ## EPIDEMIOLOGY
   - Prevalence: 5.7 million Americans; number one cause for hospitalization among Medicare patients; more hospitalizations than all cancer admissions combined
   - Cost: about $37.2 billion in 2008; about 2% of all healthcare expenditures
   - 50% rehospitalization rate in 6 months
   - Most frequent cause for hospitalization for males older than 65 yo; average LOS is 6 days
   - 75% prevalence over age 65 yo, less than 1% for age younger than 60 yo

2. ## PATHOPHYSIOLOGY
   - Inciting factors decrease myocardial function
     - Acute: myocardial infarction, viral infection
     - Chronic: hypertension, volume overload, inherited cardiomyopathy, toxic exposures
   - Progression to symptomatic heart failure depends on compensatory mechanisms that ultimately result in maladaptive remodeling of myocardium
     - Activation of renin–angiotensin–aldosterone system
     - Increased adrenergic tone
     - Release of vasodilatory hormones and cytokines (ANP, BNP, prostaglandins, NO)
   - Left ventricular systolic dysfunction
     - Neurohormonal stimulation and volume overload increases LV end-diastolic volume and LV wall thinning
     - Decreased excitation–contraction coupling due to decreased Ca in sarcoplasmic reticulum
     - Myocyte necrosis and apoptosis
     - Degradation of extracellular matrix with fibrosis
     - Desensitization of myocardium to adrenergic stimulation
   - Left ventricular diastolic dysfunction
     - Cardiac ischemia, hypertrophy, fibrosis, and/or tachycardia increase LV end-diastolic pressure which then decreases myocardial relaxation during diastole

3. ## CLINICAL PRESENTATION
   - Right heart failure
     - Positive hepatojugular reflux [LR+ 8.0, LR− 0.3]
     - Displaced apical impulse (lateral to midclavicular line) [LR+ 5.8, LR− 1]
     - S_3 gallop [LR+ 3.0, LR− 0.8]
     - JVD [LR+ 3.9, LR− 1]
     - Edema [LR+ 1, LR− 1]
     - Crackles [LR+ 1, LR− 1]
     - S_4 gallop [LR+ 1, LR− 1]
   - Left heart failure
     - Displaced apical impulse (lateral to midclavicular line) [LR+ 10.3, LR− 0.7]
     - JVD [LR+ 6.3, LR− 1]
     - S_3 gallop [LR+ 3.4, LR− 0.7]
     - Crackles [LR+ 1, LR− 1]
     - Edema [LR+ 1, LR− 1]
     - Murmur of mitral regurgitation [LR+ 1, LR− 1]

- Techniques for eliciting physical findings
  - Hepatojugular reflux: Position patient supine so that the top of the jugular venous pulsation is seen in the right side of the neck. Encourage patient to relax and breathe normally. Apply firm, steady pressure to the mid-abdomen for 30 seconds. Test is positive if there is a sustained 4 cm rise in the venous pressure.
  - Displaced cardiac apex: Position patient supine or left lateral decubitus. Palpate the 4th and 5th left intercostal space during expiration. Test is positive if maximal impulse is lateral to midclavicular line.
  - Gallop: Patient positioned left lateral decubitus. Listen with bell over the cardiac apex.
  - Jugular venous distention: Position patient supine at 45° angle, head turned to right. Adjust the bed until the top of the impulse is visible above the angle of the jaw. Measure the distance above the angle of Louis.
- Boston Criteria (50% sensitivity, 78% specificity for CHF)
  - Category I: History
    - Dyspnea at rest (4 points)
    - Orthopnea (4 points)
    - Paroxysmal nocturnal dyspnea (3 points)
    - Dyspnea while walking on flat ground (2 points)
    - Dyspnea while climbing (1 point)
  - Category II: Exam
    - HR greater than 90 (1 point) or greater than 110 (2 points)
    - JVD (2 points if greater than 6 cm, 3 points if greater than 6 cm plus hepatomegaly or edema)
    - Lung crackles (1 point if basilar, 2 points if more than basilar)
    - Wheezing (3 points)
    - Third heart sound (3 points)
  - Category III: Chest radiograph
    - Alveolar pulmonary edema (4 points)
    - Interstitial pulmonary edema (3 points)
    - Bilateral pleural effusion (3 points)
    - Cardiothoracic ratio greater than 0.5 (3 points)
    - Upper zone flow redistribution (2 points)
- No more than 4 points can be obtained from each of the three categories. Maximum score is 12. CHF "definite" at a score of 8 to 12 points; "possible" at a score of 5 to 7 points; and "unlikely" at a score of 4 points or fewer.
- See **Tables 4.1** and **4.2**

TABLE 4.1.   Clinical Findings in Patients with Suspected Heart Failure

Clinical Finding	Sensitivity	Specificity	Positive LR	Negative LR
Dyspnea on exertion	100%	17%	1.2	0
Paroxysmal nocturnal dyspnea	39%	80%	2	0.8
Prior MI	59%	86%	4.1	0.5
Laterally displaced cardiac apex (PMI)	66%	95%	16	0.4
Dependent edema	20%	86%	1.4	0.9
S_3 gallop	24%	99%	27	0.8
Hepatojugular reflux	33%	94%	6	0.7
Jugular venous distension	17%	98%	9.3	0.8
Pulmonary rales	29%	77%	1.3	0.9
CXR showing cardiomegaly and/or pulmonary edema	71%	92%	8.9	0.3
ECG with anterior Q waves or LBBB	94%	61%	2.4	0.1
BNP greater than 500 pg/mL	90% PPV for HF			
BNP less than 50 pg/mL	98% NPV excluding HF			
BNP less than 100 pg/mL	90% NPV excluding HF			
NT-proBNP greater than 450 pg/mL (younger than 50 yo)	95% PPV for HF			
NT-proBNP greater than 900 pg/mL (50–75 yo)	95% PPV for HF			
NT-proBNP greater than 1800 pg/mL (older than 75 yo)	95% PPV for HF			
NT-proBNP less than 300 pg/mL	98% NPV excluding HF			

Source: Adapted from AFP. 2004; 70(11): 2145–52 and Crit Care Med. 2005; 33(9): 2094–13.

TABLE 4.2.   Staging and Classification of Heart Failure

New York Heart Association (NYHA) Classification (current clinical status)		American Heart Association/American College of Cardiology Stages of Heart Failure (represents worst clinical status)	
Class 1	Asymptomatic except with very strenuous activity	Stage A	Risk factors for heart failure present; patient is asymptomatic
Class 2	Symptoms with moderate exertion	Stage B	Asymptomatic; pt has CAD, LVH, valvular heart disease, or LVEF less than 0.4
Class 3	Symptoms with activities of daily living	Stage C	Structural heart disease with mild–moderate heart failure
Class 4	Symptoms at rest	Stage D	End-stage heart failure

CAD = coronary artery disease; LVEF = left ventricular ejection fraction; LVH = left ventricular hypertrophy
Source: Adapted from ACC/AHA clinical practice guidelines on chronic heart failure in JACC, 2005; 46(6): 1116–43.

4. **DIAGNOSIS**
   - HF is a condition in which the heart is unable to deliver sufficient oxygenated blood to meet the metabolic demands of the body
   - HF may present as predominantly left-sided HF, right-sided HF, or biventricular HF

5. **DIFFERENTIAL DIAGNOSIS**
   - Pulmonary embolus
   - Pneumothorax
   - Cardiac tamponade
   - COPD exacerbation
   - Pneumonia
   - ARDS

6. **WORKUP**
   - Orthostatic vital signs, daily weights
   - ECG
   - Chest X-ray
   - 2D-echocardiogram with Doppler
   - Labs: CBC, CMP, fasting glucose and lipid panel, cardiac enzymes, BNP/NT-proBNP, TSH, SpO$_2$, UA
   - Consider a myocardial perfusion study or cardiac catheterization to evaluate for cardiac ischemia once HF exacerbation is resolved
   - Consider a nocturnal polysomnogram to evaluate for concomitant sleep disorders (e.g., OSA) in men younger than 70 yo

7. **TREATMENT**
   - Identify and treat any potential precipitating factors
   - See **Tables 4.3** and **4.4**

TABLE 4.3.   Stepwise Medication Approach for Chronic HF Therapy

Systolic HF (LVEF less than or equal to 0.4)	Diastolic HF (LVEF greater than 0.4)

1. Supplemental oxygen
2. Diuretics for volume control
3. Discontinue all meds that can cause fluid retention*
4. Afterload therapy
  • ACEI
  • ARB for ACEI-intolerant pts
  • Hydralazine plus nitrates if unable to use ACEI or ARB, or if African American add to optimal therapy
5. β-blocker† titrated to HR 55–65 once patient is euvolemic
6. Aldosterone antagonists (if crt less than 2.5 mg/dL in men or less than 2 in women and K less than 5)
  • LVEF less than 0.35 and NYHA Class 2–4 HF
7. Digoxin (keep level less than 1.1 ng/mL) for symptom control
8. Statin to keep LDL less than or equal to 100 mg/dL
9. Devices in select patients (AICD/CRT)
	1. Supplemental oxygen
	2. Diuretics for volume control
	3. BP control: ACEI, ARB, β-blocker, verapamil, or diltiazem
	4. Discontinue all meds that can cause fluid retention*
	5. Control cardiac ischemia: meds vs revascularization
	6. HR control for afib/flutter
	  • β-blocker
	  • verapamil
	  • diltiazem

* NSAIDs, thiazolidinediones, most antiarrhythmic agents, dihydropyridine calcium-channel blockers
† Carvedilol, bisoprolol, or metoprolol succinate

TABLE 4.4.   Nonpharmacological Interventions for HF Management

• 2 g/day sodium restriction	• Weight loss for obese patients
• Maintain BP lower than 130/80 mmHg	• Fluid restrict to less than 2 L/day if serum Na is less
• Smoking cessation	than 130 and to less than 1.5 L/day if serum Na is
• Drink alcohol in moderation	less than 125 MEq/L
• Vaccinations: annual influenza vaccine, pneumococcal	• Education: diet, meds, lifestyle modification
vaccine × 1	• Graded aerobic exercise

Devices to Consider in Chronic HF

- ICD if LVEF is less than or equal to 0.35 with NYHA class 2 CHF or higher **OR** any history of cardiac arrest, VF, or unstable VT and expected survival more than 1 year
- Biventricular pacemaker (CRT) if LVEF is less than or equal to 0.35 and NYHA class 3 CHF or higher on optimal med therapy, QRS duration is 120 ms or longer, and expected survival more than 1 year
  - May consider CRT-ICD if NYHA Class 2, LVEF is less than or equal to 0.3, and QRS greater than or equal to 150 ms

Management of ADHF

- See **Figure 4.1**

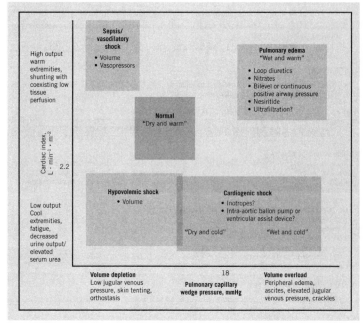

FIGURE 4.1.   Classification of Acute Decompensated Heart Failure

Source: Reproduced from American Journal of Cardiology, 96 (6A); Nohira, Anju; Mielniczuk, Lisa; Stevenson, Lynne; Evaluation and Monitoring of Patients with Acute Heart Failure: 32G-40G, with permission from Elsevier.

- **Wet/warm** (49%): IV diuretics, oxygen, morphine, and nitrates (SL or SQ)
  - Vasodilators if NL/elevated BP and poor response to diuretics and nitrates
  - Consider noninvasive ventilation for moderate–severe HF with respiratory failure
- **Wet/cold** (20%): IV diuretics, oxygen, and vasodilators
  - Consider ICU admission with central hemodynamic monitoring
  - May need inotropic therapy if very low output state
  - Mechanical assist devices for refractory hypotension or low cardiac output: IABP (not if severe AI, sepsis, or recent CVA); LVAD (bridge to transplant)
- **Dry/warm** (27%): Decrease chronic diuretic dose or cautious fluid challenge, oxygen, and afterload reduction (ACEI, ARB, or hydralazine plus nitrates)
- **Dry/cold** (4%): cautious fluid challenge, oxygen, and inotropic therapy
  - Consider ICU admission with central hemodynamic monitoring
  - Mechanical assist devices for refractory hypotension or low cardiac output (as above)
- **IV loop diuretics:** furosemide 20–40 mg, bumetanide 2–4 mg, or torsemide 10–20 mg
  - Double diuretic dose every 15–20 minutes until effective diuresis is obtained
- **Refractory diuresis**
  - Add thiazide 30 minutes before loop diuretic: chlorothiazide 500 mg IV or metolazone 10 mg PO
  - Furosemide drip: give bolus dose, then start 10–20 mg/hour infusion
  - Ultrafiltration: use if venous access, SBP is greater than 85 mmHg, and no ESRD or shock
- **Vasodilators** (if BP is greater than 90/60 mmHg)
  - Nitroglycerin: 5–10 to max 200 mcg/min; nitroprusside start 0.3–0.5 mcg/kg/min; nesiritide 2 mcg/kg bolus, then 0.01 mcg/kg/min (may increase mortality and serum creatinine)
- **Inotropes for low output states** (especially if SBP is less than 85 mmHg or cardiorenal syndrome;
  - watch for significantly increased BP)
  - Dobutamine: Start at 2.5 mcg/kg/min and titrate to max 20 mcg/kg/min
  - Milrinone: 50 mcg/kg load over 10 min, then 0.2–0.75 mcg/kg/min (causes less tachycardia)
- **β-blockers in ADHF**
  - No change to β-blocker dose in wet/warm or dry/warm ADHF
  - Hold or decrease β-blocker dose 50% in wet/cold or dry/cold ADHF
- **Indication for heart transplantation**
  - Refractory CHF, ischemia, or arrhythmias despite optimal medical therapy
  - Poor candidates: pulmonary hypertension, sepsis, CA, advanced lung disease, cirrhosis, ESRD, substance abuse, older than 60 yo, or noncompliance
- **Prognosis in ADHF**
  - CART risk analysis/risk factors (RFs): BUN greater than or equal to 43 mg/dL; crt greater than or equal to 2.75 mg/dL; SBP less than 115
    - In-hospital mortality: 22% if all 3 RFs present; 2% if no RFs present
  - Predischarge BNP: greater than 700 pg/mL has 15 × higher 6-month death or readmissions vs less than 350 pg/mL
  - Initial TnI greater than or equal to 1 mcg/L has 8% in-hospital mortality vs 2.7% if TnI normal
  - Patients with chronic NYHA class IV symptoms have an annual mortality risk of 40–60%; those with NYHA I–II have a 5–10% mortality risk

Management of Refractory End-Stage HF

- Referral for cardiac transplantation in eligible patients
- Referral to a HF center of excellence
- Consider a ventricular assist device
- Discuss options for end-of-life care: including options for hospice, inactivating an implanted defibrillator, and code status

8. COMPLICATIONS

- Arrhythmia
- Acute decompensated heart failure
- Sudden cardiac death: most commonly caused by ventricular fibrillation; can also be caused by bradyar-rhythmia or PEA
- Cardiac cachexia: condition involving reduced skeletal muscle mass, fat tissue, and bone, leading to further fatigue and weakening; associated with poor prognosis and increased mortality
- Acute renal failure: due to decreased renal blood flow from either hypervolemia (decreased cardiac output from elevated filling pressure in left ventricle) or hypovolemia (overdiuresis)
- MI/angina
- Depression

REFERENCES

American College of Cardiology Foundation/American Heart Association Task Force on Practice Guidelines Developed in Collaboration With the International Society for Heart and Lung Transplantation. 2009 Focused Update: ACCF/AHA guidelines for the diagnosis and management of heart failure in adults: a report of the American College of Cardiology Foundation/American Heart Association Task Force on Practice Guidelines. *J Am Coll Cardiol*, 2009;53(15):343–82.

McKelvie RS, Moe GW, Cheung A, et al. The 2011 Canadian Cardiovascular society heart failure management guidelines update: focus on sleep apnea, renal dysfunction, mechanical circulatory support, and palliative care. *Can J Cardiol*. 2011;27(3):319–38.

Dosh SA. Diagnosis of heart failure in adults. *Am Fam Physician*. 2004;70(11):2145-52.

Shamsham F, Mitchell J. Essentials of the diagnosis of heart failure. *Am Fam Physician*. 2000;61(5):1319–28.

CHAPTER 5

ATRIAL FIBRILLATION

1. **EPIDEMIOLOGY**
   - Prevalence is 1%; associated with structural heart disease: HTN (more than 50%), CAD (25%), HF (23–29%), valvular heart disease (17%)
   - Only 10–15% occur in absence of comorbidities

2. **PATHOPHYSIOLOGY**
   - Initiation: sleeve of atrial tissue around pulmonary veins serves as abnormal automatic focus; increased sympathetic tone (e.g., hyperthyroidism, alcohol intoxication, postop stress) also precipitates AF
   - Maintenance: structural heart disease (hypertrophy, fibrosis) creates multiple reentry loops
   - Loss of atrial contractility decreases cardiac output, especially in patients with structural heart disease who are dependent on "atrial kick"
   - Thrombus formed in left atrial appendage embolizes, leading to ischemic CVA
   - Rapid atrial impulses conducted through AV node (or worse through accessory pathway) lead to rapid ventricular rate (perceived as palpitations) and as a result, decreased left ventricular filling

3. **ETIOLOGIES OF ATRIAL FIBRILLATION (MNEMONIC IS CPR HEARTS)**
   - **C**: CAD or acute MI
   - **P**: pulmonary (COPD/obstructive sleep apnea), pheochromocytoma, and pericarditis
   - **R**: rheumatic heart disease (or valvular cardiomyopathy)
   - **H**: hypertensive/hypertrophic cardiomyopathy or severe hypoxia
   - **E**: embolus (pulmonary)
   - **A**: alcohol and amyloidosis
   - **R**: ruled out cardiopulmonary disease (if none present, then lone Afib)
   - **T**: theophylline toxicity, thyrotoxicosis, or trauma (blunt chest)
   - **S**: surgery (e.g., postcoronary artery bypass grafting), sick sinus syndrome, sarcoidosis or sympathomimetic toxicity

4. **CLINICAL PRESENTATION**
   - Often asymptomatic
   - Fatigue (most common symptom)
   - Chest pain
   - Lightheadedness
   - Dyspnea
   - Palpitations (26%)
   - Signs: irregular pulse

5. **DIAGNOSIS**
   - ECG has characteristic appearance
   - Irregularly, irregular rhythm usually with a narrow complex QRS complex (unless patient has an underlying bundle-branch block)
   - See **Figures 5.1** and **5.2**

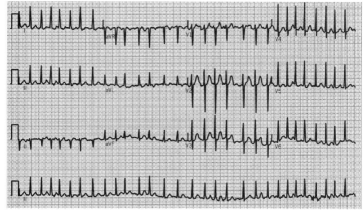

FIGURE 5.1.   ECG Demonstrating Atrial Fibrillation

Source: Courtesy of Daniel Clark, M.D., Director of Medicine and Cardiology, Ventura County Medical Center, Ventura, California.

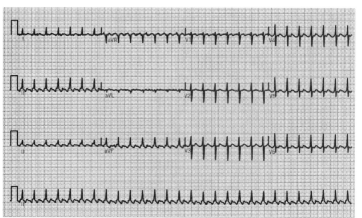

FIGURE 5.2.   ECG Demonstrating Atrial Flutter with 2:1 Block

Source: Courtesy of Daniel Clark, M.D., Director of Medicine and Cardiology, Ventura County Medical Center, Ventura, California.

6. **WORKUP OF ATRIAL FIBRILLATION**

- ECG, chest radiograph, and 2D-echocardiogram
- Labs: CBC, CHEM 7, liver panel, TSH with or without blood alcohol level, and urine drug screen
- Fecal occult blood testing prior to anticoagulation
- Electrophysiologic study (EPS) to determine the etiology of wide-complex tachycardias or for curative atrial or AV nodal ablation in refractory, symptomatic chronic, or paroxysmal Afib/aflutter
- Noninvasive testing to rule out cardiac ischemia if clinically indicated

7. <u>**TREATMENT**</u>

Antithrombotic Therapy to Minimize Cardioembolic Stroke Risk

- Therapy indicated for persistent, permanent, or recurrent paroxysmal Afib
- Chronic anticoagulation with warfarin titrated to INR 2.5 (range 2–3) indicated for $CHADS_2$ or $CHAD_2$-VASc score 2 or higher; valvular Afib; history of prior cardioembolic stroke/TIA/arterial embolus; prosthetic heart valve; age 75 yo or older; LVEF less than or equal to 0.35; atrial thrombus; DM; or CHF
  - Dabigatran is an alternative only in nonvalvular Afib, and CrCl greater than 15 mL/min
    - Dabigatran 150 mg PO bid had a lower rate of stroke and CNS bleeding, and same rate of major bleeding compared with warfarin in RE-LY trial; does require twice daily dosing; this may increase nonadherence; no specific reversal agent available for overdose
  - Clopidogrel plus aspirin another alternative to warfarin if pt unsuitable for anticoagulation; the small benefit in decreased embolism is offset by increased bleeding risk
- Aspirin 81–325 mg PO daily if nonvalvular Afib with $CHADS_2$ or $CHAD_2$-VASc score 1 or lower
  - European Society of Cardiology recommends $CHAD_2$-VASc score, which is more aggressive toward warfarin therapy
- In nonvalvular Afib, warfarin reduces stroke risk 64%, and aspirin reduces risk 22%
- Warfarin increases risk of serious intracranial hemorrhage 0.2%/year versus aspirin
- Warfarin contraindications: fall risk, noncompliance, active drug or alcohol abuse, unstable psychiatric conditions, hemorrhagic diathesis, severe thrombocytopenia, recent neurosurgery, ophthalmologic or trauma surgery, active bleeding, pericarditis, endocarditis, history of intracranial hemorrhage, regional anesthesia, pregnancy, or threatened abortion

Atrial Fibrillation Rate Versus Rhythm Control

- Rate control plus antithrombotic therapy is preferred over rhythm control in elderly patients with advanced heart disease
  - Desired resting rate 60–80 and 90–115 with exercise or during 6-minute walk test
  - Acceptable if resting rate less than 110 in persistent Afib with LVEF greater than 0.4 and tolerable symptoms
- Consider rhythm control in younger patients with minimal heart disease, for disabling symptoms, or poor exercise capacity in those with advanced heart disease
- Catheter ablation of atrial focus for paroxysmal Afib with refractory symptoms or poor rate control on meds who have failed antiarrhythmic therapy and have only mildly dilated LA, normal LVEF, and no severe lung disease
  - Catheter-directed pulmonary vein isolation procedure
  - The "Maze" procedure is an option during concomitant cardiac surgery
  - Continue anticoagulation for 4 weeks postablation

- See **Figure 5.3** and **Tables 5.1, 5.2, 5.3,** and **5.4**

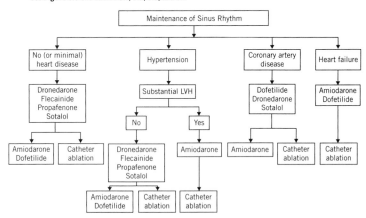

FIGURE 5.3.   Therapy to Maintain Sinus Rhythm in Patients with Recurrent Paroxysmal or Persistent Atrial Fibrillation
Drugs are listed alphabetically and not in order of suggested use. The seriousness of heart disease progresses from left to right, and selection of therapy in patients with multiple conditions depends on the most serious condition present. LVH indicates left ventricular hypertrophy.

Source: Curtis, Craig et al. 2011 ACCF/AHA/HRS Focused Update. Circulation; 123(1): 104–123. Printed with permission from Wolters Kluwer Health.

TABLE 5.1.   CHADS₂* Score to Determine the Embolic Risk for Stroke in Nonvalvular Afib

CHADS$_2$ Score	Adjusted Stroke Rate†	CHADS$_2$ Stroke Risk
0	1.9	Low level
1	2.8	Low level
2	4.0	Moderate level
3	5.9	Moderate level
4	8.5	High level
5	12.5	High level
6	18.2	High level

* CHADS$_2$ Score = 1 point each for **C**HF exacerbation in last 100 days, **H**TN, **A**ge older than 75 yo, and **D**M; 2 points for history of **S**troke/TIA.
Warfarin recommended for CHADS$_2$ 2 or higher; aspirin recommended for CHADS$_2$ 0–1.
† number of strokes per 100 patient-years from the National Registry of Atrial Fibrillation
Source: Adapted from *Annals Intern. Med.* 2003; 139(12): 1009–17.

TABLE 5.2.   CHADS$_2$-VASc Score to Assess Embolic Risk for Stroke in Nonvalvular Afib

CHADS$_2$-VASc Score*	Adjusted Stroke Rate (%/year)	CHADS$_2$ Stroke Risk
0	0	Low level
1	1.3	Low level
2	2.2	Moderate level
3	3.2	Moderate level
4	4.0	Moderate level
5	6.7	Moderate level
6	9.8	High level
7	9.6	High level
8	6.7	High level
9	15.2	High level

* CHADS$_2$-VASc Score = 1 point for CHF or LVEF less than or equal to 0.4, HTN, DM, vascular disease, age 65–74 yo, female sex; 2 points for age 75 yo or older or history of stroke/TIA/arterial embolism
Source: Adapted from *Eur Heart J.* 2010; 31(19): 2369–429.

TABLE 5.3.   Agents for Afib Rate Control

Agent	Acute IV Therapy	Chronic Oral Rx	Comments
Metoprolol*	5 mg q 5 min × 3	25–100 mg bid	Good for CAD
Esmolol*	500 mcg/kg IV, then 6–200 mcg/kg/min		Caution if decreased BP, severe bronchospasm, or HF
Diltiazem*	20 mg, then 5–15 mg/h	120–360 mg daily	Caution if severe HF or hypotension
Verapamil*	5–10 mg q 15 min × 2	120–360 mg daily	
Digoxin*	0.25 mg q 4–6 h up to 1.5 mg	0.125–0.375 mg daily	Use if HF; decreases dose if CrCl less than 50 mL/min
Amiodarone	150 mg over 10 min then 1 mg/min × 6 h then 0.5 mg/min × 18 h	200–400 mg daily	Good for HF or WPW; many drug interactions

* Contraindicated if evidence of preexcitation syndrome/accessory pathway (e.g., WPW), Rx = therapy
Source: *JACC.* 2006; 48(4): e149–246.

TABLE 5.4.   HAS-BLED Risk Score for Bleeding with Warfarin Anticoagulation

HAS-BLED Score	Annual Risk of Major Bleeding
0	1.1%
1	1.0%
2	1.9%
3	3.7%
4	8.7%
5	12.5%

H = hypertension, A = abnormal renal/liver function (each 1 point), S = prior stroke, B = bleeding history or predisposition, L = labile INR, E = elderly (older than 65 yo), and D = drugs/alcohol (each 1 point); the maximum possible score is 9—with 1 point for each of the components
Source: Information from *Chest* 2010; 138(5):1093–100.

Synchronized Electrical or Chemical Cardioversion

- Timing of electrical or chemical cardioversion
  - Immediately if hemodynamically unstable (chest pain, CHF, or shock)
  - If negative transthoracic echocardiogram and Afib duration less than 48 hours, **OR**
  - Negative transesophageal echocardiogram and heparin anticoagulation started, **OR**
  - After 3 weeks of adequate warfarin anticoagulation
- Biphasic shock using anterior and posterior placement of pads has the highest rate of successful electrical cardioversion (nearly 100%)
- Medical cardioversion: amiodarone, dronedarone, dofetilide, flecainide, ibutilide, or propafenone
- Continue warfarin for at least 4 weeks after successful cardioversion
- Continue converting agent × 2 weeks **AND** continue a β-blocker or diltiazem/verapamil after a successful cardioversion to prevent atrial remodeling and to maintain sinus rhythm
- Avoid cardioversion if Afib more than 6 months, left atrium larger than 5 cm, or endocardial clot present

Special Circumstances

- Preexcitation syndrome/accessory pathway
  - Suggested by ventricular rate greater than or equal to 220, delta waves, or increased HR after giving AV nodal blocker
  - Rate control with amiodarone or ibutilide or DC cardioversion
  - Once stabilized, catheter ablation for Afib with an accessory pathway is required
- Acute MI
  - β-blocker, diltiazem, or verapamil (LVEF greater than 0.35); amiodarone (LVEF less than or equal to 0.35)
- Hyperthyroidism
  - β-blocker and antithyroid medications for rate control
  - Consider acute anticoagulation depending on comorbid conditions
- Pregnancy
  - Digoxin, β-blocker, verapamil, or diltiazem are safe for rate control
  - Subcutaneous UFH, LMWH, and aspirin are safe antithrombotic medications
- Tachy-brady syndrome
  - AV-sequential pacemaker insertion, then aggressive AV nodal blocker therapy

8. PROGNOSIS

- CHADS$_2$ score (see Table 5.1) predicts the risk of a cardioembolic event in nonvalvular Afib
- Average risk of stroke with CHADS$_2$ score 2 or higher *without* warfarin (Coumadin): 5% risk of stroke per year
- Average risk of stroke with CHADS$_2$ score 2 or higher *with* warfarin (Coumadin): 1% risk of stroke per year
- HAS-BLED score (see Table 5.4): identifies patients with high risk of major bleeding with oral anticoagulation

9. COMPLICATIONS

- Stroke/systemic embolization
- Heart failure: especially if ventricular rate not controlled
- Hemorrhagic events with anticoagulation: ASA less effective than ASA plus clopidogrel, which is equivalent to warfarin

REFERENCES

Circulation, 2011;123(1):104–23; *Ann Intern Med*, 2007;146(12):857–67; *J Am Coll Cardiol*, 2011;57(11):1330–37.

CHAPTER 6

BRADYARRHYTHMIAS

1. **EPIDEMIOLOGY**
   - Idioventricular pacer (ventricular) at 20–40 bpm; sudden cardiac arrest more than 30% of time

2. **PATHOPHYSIOLOGY**
   - Abnormal impulse generation indicates SA node dysfunction
   - Extrinsic causes due to suppressed automaticity: carotid sinus hypersensitivity, medications (antiadrenergics, antiarrhythmics), hypothyroidism, hypoxia, vagal stimulation, hypothermia, elevated ICP
   - Intrinsic causes due to degenerative fibrosis: sick sinus syndrome, MI, pericarditis, myocarditis, postoperative, trauma, familial
   - Abnormal impulse conduction indicates AV node dysfunction
   - Autonomic causes: carotid sinus hypersensitivity, vasovagal response
   - Medication-related causes: β-blockers, calcium channel blockers, digitalis, adenosine, antiarrhythmics, lithium
   - Inflammatory/infiltrative causes: endocarditis, Lyme disease, Chagas disease, syphilis, TB, diphtheria, SLE, RA, MCTD, scleroderma, amyloidosis, sarcoidosis, hemochromatosis
   - Congenital causes: congenital heart disease, maternal SLE, myotonic dystrophy
   - Miscellaneous causes: trauma, MI, radiation, neoplasm

3. **CLINICAL PRESENTATION**
   - Fatigue
   - Weakness
   - Lightheadedness
   - Syncope
   - Sinus bradycardia: first heart sound has same intensity with each beat, no ventricular contractions between radial pulses
   - Complete heart block: changing intensity of first heart sound, intermittent "cannon" a waves on CVP monitor

4. **DIAGNOSIS**
   - **Symptomatic bradycardia**: any documented bradyarrhythmia that is directly responsible for the development of syncope, near syncope, lightheadedness, or transient confusional states from cerebral hypoperfusion
   - **Sick sinus syndrome**: inappropriate sinus bradycardia, sinus pauses longer than 2 seconds, or chronotropic incompetence
   - **Atrioventricular block (AVB)**
     - **First-degree AVB:** PR interval longer than 0.2 seconds
     - **Mobitz I second-degree AVB (Wenckebach):** progressive prolongation of PR interval until dropped beat; QRS typically narrow
     - **Mobitz II second-degree AVB:** fixed PR interval with dropped beats; QRS typically wide
     - **Third-degree AVB:** complete AV dissociation; narrow QRS complex indicates a junctional escape; wide QRS complex indicates a ventricular escape rhythm
   - See **Figures 6.1** through **6.4**

First-Degree AVB

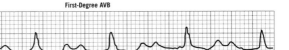

FIGURE 6.1. Rhythm Strip of First-Degree AV Block

Source: Courtesy of Daniel Clark, M.D., Director of Medicine and Cardiology, Ventura County Medical Center, Ventura, California.

Type 1 Second-Degree AVB

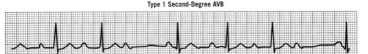

FIGURE 6.2. Rhythm Strip of Mobitz I Second-Degree AV Block (Wenckebach)

Source: Courtesy of Daniel Clark, M.D., Director of Medicine and Cardiology, Ventura County Medical Center, Ventura, California.

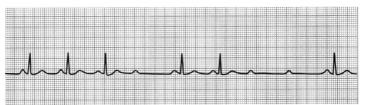

FIGURE 6.3. Rhythm Strip of Mobitz II Second-Degree AV Block

Source: Courtesy of Daniel Clark, M.D., Director of Medicine and Cardiology, Ventura County Medical Center, Ventura, California.

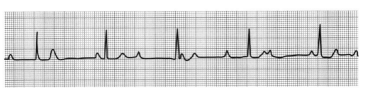

FIGURE 6.4. Rhythm Strip of Third-Degree AV Block (Complete Heart Block)

Source: Courtesy of Daniel Clark, M.D., Director of Medicine and Cardiology, Ventura County Medical Center, Ventura, California.

5. **WORKUP**
   - CBC, CMP, TSH, urine drug screen, cardiac enzymes, SpO$_2$
   - ECG
   - Check medication list and discontinue all offending medications

6. **TREATMENT**
   - Symptomatic bradycardia can be stabilized with medications or transcutaneous pacing until a definitive transvenous pacemaker is inserted
   - Atropine 0.5 mg IVP q 3 min (max 3 mg) for symptomatic bradycardia from AV nodal block
   - Dopamine 2–10 mcg/kg/min for symptomatic bradycardia from infranodal block or for shock
   - Glucagon 3–5 mg IVP and may repeat in 10 min, then drip at 0.07 mg/kg/h for symptomatic bradycardia/hypotension from β-blocker overdose
   - Discontinue all AV nodal blocking medication, correct electrolytes, maintain normothermia, treat hypoxia if present, treat hypothyroidism if present

7. **ACC/AHA INDICATIONS FOR PACEMAKER INSERTION**
   - Pacing for acquired atrioventricular (AV) block
     - Reversible causes of AV block have been ruled out (e.g., MI, abnormal electrolytes, and medications).
     - Type II second-degree AV block (especially if a wide QRS or symptoms are present)
     - Third-degree AV block (complete heart block [CHB]), excluding congenital CHB
     - Can consider for first-degree AV block (PR longer than 0.30 seconds) or Type I second-degree AV block with symptomatic bradycardia
   - Pacing for chronic bifascicular or trifascicular block
     - If ambulatory ECG monitoring reveals intermittent Type II second-degree AV block or third-degree AV block
   - Pacing in sinus node dysfunction
     - Symptomatic sinus pauses (3 seconds or longer)
     - Symptomatic chronotropic incompetence
   - Pacing in carotid sinus syndrome and neurocardiogenic syncope
     - Documented asystole longer than 3 seconds with minimal carotid sinus pressure
     - Recurrent neurocardiogenic syncope associated with bradycardia
   - Pacing in tachy-brady syndrome
     - Pacemaker inserted to prevent symptomatic bradycardia when AV nodal blocking agents used to rate control rapid atrial fibrillation/flutter
   - Pacemaker tips
     - Chronic ventricular pacing can lead to ventricular dyssynchrony and increase the risk of CHF; attempt to adjust pacemaker to maximize atrial pacing and minimize ventricular pacing (set a slow back-up ventricular rate and a long PR interval)
   - See **Figures 6.5 through 6.11**

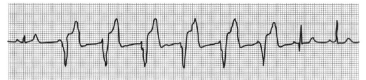

FIGURE 6.5   VVIR Pacemaker Capturing and Sensing Properly

Source: Courtesy of Daniel Clark, M.D., Director of Medicine and Cardiology, Ventura County Medical Center, Ventura, California.

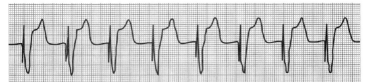

FIGURE 6.6.   VVIR Pacemaker Capturing

Source: Courtesy of Daniel Clark, M.D., Director of Medicine and Cardiology, Ventura County Medical Center, Ventura, California.

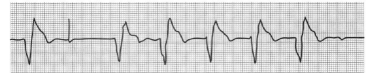

FIGURE 6.7.   VVIR Pacemaker with Failure to Capture

Source: Courtesy of Daniel Clark, M.D., Director of Medicine and Cardiology, Ventura County Medical Center, Ventura, California.

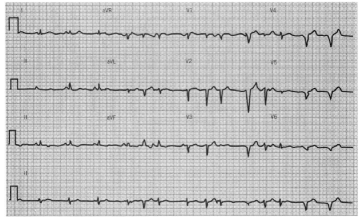

FIGURE 6.8.   VVIR Pacemaker with Failure to Sense

Source: Courtesy of Daniel Clark, M.D., Director of Medicine and Cardiology, Ventura County Medical Center, Ventura, California.

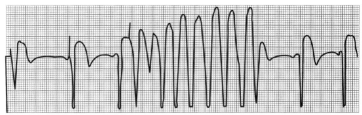

FIGURE 6.9.   VVIR Pacemaker with Undersensing

Source: Courtesy of Daniel Clark, M.D., Director of Medicine and Cardiology, Ventura County Medical Center, Ventura, California.

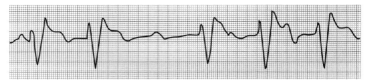

FIGURE 6.10.   VVIR Pacemaker with Oversensing

Source: Courtesy of Daniel Clark, M.D., Director of Medicine and Cardiology, Ventura County Medical Center, Ventura, California.

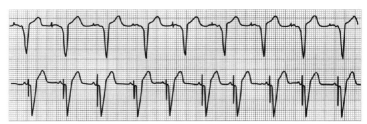

FIGURE 6.11.   DDD Pacemaker with Atrial Pacing and Ventricular Tracking

Source: Courtesy of Daniel Clark, M.D., Director of Medicine and Cardiology, Ventura County Medical Center, Ventura, California.

8. <u>**PROGNOSIS**</u>
   - 5-year survival rates in patients with sick sinus syndrome are 47–69%

9. <u>**COMPLICATIONS**</u>
   - Sinus bradycardia
     - Syncope
     - Heart failure
     - Sudden cardiac arrest/death

- Sick sinus syndrome
  - Complete SA node arrest (usually evolves slowly over time, between 7 and 29 years)
  - Conversion to other conduction disturbances such as tachy-brady syndrome, high-grade AV-block
  - Syncope
  - Heart failure
  - Atrial arrhythmias
  - Thromboembolic event (especially in atrial fibrillation with tachy-brady syndrome)
- AV block
  - First degree: mostly benign; however compared to normal PR interval, incidence of atrial fibrillation and all-cause mortality higher if PR interval 200 ms or longer
  - Second degree: hypoperfusion from decreased cardiac output/heart failure especially with significant bradycardia or decreased conducted beats (i.e., 2:1 or 3:2 block)
- Third degree/complete heart block: syncope, hypotension, development of polymorphic ventricular tachycardia in presence of severe bradycardia, sudden cardiac arrest/death

REFERENCES

J Am Coll Cardiol, 2002;40(9):1703–19; *J Am Coll Cardiol*, 2004;43(2):1145–8; *Crit Care Med*, 2010; 38 (Suppl 6):S188–197; *J Am Coll Cardiol*, 2008;51(21):e1–62.

CHAPTER 7

ACUTE PERICARDITIS

1. **PATHOPHYSIOLOGY**
   - Adjacent inflamed parietal pleura (e.g., infectious pericarditis)
   - Pericardium is devoid of pain fibers; thus pain is due to inflammation of adjacent parietal pleura
     * Noninflammatory causes of pericarditis (e.g., uremia or post-MI) are generally painless

2. **ETIOLOGIES**
   - Excluding patients with known CA, ESRD, trauma, and postradiation, 90% of cases are idiopathic or of viral etiology
   - Other causes: neoplastic, infectious (tuberculous, bacterial, fungal, rickettsial, or fungal), Dressler's syndrome (post-MI), postirradiation, chest trauma, uremia, postpericardiotomy, hypothyroidism, connective tissue diseases (systemic lupus erythematosus, scleroderma, and rheumatoid arthritis) and meds (hydralazine, isoniazid, methyldopa, phenytoin, and procainamide)

3. **CLINICAL PRESENTATION**
   - Sudden onset of constant, sharp, or stabbing retrosternal chest pain
   - Exacerbating factors: deep inspiration, lying down, and possibly swallowing
   - Alleviating factors: improved with leaning forward
   - Radiation pattern: neck, arms, shoulders, trapezius muscle ridges, or epigastrium
   - Classically, there is no improvement with nitroglycerin
   - Associated symptoms: malaise, myalgias, dry cough, and dyspnea are common
   Physical Exam
   - Pericardial rub in 85% of patients: harsh, high-pitched, scratchy sound best heard at end expiration at cardiac apex with the patient leaning forward using the stethoscope's diaphragm
     * Classic rub with 3 components best heard at the apex: ventricular systole, early diastole, and atrial systole; 50% of rubs triphasic, 33% biphasic, and the rest are monophasic
   - Signs of cardiac tamponade: muffled heart sounds, hypotension, tachycardia, jugular venous distension, and pulsus paradoxus (fall in systolic blood pressure greater than 10 mmHg with inspiration)
   - Temperature higher than 38°C uncommon except in purulent pericarditis

4. **DIAGNOSIS**
   - Characteristic clinical findings and ECG changes
   Electrocardiographic Changes (seen in 90% of patients)
   - **Stage 1:** diffuse, *upward concave* ST segment elevations and PR segment depressions in all leads (especially leads I, II, aVL, aVF, and V3–V6), except lead aVR where ST segment depression and PR-segment elevation occurs; no T wave inversions
   - **Stage 2:** ST and PR segments normalize and T waves progressively flatten
   - **Stage 3:** diffuse T wave inversions
   - **Stage 4:** normalization of the T waves
   - Electrical alternans may be seen if a large pericardial effusion exists
   - A ratio of ST segment elevation (in millimeters) to T wave amplitude (in millimeters) greater than 0.24 in lead V6 is highly specific for acute pericarditis
   - Diffuse T wave inversions AND concave ST elevations and PR depressions suggests myopericarditis
   - See **Figure 7.1**

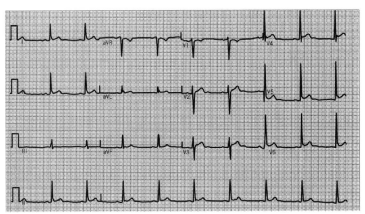

FIGURE 7.1.   ECG Demonstrating Acute Pericarditis

Source: Courtesy of Daniel Clark, M.D., Director of Medicine and Cardiology, Ventura County Medical Center, Ventura, California.

5. **DIFFERENTIAL DIAGNOSIS**

   - Aortic dissection
   - Pericarditis
   - Pulmonary embolus
   - Esophageal spasm
   - Pneumothorax
   - Costochondritis
   - Panic attack

6. **WORKUP OF ACUTE PERICARDITIS**

   - Labs: complete blood count, renal panel, cardiac enzymes with or without ANA, RF, and PPD
   - If Tb or malignant effusion suspected, pericardial fluid should be sent for cytology, CEA (level greater than or equal to 5 ng/mL is 75% sensitive/100% specific for malignancy), and *mycobacterium tuberculosis* RNA by polymerase chain reaction assay and adenosine deaminase activity (more than 30 units/L suggests Tb pericarditis)
     - Equivocal fluid analysis may require a pericardial biopsy for malignancy or Tb
   - Chest radiograph
   - Echocardiogram is indicated in all patients with suspected pericarditis

7. **TREATMENT OF ACUTE PERICARDITIS**

   - Oral indomethacin 75–225 mg/day or ibuprofen 1600–3200 mg/day × 7–14 days
     - Colchicine 0.6 mg PO bid can be added if symptoms persist for more than 2 weeks or for recurrent pericarditis and continue 0.6 mg PO daily–bid for up to 6 months
   - Prednisone 1–1.5 mg/kg/day orally × 1 month then taper over several months only for severe, recurrent pericarditis or if due to a connective tissue disease or tuberculous pericarditis
   - Avoid full anticoagulation, which increases the risk of a hemopericardium
   - Pericardiocentesis: therapeutic for clinical evidence of tamponade or diagnostic for possible tuberculous, bacterial, or neoplastic pericarditis
     - Fluid for cell count, culture, Gram stain, protein, LDH, glucose with or without cytology
   - Pericardial window or pericardiectomy for recurrent large effusions

8. <u>PROGNOSTIC FACTORS WARRANTING ADMISSION TO HOSPITAL</u>

- Fever above 38°C, subacute onset over weeks, immunocompromised, history of trauma, anticoagulant therapy, myocarditis, elevated troponin I, evidence of cardiac tamponade, or a large pericardial effusion (echo-free space greater than 2 cm)

9. <u>COMPLICATIONS</u>

- Shock
- Cardiac arrest
- Arrhythmias
- MI

REFERENCES

N Engl J Med, 2004;351,(21):2195–202, *Lancet*, 2004;351:2195; *Circulation*, 2003;108(9):1146–62.

CHAPTER 8

VALVULAR HEART DISEASE

1. **EPIDEMIOLOGY**
   - Aortic stenosis is a disease of people older than 50 yo; 25% over age 65 yo and 35% over age 70 yo have echo evidence of AS; 10–20% of these will progress to hemodynamically significant AS over 10–15 years
   - Mitral regurgitation: diagnosed in up to 10% of healthy females
   - Mitral stenosis: Afib develops in 50–80% of these pts, pulmonary hypertension
   - Tricuspid stenosis: exclusively of rheumatic origin, rare in developed countries
   - Tricuspid regurgitation: mostly a functional problem

2. **PATHOPHYSIOLOGY**
   Aortic Stenosis
   - Aortic orifice area less than 1 cm^2: LV outflow obstruction leads to compensatory LV concentric hypertrophy, then diastolic dysfunction
   - Decreased LV compliance results in failure to increase cardiac output with exertion (even if normal at rest)
   - Myocardial oxygen demand that is greater than coronary supply results in ischemia

   Aortic Insufficiency
   - Total stroke volume (which equals effective forward stroke volume plus regurgitant volume) is delivered into high-pressure aorta, increasing LV end-diastolic volume (preload) and leading to LV dilation/eccentric hypertrophy
   - Increased myocardial oxygen demand from LV hypertrophy plus decreased coronary blood supply from low diastolic pressure leads to ischemia

   Mitral Stenosis
   - When mitral valve orifice area reaches 2 cm^2 (normal 4–6 cm^2), increased LA pressure is required for blood to flow into LV and maintain cardiac output, resulting in increased LA pressure, then ultimately increased PA pressure and thus, exertional dyspnea
   - As HR increases, diastole shortens more than systole decreasing the time available for flow across valve and thus worsening the pressure gradient
   - In severe mitral stenosis, can have secondary right-sided CHF from increased PA pressure

   Mitral Regurgitation
   - Regurgitant volume greater than 60 mL/beat: decreased LV afterload decreases LV tension, resulting compensatory increased LV emptying
   - As LVEF increases, LV volume increases, leading to LA enlargement if chronic

3. **CLINICAL PRESENTATION**
   - Murmurs by location (AParTMent)
     - **A**: right upper sternal border, 2nd intercostal space: aortic stenosis (systolic, radiating to R carotid)
     - **P**: left upper sternal border, 2nd intercostal space: pulmonic regurgitation (diastolic)
     - **T**: left lower sternal border: tricuspid regurgitation (systolic)
     - **M**: apex (usually 5th–6th intercostal space): mitral regurgitation (systolic, radiating to axilla)
   - Grading of murmurs
     - Grade I: only heard after a few seconds of focusing
     - Grade II: heard relatively easily on auscultation
     - Grade III: loud murmur without thrill
     - Grade IV: thrill
     - Grade V: thrill; audible with one edge of stethoscope on chest
     - Grade VI: thrill; audible with stethoscope held off the chest

- "Significant" murmurs (*moderate–severe AS or MR, congenital shunt, or intraventricular pressure gradient*)
  - Systolic thrill [LR+ 12, LR– 0.7]
  - Holosystolic murmur [LR+ 8.7, LR– 0.2]
  - Loud murmur (higher than grade II) [LR+ 6.5, LR– 0.08]
  - Plateau shaped [LR+ 4.1, LR– 0.5]
  - Loudest at the apex [LR+ 2.5, LR– 0.8]

Aortic Stenosis

- Symptoms: angina, syncope, dyspnea
- Murmur: mid- or long-systolic (NOT early); loudest at R 2nd intercostal space; sounds harsh, *not* blowing; radiates to carotids
- Other signs: sustained apical impulse [LR+ 4.1, LR– 0.3], delayed carotid pulse [LR+ 3.3, LR– 0.4], delayed brachioradial pulse [LR+ 2.5, LR– 0.04], diminished S2 [LR+ 3.1, LR– 0.4], S4 [LR+ 2.5, LR– 0.3]

Aortic Insufficiency

- Murmur: early diastolic, blowing, high frequency, decrescendo; heard best at L sternal boarder 3rd or 4th intercostal space, with diaphragm of stethoscope pressed firmly; if heard best at the R sternal, consider AI related to dilated aortic root; louder if they sit up, lean forward, and hold breath in exhalation
- Austin Flint murmur: end-diastolic low-pitched rumbling, heard at the apex; "presystolic rumbling if in sinus rhythm;" only heard with bell, patient in left lateral decubitus [LR+ 4.0, LR– 0.8]
- S_3 gallop [LR+ 5.9, LR– 0.8]
- Widened pulse pressure [pulse pressure greater than 80 mmHg: LR+ 10.9; diastolic BP less than 50 mmHg: LR+ 19.3, diastolic BP greater than 70 mmHg: LR+ 0.2]
- Water hammer pulse (AKA Corrigan pulse), a pounding sensation caused by collapsing diastolic pressure and increased filling of LV [LR+ 1, LR– 0.7]
- Other aortic regurgitation eponyms: Quincke's capillary pulsations (nail beds pulsate after being blanched), de Musset's sign (bobbing of the head in time with the pulse), Lighthouse sign (alternate blanching and flushing of the face), Müller's sign (pulsation of the uvula), Becker's sign (pulsation of the retinal arteries), Oliver-Caravelli's sign (pulsation of the larynx), Sailer's sign (pulsation of the spleen), Dennison sign (pulsation of the cervix)

Mitral Stenosis

- Murmur: low-frequency, rumbling mid-diastolic murmur; listen with bell lightly applied to apex; may only be heard with patient in L lateral decubitus position; sounds like "distant thunder" or "the absence of silence"
- Mitral valve opening snap (OS) heard after S2, loud S1; both heard with diaphragm

Mitral regurgitation

- Murmur: late or holosystolic, high frequency, loudest at apex; radiates to axilla, inferior angle of L scapula [LR+ 4.4, LR– 0.2]
- S_3, split S_2 common, S1 is often soft

4. <u>GENERAL COMPLICATIONS OF VALVULAR HEART DISEASE</u>

- Heart failure
- Cor pulmonale results in ascites, peripheral edema (due to decreased cardiac output, increased pulmonary hypertension and development of right-sided heart failure)
- Arrhythmia (i.e., atrial fibrillation) leads to increased risk of systemic thromboembolism
- Poor exercise tolerance (due to decreased cardiac output)
- Infective endocarditis (risk factors and requirement for antibiotic prophylaxis as follows): prosthetic valves or material, prior IE, unrepaired cyanotic congenital heart disease (including shunts and conduits), complete congenital heart disease repair within previous 6 months, repaired congenital heart disease with residual defects, valve regurgitation due to structural abnormalities in cardiac transplant patients

AORTIC STENOSIS

- See **Table 8.1**

TABLE 8.1. Echocardiographic Features of Aortic Stenosis

Characteristic	Mild AS	Moderate AS	Severe AS
Mean gradient (mmHg)	Less than 25	25–40	Greater than 40*
Valve area (cm²)	Greater than 1.5	1–1.5	Less than 1†
Jet velocity (m/sec)	Less than 3	3–4	Greater than 4

* If left ventricular ejection fraction is less than 0.4, may have severe AS with only a moderate gradient of 25–40 mmHg
† Valve area index (cm² per m²) less than 0.6 also indicates severe AS
Source: Adapted from *JACC.* 2008; 52(13): e1–e142.

1. **WORKUP**
   - Echocardiogram
   - ECG and CXR
   - Cardiac catheterization indicated:
     - Prior to an AVR, to assess for CAD in patients at risk or if considering a pulmonary allograft
     - To assess severity of AS when noninvasive studies are inconclusive or not consistent with clinical findings

2. **TREATMENT**
   Medical Therapy
   - Indicated primarily to bridge patients until they have an AVR
   - Heart failure
     - Mild–moderate: judicious diuretics; control BP with ACEI; and digoxin for LVEF less than 0.4
     - Severe HF with a normal BP and LVEF less than or equal to 0.35: nitroprusside with central hemodynamic monitoring titrated to MAP 60–70 mmHg
   - Atrial fibrillation: digoxin for ventricular rate control
   - Angina: avoid β-blockers, diltiazem, verapamil, and nitrates
   Indications for Surgical Treatment
   - Aortic valve replacement (AVR) for severe aortic stenosis and any of the following:
     - Undergoing CABG or other heart surgery (may also consider AVR for moderate AS)
     - Symptomatic aortic stenosis
     - Left ventricular ejection fraction less than 0.5
     - Consider for hypotension during a supervised exercise test
     - Consider if severe AS with AVA less than 0.6 cm², mean gradient greater than 60 mmHg, aortic jet greater than 5 m/s
   - Aortic balloon valvotomy reasonable option for:
     - Hemodynamically unstable or pregnant patients with severe AS at high risk for an AVR
     - Palliation for severe AS in patients who are not candidates for an AVR
     - May consider TAVI surgery (trans-aortic AV replacement) in high-risk surgical patients

3. **PROGNOSIS**
   - Presence of symptoms determines life expectancy in patients with AS
     - Angina: 5 years
     - Syncope: 3 years
     - CHF: 2 years

4. **SPECIFIC COMPLICATIONS**
   - Exercise-induced hypotension or brady/tachyarrhythmia results in syncope
   - Left ventricular hypertrophy (LVH)
   - Heart failure
   - Arrhythmias (especially ventricular arrhythmias)
   - Sudden cardiac death (incidence 0–5% asymptomatic AS, 8–34% symptomatic AS)
   - Left ventricular systolic dysfunction (rare complication)
   - Bleeding (from acquired von Willebrand syndrome)
   - Stroke (from calcium emboli)

AORTIC INSUFFICIENCY

1. **WORKUP**
   - Echocardiogram: severe AI with Doppler jet width greater than 65%, left ventricular outflow tract and vena contracta width greater than 0.6, LV systolic diameter larger than 55 mm, or LV diastolic diameter larger than 75 mm
   - ECG and CXR
   - Radionuclide ventriculography or cardiac MRI if LV function equivocal by echocardiogram
   - Cardiac catheterization indicated if noninvasive tests are equivocal or discordant with clinical symptoms, or to evaluate for CAD in patients at risk
     - Severe AI if regurgitant volume greater than or equal to 60 mL/beat, regurgitant fraction greater than or equal to 50%, regurgitant orifice area 0.3 cm^2 or larger, and/or dilated left ventricle

2. **TREATMENT**
   Medical Treatment
   - Vasodilators (ACEI, nifedipine ER, amlodipine, felodipine, or hydralazine) for severe chronic AI or LVEF less than 0.4
   - Loop diuretics indicated for volume control in CHF
   - Acute severe AI: nitroprusside with or without dobutamine as bridge to urgent AVR
     - Intra-aortic balloon pump and vasoconstrictors are contraindicated
   Indications for AVR
   - Symptomatic severe AI
   - Left ventricular ejection fraction less than or equal to 0.5
   - Left ventricular end-systolic dimension larger than 55 mm or end-diastolic dimension greater than 75 mm
   - Severe AI in patients undergoing a CABG or other surgery on the heart or aorta

3. **PROGNOSIS**
   - The presence of symptoms predicts yearly mortality risk
     - Asymptomatic, 2.8% yearly mortality risk
     - NYHA Class I, 3.0% yearly mortality risk
     - NYHA Class II, 6.3% yearly mortality risk
     - NYHA Class III-IV, 24.6% yearly mortality risk

4. **SPECIFIC COMPLICATIONS**
   - Atypical chest pain
   - Aortic root dilation leads to dissecting/saccular aneurysm
   - Heart failure

MITRAL STENOSIS

- See **Table 8.2**

TABLE 8.2.   Echocardiographic Features of Mitral Stenosis

Characteristic	Mild MS	Moderate MS	Severe MS
Mean gradient (mmHg)	Less than 5	5–10	Greater than 10
Pulmonary artery systolic pressure (mmHg)	Less than 30	30–50	Greater than 50
Valve area (cm²)	Greater than 1.5	1–1.5	Less than 1

Source: Adapted from *JACC.* 2008: 52(13); e1–142.

WORKUP

- Echocardiogram
- ECG and CXR
- Cardiac catheterization indicated
  - Noninvasive testing is equivocal or discordant with clinical symptoms
  - Hemodynamic evaluation when echocardiogram reveals discrepancy between MV gradient and MV area
  - To assess cause of pulmonary hypertension when noninvasive testing is inconclusive

TREATMENT

Medical Therapy

- Atrial fibrillation: anticoagulation with heparin/warfarin; rate control with digoxin, β-blocker, verapamil, or diltiazem; DC cardioversion for severe hemodynamic instability
- Heart failure: sodium restriction, judicious diuresis, Afib rate control, and avoid tachycardia
- Chronic anticoagulation if: chronic or paroxysmal Afib/aflutter, prior embolization, severe mitral stenosis with left atrium (LA) greater than 5.5 cm or presence of LA clot

Surgical Therapy

- Indications for percutaneous mitral balloon valvulotomy (PMBV)
  - Moderate–severe mitral stenosis with NYHA Class II–IV CHF
  - Moderate–severe mitral stenosis and pulmonary artery systolic pressure greater than 50 mmHg (rest) or greater than 60 (exercise)
- Contraindications for PMBV: LA clot, moderate–severe MR, or MV morphology not suitable
- Indications for MV replacement or repair
  - Moderate–severe mitral stenosis with NYHA Class III–IV CHF and PMBV contraindicated
  - Moderate–severe mitral stenosis with NYHA Class I–II CHF and pulmonary artery systolic pressure greater than 60 mmHg who are not candidates for PMBV

PROGNOSIS

- Severe mitral stenosis occurs with a valve area of less than 1 cm²
  - Hemoptysis, atrial fibrillation, pulmonary hypertension, and thromboembolism may occur

SPECIFIC COMPLICATIONS

- Hypotension from decreased stroke volume/cardiac output
- Pulmonary hypertension
- Hemoptysis
- Atrial fibrillation
- Thromboembolism
- Ortner's syndrome/cardiovocal syndrome
  - Hoarseness from compression of recurrent laryngeal nerve or cough

MITRAL REGURGITATION

- See **Table 8.3**

TABLE 8.3. Echocardiographic Features of Mitral Regurgitation (MR)

Characteristics	Mild MR	Moderate MR	Severe MR
Doppler jet area	Less than 20% LA area	20–40% LA area	Greater than 40% LA area*
Doppler vena contracta width	Less than 0.3 cm	0.3–0.69 cm	Greater than 0.7 cm

* Severe MR also if any LA swirling or if jet impinges on LA wall
Source: Adapted from JACC, 2008; 52(13): e1–142.

1. **WORKUP**
   - Echocardiogram
   - ECG and CXR
   - Cardiac catheterization indicated
     - LV hemodynamic evaluation when echocardiogram is equivocal or discordant with clinical findings or displays a discrepancy between MR severity and elevated pulmonary artery pressures
     - Evaluate for CAD in patients at risk

2. **TREATMENT**
   Medical Therapy
   - Heart failure: sodium restriction, diuretics, nitrates, and afterload reduction (ACEI, ARB, or hydralazine nitrates); add β-blocker if LVEF is less than 0.4
   - Atrial fibrillation: anticoagulation with heparin/warfarin; rate control with digoxin, β-blocker, verapamil, or diltiazem; DC cardioversion for severe hemodynamic instability
   - Acute MR with normal BP: nitroprusside with central hemodynamic monitoring
   - Acute MR with hypotension: nitroprusside and dobutamine with or without IABP; avoid vasoconstrictors then an urgent MVR
   Indications for Mitral Valve Repair or Replacement
   - Acute symptomatic severe MR
   - Chronic severe MR with NYHA Class II–IV CHF and:
     - LVEF 0.3–0.6 or LV end-systolic dimension (LVESD) greater than or equal to 40 mm
     - Consider if LVEF greater than 0.6, LVESD less than 40 mm, and new-onset Afib or pulmonary HTN with concomitant Maze procedure
     - Patients undergoing CABG with moderate–severe MR

3. **PROGNOSIS**
   - Can lead to atrial fibrillation secondary to dilatation
   - LV dysfunction and heart failure can occur with progressive disease

4. **SPECIFIC COMPLICATIONS**
   - Pulmonary hypertension
   - Heart failure
   - Atrial fibrillation
   - Thromboembolism

REFERENCES

Circulation, 2003;108(20):2432–8; *Circulation,* 2005;112(3):432–7; *J Am Coll Cardiol,* 2008;52(13):e1–142;
N Engl J Med, 2003;348(18):1756–63; *N Engl J Med,* 2004;351(16):1627–34; *N Engl J Med,* 2005;353(13):1342–9.

Choudhry N. Does this patient have aortic regurgitation? In: *Simel DL, Rennie D, eds. The Rational Clinical Examination.* New York, NY: McGraw-Hill; 2009:419–32.

Etchells E. Does this patient have an abnormal systolic murmur? In: *Simel DL, Rennie D, eds. The Rational Clinical Examination.* New York, NY: McGraw-Hill; 2009:433–42.

McGee S. Aortic regurgitation. In: *McGee S. Evidence Based Physical Diagnosis.* 3rd ed. Philadelphia, PA: Saunders-Elsevier; 2012:379–87.

McGee S. Aortic stenosis. In: *McGee S. Evidence Based Physical Diagnosis.* 3rd ed. Philadelphia, PA: Saunders-Elsevier; 2012:373–8.

CHAPTER 9

PERIOPERATIVE CARDIOVASCULAR EVALUATION

Active Cardiac Conditions
- Unstable or CCS III–IV angina
- Recent MI: more than 7 days or within 30 days
- Decompensated CHF
- 2nd- or 3rd-degree AV block
- Ventricular arrhythmias
- Uncontrolled Afib/SVT

Coronary Revascularization Indicated before Nonurgent Surgery
- Stable angina with either severe left main, 3-vessel, or proximal LAD stenosis
- High-risk unstable angina or NSTEMI
- Acute STEMI

Clinical Risk Factors (Revised Cardiac Risk Index – [RCRI])
- History of CAD
- History of CHF
- History of CVA/TIA
- Diabetes
- CKD (crt greater than 2 mg/dL)

Cardiac Risk for Noncardiac Surgical Procedures (incidence of death or nonfatal MI)		
Vascular surgery (more than 5%)	Intermediate risk (1–5%)	Low risk (less than 1%)
• Aortic surgery	• Intraperitoneal, intrathoracic	• Endoscopic, superficial
• Peripheral vascular surgery	• Carotid endarterectomy, orthopedic	• Breast, cataract
• Other major vascular surgery	• Head/neck surgery, prostate surgery	• Ambulatory surgery

1–4 METS Functional Level	4 METS Functional Level	4–10 METS Functional Level
ADLs	Light housework	Scrub bing or mopping floors
Walk 2 blocks on level ground at 2–3 mph	Walk up a hill/flight of stairs	Dancing, doubles tennis, golfing
	Walk level ground at 4 mph	Bowling, moving heavy furniture

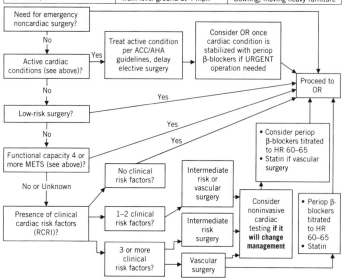

FIGURE 9.1. Preoperative Cardiac Evaluation for Noncardiac Surgery

Source: Adapted from *Circulation*, 2009; 120(21): e169–276 and *JACC*, 2007; 50(17): e159–241.

TABLE 9.1.   Recommendations for Testing Prior to Non-emergent Surgery

Test	Indications for Preoperative Laboratory Testing
White blood count	Symptoms to suggest infection, myeloproliferative disorder, or use of myelotoxic drugs
Hemoglobin	Anticipated large blood loss, symptoms/history of anemia, renal disease, liver disease, hematologic disorders, bleeding diathesis, extremes of age, anticoagulant use
Electrolytes	Renal disease, CHF, DM, adrenal disease, liver disease, HTN, meds that can affect electrolytes
Glucose	Diabetes, metabolic syndrome, or morbid obesity
Renal panel	Age older than 50 yo, HTN, heart disease, diabetes, liver disease, malnutrition, major surgery, meds that can affect kidneys
Liver panel	Chronically ill, malnourished, liver disease, major surgery, endocrine disease, renal disease, meds that can affect liver
PT/PTT/Platelet	Bleeding diathesis, liver disease, myeloproliferative disorder, malnutrition, anticoagulant use, recent antibiotic use, renal disease, planned major surgery
ECG	DM, CKD, CAD, PVD, CVA, CHF, AAA, carotid artery disease, unexplained chest pain or dyspnea, planned major surgery
Chest X-ray	Age older than 50 yo, known cardiac or pulmonary disease, active cardiac or pulmonary symptoms, abnormal lung exam, morbid obesity
2D-Echocardiogram	Unexplained dyspnea, clinical signs of heart failure, history of CHF with worsening dyspnea or deterioration in clinical status
Urinalysis	Urinary tract symptoms or genitourinary procedure
Urine pregnancy test	Any woman of childbearing age undergoing surgery

CHF = congestive heart failure, DM = diabetes mellitus, HTN = hypertension, PT = prothrombin time, PTT = partial thromboplastin time, ECG = electrocardiogram, CKD = chronic kidney disease, CAD = coronary artery disease, PVD = peripheral vascular disease, CVA = cerebrovascular accident (stroke), AAA = abdominal aortic aneurysm
Source: Adapted from *Anesthesiology.* 2002; 96(2): 485–96, *Med Clin N Amer.* 2003; 87(1): 7–40 and *JACC.* 2007; 50(17): e159–241.

TABLE 9.2.   Perioperative Anticoagulation Based on Risk of Thromboembolism

Perioperative Risk of Thromboembolic Event	Conditions	Management
Low (less than 5%/year)	• Nonvalvular Afib with CHADS$_2$ score* 3 or lower • St. Jude valve—aortic position • VTE more than 90 days ago • Nonrecurrent stroke/TIA	• Stop warfarin 5 days prior to surgery • Proceed with surgery if INR is less than 1.5 on day of surgery
Intermediate (5–10%/year)	• VTE 30–90 days ago • History of 2 or more strokes/TIAs • St. Jude valve—mitral position • Older mechanical aortic valve	• Stop warfarin 5 days prior to surgery • Start enoxaparin† 1 mg/kg SQ q 12 h 36 h after last warfarin dose • Stop enoxaparin 24 h preop • Restart enoxaparin 1 mg/kg SQ q 12 h on POD#1 • Overlap enoxaparin and warfarin at least 5 days and until INR 2–3 × 24 h
High (greater than 10%/year)	• VTE in last month • Valvular Afib • Cardioembolism from Afib or a mechanical heart valve • Hypercoagulable state • Acute intracardiac thrombus • Older mechanical mitral valve	

* See Table 5.1, Afib = Atrial fibrillation, VTE = venous thromboembolism, TIA = transient ischemic attack, INR = international normalized ratio
† Use unfractionated heparin for wt greater than 155 kg; dose adjust for CrCl 15–30, and avoid if CrCl is less than 15 mL/min
Source: Adapted from *Clev Clin J Med,* 2005; 72(2): 157–63.

TABLE 9.3.   Perioperative Management of Patients Taking Chronic Steroids*

Operation	Recommended Management
Minor	• Hydrocortisone† 25 mg/day divided bid × 1 day, then resume regular dose
Moderate	• Hydrocortisone† 25 mg IV q 8 h × 24 h, then 25 mg IV q 12 h × 24 h, then regular dose
Major	• Hydrocortisone† 50 mg IV q 8 h × 24 h, then wean to regular dose over 2–3 days

* Indicated for use of prednisone 20 mg/day or more for at least 3 weeks or more than 5 mg/day chronically
† Give first dose within 1–2 hours of the operation start time
Source: Adapted from *J Amer Coll Surg,* 2001; 193(6): 678–86.

Perioperative Management of the Diabetic Patient
- Minor surgery in Type II DM patients controlled with oral agents
  - Hold oral agents on day of surgery
  - Cover glucose greater than 180 mg/dL with controlled-dose insulin
- Minor surgery in Type II DM patients controlled with insulin
  - Normal insulin glargine the night prior or ½ dose NPH insulin the morning of surgery
  - Restart the normal insulin regimen once patient is eating well after surgery
- Major surgery in Type II DM patients
  - Hold oral agents or give ½ dose of NPH insulin the morning of surgery
  - Start continuous insulin infusion prior to surgery and continue perioperatively
- Surgery in Type I DM patients
  - Start 5% dextrose fluids at 100–125 mL/h the morning of surgery
  - Control glucose with a continuous insulin infusion perioperatively

Postoperative Diabetic Management
- Target glucose levels 70–150 mg/dL for 48 hours using an insulin infusion after major surgery
  - Fewer infectious complications and lower mortality if glucose is less than 220 mg/dL
- Transition to subcutaneous insulin once patient is tolerating oral intake

REFERENCES
Diabetes Care, 2004;27(2):553–91; *N Engl J Med,* 2006;355(18):1903–11; *Diabetes Care,* 2008; 31 *Suppl:*S12–S54.

CHAPTER 10

HYPERTENSION

1. EPIDEMIOLOGY

- Essential hypertension applies to 95% of cases
- Onset usually between 25–55 yo; onset before 20 yo is rare
- Risks for secondary HTN: early age of onset, onset over age 50, previous well-controlled HTN suddenly becomes refractory
- Antihypertensive therapy reduces stroke incidence by 30–50%, heart failure by 40–50%, and decrease in CAD mortality by 10–15%
- Ambulatory BP is superior to office BP in predicting risk of end-organ damage
- LVH, a risk factor for heart failure, is found in 15% of chronic HTN. LVH is a risk factor for heart failure. Antihypertensives that reduce SBP can reduce this risk by 50%
- 60–70% of HTN patients are overweight based on the Framingham data

2. PATHOPHYSIOLOGY

- Mechanisms
  - Volume dependent: impaired ability of kidney to excrete Na, which is the primary determinant of intravascular volume
  - Hyperadrenergic state: $\alpha 1$ causes peripheral vasoconstriction, $\beta 1$ causes positive inotropy and positive chronotropy plus renin release
  - Renin-angiotensin-aldosterone upregulation: renal hypoperfusion increases renin, which then increases angiotensin I/II, which then increases aldosterone, resulting in Na retention.
  - Vascular: decreased arterial compliance and/or decreased lumen diameter leading to increased resistance, impaired endothelial function relaxation by NO and endothelin (e.g., coarctation of the aorta, isolated systolic hypertension of the elderly)

3. CLINICAL PRESENTATION

- Presentation: asymptomatic
- Hypertensive urgency is BP greater than 180/120
- Hypertensive emergency is BP greater than 180/120 with end-organ dysfunction (encephalopathy, stroke, myocardial infarction, pulmonary edema, aortic dissection, renal failure)
- Look for sequelae of chronic HTN: hypertensive retinopathy (hemorrhages, exudates, papilledema)
- Secondary causes of HTN
  - Coarctation (arm:leg BP 20 mmHg difference; delayed femoral pulse; rib notching on chest x-ray)
  - Renal artery stenosis (renal bruit; increase in creatinine after starting ACEI)
  - Thyroid disorders (bradycardia/tachycardia, cold/heat intolerance, constipation/diarrhea, menstrual irregularities)
  - Hyperaldosteronism (hypokalemia)
  - Obstructive sleep apnea (apnea while asleep, daytime sleepiness, snoring)
  - Pheochromocytoma (flushing, headaches, labile BPs, orthostatic hypotension, sweating, palpitations, syncope)
  - Cushing syndrome (buffalo hump, central obesity, moon facies, striae)

- See **Tables 10.1** and **1.2**

TABLE 10.1.   Risk Stratification for Hypertensive Patients

Risk Factors	End-Organ Damage
Cigarette smoking	Heart disease
Obesity (body mass index 30 kg/m² or greater)	• Left ventricular hypertrophy • Coronary artery disease
Family history of cardiovascular disease ♀ younger than 65 years or ♂ younger than 55 years	• Congestive heart failure
Dyslipidemia	Stroke or transient ischemic attack
Diabetes mellitus	Nephropathy (microalbuminuria or creatinine clearance less than 60 mL/minute)
Very sedentary lifestyle	
Age older than 55 yo (♂) or older than 65 yo (♀)	Peripheral vascular disease
Men or postmenopausal women	Retinopathy

TABLE 10.2.   Causes of Secondary Hypertension

Features of Secondary Hypertension	Possible Etiologies
Sudden onset of severe hypertension or newly diagnosed in those younger than 30 or older than 60 yo	Renal vascular disease **or** renal parenchymal disease
Abnormal urinalysis	Renal parenchymal/glomerular disease
Hypokalemia and ARR greater than 66.9 ng/dL*	Primary hyperaldosteronism
Hypercalcemia	Hyperparathyroidism
Fine tremor, heat intolerance, decreased TSH, increased fT₄	Hyperthyroidism
Paroxysmal severe HTN, palpitations, HA	Pheochromocytoma
Abdominal mass	Polycystic kidney disease
Flank bruit	Renal artery stenosis
Elevated glucose, striae, truncal obesity, etc.	Cushing syndrome
Resistant hypertension on three meds	Renal vascular/parenchymal disease
Markedly decreased femoral pulses	Coarctation of aorta
Central obesity, loud snoring, daytime hypersomnolence, nonrestorative sleep	Obstructive sleep apnea

* ARR = aldosteron/renin ratio after 30 minutes sitting greater than 66.9 ng/dl confirms with 100% specificity and ARR less than 23.6 ng/dl excludes 97% of cases of primary hyperaldosteronism

4.   INITIAL WORKUP FOR HYPERTENSION

- Blood work: complete blood count, electrolytes, calcium, fasting lipid and renal panels
- Other studies: urinalysis, ECG, eye exam, and a chest X-ray if signs of CHF
- Evaluate for secondary HTN if: onset younger than 30 or older than 60 yo; accelerated, resistant, or paroxysmal HTN; abnormal UA or increased creatinine; unprovoked decreased K/increased Ca; Cushing syndrome; abdominal mass/bruit

5. TREATMENT

Educate About Therapeutic Lifestyle Changes (TLC)

- Weight reduction (aiming for BMI less than 25 kg/m^2): decreases SBP 5–20 mmHg
- Less than 2 drinks of alcohol/day (for men) and 1 drink or less per day (for women): decreases SBP 2–4 mmHg
- Aerobic exercise (at least 30 minutes/day at least 4 days/week): decreases SBP 4–9 mmHg
- Less than 2.3 grams sodium/day: decreases SBP 2–8 mmHg
- Diet: dietary approaches to stop hypertension (DASH) diet (decreased SBP 8–14 mmHg); adequate potassium, magnesium, calcium; low in saturated fat, high in fiber, and low in cholesterol
- Smoking cessation

Medications/Herbs That Cause Elevated Blood Pressure (discontinue if possible)

- Anabolic steroids and corticosteroids, bevacizumab, bromocriptine, bupropion, buspirone, clozapine, cyclosporine, darbepoetin, ephedra, epoetin-α, estrogens, fludrocortisone, MAOIs, metoclopramide, nicotine, NSAIDs, phentermine, pseudoephedrine, sibutramine, sorafenib, sunitinib, sympathomimetics, tacrolimus, and venlafaxine
- Herbs: aniseed, bayberry, blue cohosh, capsaicin, ephedra, gentian, ginger, ginseng, guarana, licorice, Ma Huang, Pau de Arco, parsley, and St. John's wort

Clinical Conditions That Can Cause Elevated Blood Pressure in Hospitalized Patients

- Important to exclude and address these causes of blood pressure elevation: pain, anxiety, alcohol/drug withdrawal, elevated intracranial pressure, renal failure, excess sodium administration (watch IV fluids), or excessive bladder or bowel distension

Initial Drug Therapy for Uncomplicated Hypertension

- BP goals: BP less than or equal to 130/80 for DM, CAD, or CKD; BP less than or equal to 125/75 for proteinuria more than1 g/day
- Initial therapy in patients with no compelling indications for specific drug classes
  - Thiazides (drug of choice for most patients if creatinine is less than 2 mg/dL or CrCl is greater than 35 mL/min/1.73 m^2) despite the small increase in risk of new-onset diabetes
  - Alternative options are: ACEI, CCBs, and ARBs (if ACEI-intolerant)
  - β-blockers not the best monotherapy for HTN if no compelling indications
  - Stage 2 hypertension usually requires at least 2 drugs
- See **Tables 10.3** and **10.4**

TABLE 10.3. Mechanism of Action of Various Antihypertensive Medications

Diuretics	Negative Inotropic	Sympatholytics	Renin-Angiotensin-Aldosterone Blockers	Vasodilators
• Furosemide (preferred over thiazides if serum creatinine is 2.5 mg/dL or higher)	• β-blockers • Verapamil • Diltiazem	• β-blockers • Clonidine • Methyldopa • Guanethidine	• β-blockers • Angiotensin receptor blockers • Angiotensin converting enzyme inhibitors • Direct renin inhibitors • Aldosterone antagonists	• Hydralazine • α₁-blockers • Minoxidil • Dihydropyridine CCBs • Thiazides (creatinine less than 2.5 mg/dL)

TABLE 10.4. Compelling Indications for Specific Antihypertensive Drug Therapy

Indication	Drug Class
Diabetes with proteinuria	ACEI*, ARB*, verapamil, or diltiazem
Congestive heart failure	ACEI*, ARB*, β-blockers, diuretics, or AA
Diastolic dysfunction	β-blocker, verapamil, diltiazem, thiazides, ACEI*
Isolated systolic hypertension	Thiazides, dihydropyridine CCB, β-blocker, ACEI*, or nitrates
Postmyocardial infarction	β-blocker, ACEI*, or AA
Angina	β-blocker or calcium channel blocker
Atrial fibrillation	β-blocker, verapamil, or diltiazem
Dyslipidemia	ACEI, β-blocker, or thiazides
Essential tremor	β-blocker
Hyperthyroidism	β-blocker
Migraine	β-blocker, verapamil, or diltiazem
Osteoporosis	Thiazides
Pregnancy	Methyldopa, hydralazine, or labetalol
Benign prostatic hyperplasia	α_1-blockers† in combination with other agents
Erectile dysfunction	ACEI, ARB, or CCB
Renal insufficiency	ACEI* or ARB*
Cerebrovascular disease	Thiazides, ACEI, ARB, or amlodipine
Obstructive sleep apnea	CPAP therapy, AA, thiazides, CCB at bedtime
African American race	Thiazides (first-line), CCB, or ACEI*
Aortic dissection	Labetalol, β-blocker, or diltiazem
Refractory hypertension	Minoxidil + loop diuretics + β-blocker or CCB
Primary hyperaldosteronism‡	ARB

AA = aldosterone antagonist, ACEI = angiotensin converting enzyme inhibitor, ARB = angiotensin receptor blocker, CCB = calcium channel blocker,
CPAP = continuous positive airway pressure
* Caution with ACEI or ARB use if creatinine is greater than 3 mg/dL
† Never use as monotherapy for HTN
‡ ARR = aldosterone/renin ratio after 30 minutes sitting greater than 66.9 ng/dL confirms with 100% specificity and ARR less than 23.6 ng/dL excludes
97% of cases of primary hyperaldosteronism

Treatment of Hypertensive Urgency (BP greater than 180/110 mmHg without end-organ damage)

- Need to exclude chronic, poorly controlled hypertension (outpatient management)
- Goal is to reduce BP to a safe range in several hours and normalize BP within several days
- Oral agents titrated to effect: clonidine 0.2 mg × 1, then 0.1 mg q 1 h × 6; captopril 25 mg q 1 h × 4; labetalol 200–400 mg q 2–3 h; or nifedipine XL 30 mg × 1
- IV agents if pt NPO: metoprolol 5 mg q 15 min × 3; labetalol 20–40 mg q 10–15 min (max 300 mg/day); hydralazine 5–10 mg q 30 min; enalaprilat 1.25 mg q 6 h; diltiazem 20 mg, then 5–15 mg/h

Treatment of Hypertensive Emergency

- Definition: markedly elevated blood pressure associated with acute end-organ damage
- Examples: hypertensive encephalopathy (headache, confusion, and papilledema); CHF; acute coronary syndrome; ARF; aortic dissection; ischemic or hemorrhagic stroke; preeclampsia or eclampsia
- Treatment of HTN emergency is to cautiously decrease MAP 25% with IV meds in the ICU
- See **Table 10.5**

TABLE 10.5.   Management of Hypertensive Emergencies

Medication	IV Dosages	Special Indications	Cautions
Nitroprusside	0.25–10 mcg/kg/min	CHF or refractory HTN in stroke or aortic dissection, with or without for encephalopathy	Increased ICP, cyanide or thiocyanate toxicity*
Labetalol	20–80 mg IV q 10 min, then 0.5–2 mg/min IV	Encephalopathy, ACS[†], aortic dissection, acute stroke, pre-eclampsia or pheochromocytoma (pheo)	Bradycardia or heart block, severe bronchospasm, severe CHF
Nitroglycerin	5–200 mcg/min	ACS or CHF	Headache (HA)
Nicardipine	5–15 mg/h	Acute stroke or pre-eclampsia	Tachycardia, ACS
Hydralazine	10–20 mg IV q 20 min	Pre-eclampsia, CHF	Tachycardia, HA
Enalaprilat	0.625–1.25 mg IV q 6 h	CHF	Decreased renal function, elevated K
Esmolol	500 mcg/kg load, then 50–300 mcg/kg/min	ACS[†], aortic dissection or adjunct for pheo	Bradycardia or heart block
Fenoldopam	0.1–0.3 mcg/kg/min	CHF, ACS, or acute kidney injury	Tachycardia or glaucoma

CHF = congestive heart failure, HTN = hypertension, ICP = intracranial pressure, ACS = acute coronary syndrome, pheo = heochromocytoma, HA = headache, K = potassium
* Risk higher with prolonged use longer than 24 hours and with severe renal or hepatic impairment
† Avoid if ACS secondary to cocaine or methamphetamine abuse, treat with nitrates and benzodiazepines
Source: Information from *Chest,* 2007; 131(16): 1949–62 and *Circulation,* 2008; 117(14): 1897–907.

6. PROGNOSIS

- In adults, for every 20 mmHg systolic or 10 mmHg diastolic increase in BP above 115/75 mmHg, the mortality rate for both ischemic heart disease and stroke doubles

7. COMPLICATIONS

- Neuro: cerebrovascular disease (i.e., hemorrhagic/ischemic stroke, vascular dementia, Alzheimer's disease, acceleration in cognitive decline)
- Cardiovascular: CAD (i.e., MI, angina), left ventricular remodeling/dysfunction (i.e., LVH, heart failure), arrhythmia (i.e., atrial fibrillation), sudden cardiac death (i.e., from arrhythmia), aortic and peripheral arterial disease (i.e., AAA, thoracic aortic aneurysm, aortic dissection, occlusive PAD)
- Renal: hypertensive nephrosclerosis may lead to ESRD
- Ophthalmologic diseases (hypertensive retinopathy, retinal artery occlusion, nonarteritic anterior ischemic optic neuropathy, macular degeneration)

REFERENCES

JAMA, 2003:289:2560–72; *N Engl J Med,* 2003;348(7):610–7; *JAMA,* 2002;288(23):2981–97; *J Clin Hypertens (Greenwich),* 2007;9(10):760–9; *Circulation,* 2007;115(21): 2761–88; *Cochrane Database Syst Rev,* 2008;(1):CD003653; *Chest,* 2007;131(16):1949–62.

CHAPTER 11

PERIPHERAL ARTERIAL DISEASE

1. ## EPIDEMIOLOGY
   - Type I (10–15%) limited to aorta and common iliac arteries found most commonly in ages 40–45 yo who are heavy smokers or with hyperlipidemia
   - Type II (25%) involves aorta, common iliacs, and external iliac arteries
   - Type III (60–75%) is a multilevel disease involving aorta, iliac, femoral, popliteal, and tibial arteries
   - Type II and III risk factors are old age, male, DM, and HTN. They have 2.5 × higher risk factor for cardiac event and 30% have triple vessel disease at time of peripheral artery bypass.
   - Lipid-lowering agents reduce claudication symptoms by about 40%
   - Patients with claudication have 50% 5-year survival rate from cardiovascular mortality
   - 90% of pts with PAD also have CAD
   - 30% of pts with PAD also have cerebrovascular disease in more than 70% of brain regions
   - Claudication has a 2% per year gangrene risk and 1% per year amputation risk

2. ## PATHOPHYSIOLOGY
   - Most commonly due to atherosclerosis of medium and large vessels
     - Plaques with deposition of calcium, thrombi made of platelets and fibrin
     - Localized to aorta and iliac, femoral, popliteal, tibial, and peroneal arteries
     - Branch points create turbulence, leading to arterial injury, then atherosclerosis
   - Other etiologies: thrombosis, embolism, vasculitis, fibromuscular dysplasia

3. ## CLINICAL PRESENTATION
   - Absence of both dorsalis pedis and posterior tibial pulses (either can be absent in up to 10% of normal individuals) [LR+ 14.9, LR– 0.3].
   - Other signs including toe/foot ulcers [LR+ 7.0, LR– 1], impaired nail growth, atrophic skin with absent hair [LR+ 1.7, LR– 1], foot pallor with elevation [LR+ 2.0, LR– 0.7], asymmetrically cool feet [LR+ 6.1, LR– 0.9]
   - Buerger's test: observe the color of leg when elevated, then when lowered; a positive test is pallor with elevation and rubor in the dependent position
   ### Acute Arterial Insufficiency
   - Most common cause is a cardioembolic event
   - Ischemic complication rate significantly increases if time from symptom onset to embolectomy is more than 6 h:
     - 10% if interval is less than 6 h; 20% if interval is 8 h; and 33% if interval is 24 h
   - Clinical features of arterial insufficiency (6 Ps)
     - Pain, pallor, pulseless, paresthesias, paralysis, and poikilothermia (cold)
     - Sudden onset of symptoms favors an embolic event
   - Treatment
     - Therapeutic IV heparin, then catheter-directed thrombolysis or embolectomy
   ### Chronic Arterial Insufficiency
   - Clinical features of peripheral arteriosclerotic disease
     - Intermittent claudication described as cramping discomfort, pain, or fatigue of muscles with ambulation (graded by distance walked) and relieved by rest
     - Aortoiliac disease: thigh/buttock claudication with or without impotence (Leriche syndrome)
     - Femoropopliteal disease: thigh and calf claudication

- ○ Tibial or peroneal artery disease: foot claudication
- ○ Signs: dystrophic nails, bruits, absent/weak peripheral pulses, loss of hair on and cool distal extremity, shiny skin, dependent rubor, decreased capillary refill
- Risk factors: tobacco smoking, positive family history, hyperlipidemia, diabetes, hypertension, hyperhomocysteinemia, and age 50 yo or older
- PAD pts: 60–80% have significant CAD and 25% have significant carotid artery stenosis
- PAD pts: 5-year combined event rate of MI, stroke, or vascular death is 35–50%

4. DIAGNOSIS

- Diagnosis: ankle-brachial index less than 0.91. 0.4 or lower suggests limb-threatening ischemia
- Doppler ultrasound of lower extremity arteries
- Angiogram of aorta with peripheral runoff

5. WORKUP OF PAD

- See **Table 11.1**

TABLE 11.1. Ankle-Brachial Index (ABI) to Assess for Lower Extremity PAD

ABI	Interpretation
1.3 or higher	Noncompressible vessel
0.91–1.29	Normal
0.61–0.9	Mild peripheral arterial disease
0.41–0.6	Moderate peripheral arterial disease
0.4 or lower	Severe peripheral arterial disease

- Conditions with falsely elevated ABI (usually ABI greater than 1.3): DM, very elderly, and CKD
  - ○ Toe-brachial index less than 0.7 suggests significant PAD in these patients
- Duplex ultrasound of arterial system and segmental limb pressures: good noninvasive studies to estimate degree of lower extremity arterial obstruction
- Catheter angiogram, CT angiogram, or MR angiogram with 3D reconstruction all perform well to assess for aortic and/or lower/upper extremity arterial stenosis
- Complete blood count, fasting lipid profile and glucose, basic metabolic panel, and ECG
- Consider renal artery imaging to rule out RAS if resistant HTN or renal bruit present

Medical Treatment of PAD

- Lifestyle modification: smoking cessation, graded aerobic exercise program 30 min at least 3 times/ week, and weight reduction if BMI greater than 25
- Lipid control with a statin: LDL less than 100 mg/dL (possibly less than 70 mg/dL in very high-risk patient* DM with CAD or CAD risk equivalent), triglycerides less than 150 mg/dL, and HDL greater than 40 mg/dL
- Tight diabetic (glycohemoglobin less than 7%) and blood pressure control (BP less than 130/85)
- Dual antiplatelets: aspirin 81 mg PO daily *and* clopidogrel 75 mg PO daily
  - ○ Decreased rate of MI and hospitalization for ischemic events compared with ASA alone
- Cilostazol 100 mg PO bid can improve claudication symptoms and exercise capacity, and is superior to pentoxifylline (avoid if symptoms of or history of CHF)
- Pentoxifylline 400 mg PO tid (alternative to cilostazol) modestly increase exercise capacity
- β-blockers and ACEI protect against cardiovascular events in patients with PAD
- No benefit of warfarin to decrease reocclusion rates of arterial grafts or to reduce claudication

---

*Known coronary artery disease or coronary artery disease risk equivalent and additional risk factors

Surgical Treatment or Percutaneous Interventional Therapies for PAD

- Arterial bypass or endovascular revascularization of LE PAD indicated for disabling claudication, rest pain, gangrene, Leriche syndrome, or nonhealing, ischemic ulcers
  - Angioplasty: increases success in proximal, large arteries with localized stenosis less than 10 cm
  - Surgery preferred if multiple, diffuse stenoses; complete occlusion of artery; bilateral iliac or femoral arteries or aortoiliac disease; or aneurysm surgery also needed
    - Grafts, 5-year patency: aortobifem (90%), fem-pop (80%), infrapopliteal (60%)
- Indications for angioplasty subclavian/brachiocephalic arteries: UE claudication; subclavian steal; subclavian stenosis greater than 50% plus ipsilateral dialysis shunt; before CABG with LIMA to LAD

6. **COMPLICATIONS**

- Claudication results in impaired walking performance/exercise capacity
- Limb ischemia causes limb necrosis necessitating amputation
- Stroke
- MI

REFERENCES

Circulation, 2006;113(11):e463–654; *JAMA,* 2006;295(5):547–53; *J Am Coll Cardiol,* 2007;50(6):473–90; *Circulation,* 2007;116(19):2203–15; *Prog Cardiovasc Dis,* 2011;54(1):2–13; *Eur Heart J,* 2009;30(2):192–201; *South Med J,* 2009;102(11):1141–9.

CHAPTER 12

SHOCK

1. DEFINITION OF SHOCK

- A medical condition in which tissue perfusion and oxygen delivery is insufficient for the metabolic demands of the body

2. PATHOPHYSIOLOGY

- Cellular response
  - Metabolism shifts from aerobic to anaerobic due to uncoupling of oxidative phosphorylation in mitochondria
  - Lactic acidosis then promotes vasodilation, which then worsens perfusion
  - Decreased ATP leads to failure of Na/K pump causing cellular swelling, then extracellular Ca floods into cells causing apoptosis
- Vascular response
  - Systemic vascular resistance determined by arteriolar diameter, which is controlled by vascular smooth muscle; perfusion is a balance between vasoconstriction and vasodilation
- Neurohormonal response
  - Hypotension causes adrenergic response leading to peripheral vasoconstriction, increased inotropy, increased chronotropy, increased glycogenolysis, and increased gluconeogenesis
  - Stress increases ACTH, which then increases cortisol, which then increases gluconeogenesis
  - Upregulation of renin-angiotensin-aldosterone system results in vasoconstriction and Na retention
  - Vasopressin release causes vasoconstriction
- Cardiac response
  - Cardiac output determined by heart rate and stroke volume
  - Stroke volume determined by preload (LV end-diastolic volume), contractility (inotropy), and afterload (systemic vascular resistance)
  - Decreased myocardial compliance plus hypotension decreases preload
  - Compensatory increased heart rate (limited by maximal heart rate and coronary blood flow)
  - Impaired contractility due to sepsis, ischemia, trauma, acidosis
- Pulmonary response
  - Hypoxia results in tachypnea, which leads to respiratory alkalosis
  - Reperfusion injury leads to ALI, ARDS causing pulmonary edema
- Renal response
  - Hypoperfusion results in acute tubular necrosis
  - Increased aldosterone and vasopressin decreases urine output
- Inflammatory response
  - Innate immune system activation
  - Complement cascade results in cell damage
  - Coagulation cascade results in microvascular thrombosis and fibrinolysis, which then leads to ischemic and reperfusion injury
  - Prostaglandins and leukotrienes result in vasoconstriction and vasodilation
  - Cytokines cause inflammatory response, leading to reactive oxygen species, then free-radical-mediated tissue damage
- Shock states (**boldfaced** parameter is primary insult)
  - Hypovolemic: decreased **preload**, decreased cardiac output, increased systemic vascular resistance

- Cardiogenic, obstructive: increased preload, decreased **cardiac output**, increased systemic vascular resistance
- Septic (warm/vasodilatory), anaphylactic: decreased preload, increased cardiac output, decreased **systemic vascular resistance**
- Neurogenic: decreased **preload,** decreased **cardiac output,** decreased **systemic vascular resistance**

3. **CLINICAL PRESENTATION**
   - Cardinal signs
     - Hypotension (absolute or relative)
     - Oliguria (renal blood flow shunted to other organs)
     - Changes in mental status (agitation leads to delirium, then coma)
     - Cool, clammy skin (compensatory vasoconstriction to assist central perfusion)
     - Metabolic acidosis (decreased clearance of lactate)

4. **COMPLICATIONS**
   - 35–60% mortality rate within a month in septic shock
   - 60–90% mortality rate in cardiogenic shock
   - Shock causes prolonged oxygen deprivation leading to cellular hypoxia, then derangement of ion exchange across cell membranes, causing disturbances in pH regulation and stimulation of inflammatory cascade resulting in cell death, end-organ dysfunction/damage and finally, multisystem organ failure, coma, and death
   - Refractory hypoperfusion leads to organ ischemia, which results in organ failure
   - See **Figure 12.1** and **Tables 12.1** through **12.3**

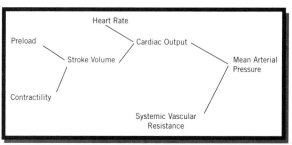

FIGURE 12.1.   **Determinants of Blood Pressure and Cardiac Output**

TABLE 12.1. Classification of Shock States

Shock Type	PCWP	Cardiac Index	SVRI
Cardiogenic (CI less than 2.0 L/min)	Elevated	Decreased	Elevated
Hypovolemic	Decreased	Decreased	Elevated
Distributive (sepsis, anaphylactic or spinal shock)	Normal or decreased	Elevated (unless SIRS-related myocardial dysfunction or underresuscitated patient)	Decreased
Obstructive (tension PTX, massive PE*, or tamponade†)	Elevated (tamponade) NL/elevated (PE or PTX)	Decreased	Elevated

* Massive PE associated with elevated PA, RA, and CVP pressures, PAD greater than PCWP, profound hypoxemia, and right heart strain on ECG and echocardiogram

† Tamponade will show equalization of RA, RV, PAD, and PCWP pressures

PCWP = pulmonary capillary wedge pressure, SVRI = systemic vascular resistance index, CI = cardiac index, PTX = pneumothorax, CVP = central venous pressure, PAD = pulmonary artery diastolic pressure

TABLE 12.2. Treatment of Shock States

Shock	Treatment
Hypovolemic	Aggressive fluid resuscitation
Cardiogenic	Dobutamine, IABP or LVAD, possible revascularization or transplantation
Septic shock	See pages 000
Spinal shock	Judicious fluids, dopamine for decreased HR and decreased BP, with or without surgical decompression
Anaphylaxis	Fluids, H₁-blocker, H₂-blocker, corticosteroids, epinephrine 1 mg IM
Tamponade	Pericardiocentesis
Tension PTX	Needle decompression 2nd ICS midclavicular line, tube thoracostomy
Massive PE	Support airway and breathing, fluids, thrombolytics and antithrombotics

TABLE 12.3.   Vasopressors

Medication	Dose	Inotropy	Chronotropy	Receptors
Dopamine	5 mcg/kg/min or less	Vasodilation effect		Dopamine rec.
	5–10 mcg/kg/min	Yes	Yes	$\alpha = \beta$
	more than 10 mcg/kg/min	Vasoconstriction effect		$\alpha > \beta$
Dobutamine	2.5–20 mcg/kg/min	Yes	Yes	β_1 and $\beta_2 > \alpha$
		Mild vasodilatation		
Norepinephrine (Levophed)	1–30 mcg/min	Yes	+/–	$\alpha > \beta$
Vasopressin (adjunct)	0.01–0.04 units/min	Vasoconstriction, augments catecholamines		V1/V2 receptors
Phenylephrine (Neo-Synephrine)	40–80 mcg/min			α_1
Isoproterenol	2–10 mcg/min	Yes	Yes	
		Mild vasodilation		Pure β agonist

Sources: *Crit Care Med*, 2005; 33(5): 1119– 22, *Crit Care Med*, 2004; 32(3): 691–9, *JAMA*. 2005; 294(13): 1693–4 and *NEJM*, 2001; 345(19): 1368–77.

CHAPTER 13

SYNCOPE

1. EPIDEMIOLOGY

- Incidence: 30%, bimodal distribution, peak around 10–30 yo with mean peak at 15 yo and then again after 70 yo
- Etiology: neural mediated much more frequent than cardiac (especially ER visit and elderly) which is more common than orthostatics in institutionalized elderly (54–68%) vs community dweller (6%)

2. PATHOPHYSIOLOGY

- Cerebral hypoperfusion causes loss of consciousness
- Normal baroreceptor reflex: standing causes blood pooling in legs and visceral circulation, decreasing blood return to heart and thus decreased preload; baroreceptors in carotid sinus and aortic arch sense decreased pressure and activate sympathetic nervous system to increase cardiac output and systemic vascular resistance
- Decreased cardiac output: hypovolemia, increased thoracic pressure, massive PE, arrhythmias, valvular heart disease, heart failure
- Decreased systemic vascular resistance: autonomic dysfunction, sympatholytic drugs, neurally mediated syncope

3. CLINICAL PRESENTATION

- Preceding palpitations or exertional syncope suggest cardiac cause

History and Exam Findings Based on Syncope Etiologies

- CV: preceding palpitations, exertional syncope, chest pain, hypoxia, murmur, or arrhythmia on exam
- Neuro: muscle weakness, paresthesias, cranial nerve abnormalities
- Vascular: carotid bruits, history of vascular disease
- GI: diarrhea, melena, occult blood positive
- Vasovagal: preceded by N/V, fatigue, myoclonic movements, transient disorientation
- See **Table 13.1**

TABLE 13.1. Etiologies of Syncope

Neurally Mediated	Orthostatic Hypotension	Cardiac Arrhythmias	Structural Cardiopulmonary	Cerebrovascular
• Vasovagal • Carotid sinus syndrome • Situational*	• Drug induced • Autonomic failure† • Hypovolemia	• Sick sinus syndrome • AV block • SVT, VT/VF • Pacemaker malfunction	• Acute MI • Aortic stenosis • Pulmonary embolus • Obstructive cardiomyopathy	• Subclavian steal syn. • Vertebrobasilar TIA • Basilar migraine
66%	10%	11%	5%	1%
Unexplained syncope = 2% and nonsyncopal causes‡ = 5%				

* Cough, micturition, defecation, swallowing, or postprandial precipitants
† Shy-Drager syndrome or secondary to amyloidosis, diabetes, Parkinson's disease, alcoholism
‡ Hypoglycemia, hyperventilation, seizures, cataplexy, drop attacks, or psychogenic "pseudo-syncope"
SVT = supraventricular tachycardia, VT = ventricular tachycardia, VF = ventricular fibrillation, MI = myocardial infarction, TIA = transient ischemic attack
Source: Adapted from *European Heart J*, 2006; 27(1): 76–82.

History and Exam

- Neurally mediated (diagnosis can be confirmed with tilt table testing in equivocal cases)
  - Supporting features: absence of cardiac disease or a long history of recurrent syncope
  - Precipitating event: fear; pain; unpleasant sight, sound, or smell; venipuncture; prolonged standing; or crowded and hot environment
  - Prodromal symptoms: feeling hot, nausea, lightheadedness, diaphoresis, and blurred vision
  - Postevent phenomena: possible nausea, vomiting, or fatigue
- Carotid sinus hypersensitivity with head rotation and tight collar or pressure on lateral neck
  - Carotid massage (positive with decreased SBP 50 mmHg or more or asystole 3 seconds or longer)
- Orthostatic hypotension
  - Check for orthostasis (decreased 20 mmHg SBP or more or 10 mmHg DBP or more, and increased HR greater than or equal to 30 bpm from supine to standing) within 3 minutes of standing
  - Autonomic nervous system failure: amyloidosis, diabetes, alcoholism, Parkinson's disease, or Shy-Drager syndrome
  - Syncope occurring within 2 minutes of standing is suggestive of orthostasis
  - Postprandial syncope occurs via postprandial hypotension
- Cardiac syncope
  - Structural heart disease (CAD, valvular/HTN/hypertrophic cardiomyopathy)
  - Exertion related, occurring at rest or in supine location, family history of sudden death, or associated with chest discomfort, palpitations, diaphoresis, or dyspnea
- Subclavian steal syndrome
  - Occurs with arm activity; difference greater than 10 mmHg in systolic BP between arms
- Situational syncope: cough, micturition, or defecation-induced syncope
- Neuropsychiatric: seizures, vertebrobasilar insufficiency, or a conversion disorder
  - Seizures often have postictal confusion for longer than 2 minutes, tongue biting, tonic-clonic activity, eyes open during event, retrograde amnesia, and incontinence
  - Psychogenic syncope usually has eyes closed during event and no postictal confusion

4. <u>WORKUP</u>

- ECG: evidence of structural heart disease or conduction disease
- 2D-echocardiogram if cardiac dysfunction, HOCM, or aortic/mitral stenosis suspected
- Continuous cardiac monitoring to rule out an arrhythmogenic etiology
  - Positive if symptoms and sinus pause last 2 seconds or longer, sinus bradycardia is less than or equal to 40, supraventricular tachycardia is greater than or equal to 180, Type II second-degree atrioventricular block, complete heart block, or sustained ventricular tachycardia 30 seconds or longer
  - Infrequent episodes concerning an arrhythmogenic etiology should be evaluated with an implantable loop recorder or event recorder
- Labs: CBC, BMP, pregnancy test (in young women) with or without cardiac enzymes
- Tilt-table testing: recurrent unexplained syncope with negative cardiac workup
- Exercise treadmill test or myocardial perfusion study to rule out cardiac ischemia for all exertional syncope or unexplained syncope at rest
- Electrophysiologic test if unexplained syncope AND underlying CAD (especially if LVEF is less than 0.4)
- All cases of cardiac syncope should be reported to the Department of Motor Vehicles
- See **Table 13.2**

TABLE 13.2.   Indications to Hospitalize for Syncope (SAVECASH)

S	Shortness of breath
A	Age older than 60 years (with unexplained syncope)
V	Valvular heart disease (by history or exam)
E	ECG abnormal (nonsinus rhythm or new ECG changes suggesting AV block or ischemia)
C	Congestive heart failure
A	Anemia (Hct less than 30%)
S	Sudden cardiac death (family history of)
H	Hypotension (SBP less than 90 mmHg)

Source: Adapted from *Eur Heart J*, 2003; 24(9): 811–9, *Ann Emerg Med*, 2004; 43(2): 224–32, and *J Emerg Med*, 2007; 33(3): 233–9.

5. **TREATMENT**

- Vasovagal syncope
  - Assure good daily hydration (2 liters of noncaffeinated fluid daily)
  - Perform physical counterpressure maneuvers to prevent future episodes: leg crossing and gluteal clenching, sustained hand grip and forearm clenching
  - Compression stockings
  - Midodrine 10 mg PO tid
  - Refractory and frequent vasovagal syncope may require a dual-chamber pacemaker
- Orthostatic hypotension
  - Discontinue all offending medications
  - Assure good daily hydration (2 liters of noncaffeinated fluid daily)
  - Compression stockings
  - Increased dietary salt (if no hypertension and CHF)
  - Fludrocortisone 0.1–0.2 mg PO bid
  - Midodrine 10 mg PO tid
- Carotid sinus hypersensitivity
  - Avoid tight clothing around the neck
  - Rotate head slowly and avoid excessive neck turning
  - Refractory symptoms require a dual-chamber cardiac pacemaker
- Cardiac syncope is treated according to ACC/AHA guidelines of underlying problem
- Subclavian steal syndrome is treated via percutaneous angioplasty of affected artery

6. **PROGNOSIS**

- **"BBRACES"** criteria for risk stratification (the absence of all of these findings qualifies the patient as low risk; 98% NPV for serious outcomes)
  - **B**NP greater than 300 pg/mL
  - **B**radycardia less than 50
  - **R**ectal exam with occult blood
  - **A**nemia
  - **C**hest pain
  - **E**KG with Q waves
  - **S**aturation less than 94%

7. COMPLICATIONS

- Cardiovascular origin: higher incidence of sudden death and all cause total mortality (vs noncardiovascular)
  - 50% mortality rate after 5 years (30% of these within first year of syncope)
- Injury from syncope: fractures (especially in elderly)

REFERENCES

J Am Coll Cardiol, 2006;47(2):473–84; *Heart,* 2007;93(1):130–6; *Ann Emerg Med,* 2006;47(5):448–54; *Ann Emerg Med,* 2007;49(4):431–44; *Emerg Med Clin North Am,* 2010;28(3):487–500; *Brit Med J,* 2010;340:468–73; *Emerg Med Clin North Am,* 2010;28(3):471–85; *Circulation,* 2006;113(2):316–27; *Am Fam Physician,* 2011;84(6):640–50.

SECTION 2

ENDOCRINOLOGY

CHAPTER 14

INPATIENT MANAGEMENT OF DIABETES MELLITUS

1. **EPIDEMIOLOGY**
   - United States: in 2007 7th leading cause of death
   - US 2010 prevalence: 0.2% younger than 20 yo, 11.3% older than 20 yo, 26.9% older than 65 yo; male and female incidence is the same
   - In 2010, 5th leading cause of death in the world

2. **PATHOPHYSIOLOGY OF DIABETES**
   - Causes of hyperglycemia: stress from surgery, infection, trauma, or inflammation leads to increased cortisol, catecholamines, and glucagon levels, which increase glucose production and insulin resistance
   - Causes of hypoglycemia: decreased PO intake, unpredictable insulin absorption, and iatrogenic
   - DKA pathophysiology
     - Precipitants: insufficient insulin, infection, infarction, intoxication, pregnancy
     - Decreased insulin (relative or absolute) in addition to increased glucagon lead to gluconeogenesis, glycogenolysis, lipolysis
     - Decreased GLUT4 leads to muscle and fat being unable to take up glucose
     - Increased carnitine palmitoyltransferase I causes the liver to turn free fatty acids into ketone bodies, which exist as ketoacids at physiological pH
     - Loss of bicarbonate to buffer ketoacids leads to anion gap metabolic acidosis
     - Total body deficit of K, Na, Cl, PO_4, and Mg (but may not be reflected in serum concentration secondary to acidosis and dehydration)

3. **DIAGNOSIS OF DIABETES IN STABLE OUTPATIENT SETTING**
   - Fasting glucose is 126 mg/dL or higher
   - Random glucose is 200 mg/dL or higher with classic hyperglycemic symptoms
   - 2-hour glucose is 200 mg/dL or higher after 75 g anhydrous glucose challenge (OGTT)
   - HgbA1c is greater than or equal to 6.5%

4. **DIFFERENTIAL DIAGNOSIS OF HYPERGLYCEMIA IN ADULT DIABETICS PATIENTS ("5 I's")**
   - Infection
   - Infarction (acute MI or acute stroke)
   - Infant (pregnancy)
   - Intoxication (e.g., cocaine or methamphetamine abuse)
   - Insulin (lack)—noncompliance with home insulin

5. **WORKUP OF POORLY CONTROLLED DIABETES**
   - Rule out infection or infarction
   - Evaluate diabetic medication compliance
   - Labs: CBCD; BMP; UA with micro, blood, and urine cultures; HgbA1c, with or without cardiac enzymes
   - ECG
   - Consider chest X-ray for any respiratory symptoms
   - See **Figure 14.1** for DKA management

DKA Diagnostic Criteria
- Glucose greater than 250 mg/dL
- pH less than 7.3
- Bicarbonate less than or equal to 18 mEq/L
- Anion gap greater than 10
- Ketonemia

Initial Evaluation
History and physical, focused on any potential precipitants: infection, MI, stroke, or complications of substance abuse; Labs: ABG, CBCD, chemistry panel, UA, magnesium, phosphorus, ECG, chest X-ray, and cultures as needed

DKA Typical Deficits
- Water: 6 liters or 100 mL/kg of body weight
- Sodium: 7–10 mEq/kg of body weight
- Potassium: 3–5 mEq per kg of body weight
- Phosphate: 1 mmol/kg body weight

IV Fluids

Potassium/Phosphorus

Insulin

Isotonic normal saline initially 1–1.5 liters in first hour, then 500–1000 mL per hour until euvolemic

If serum potassium level less than 3.3mEq/L, DO NOT GIVE INSULIN as it will lower potassium levels further, give potassium 40 mEq IV first

If potassium level is adequate, give 0.1 Units/kg IV x 1, then start insulin drip at 0.1 Units/kg/h

Once euvolemic, change to ½ NS at 200–250 mL/

If serum potassium greater than 5.5 mEq/L, do not give potassium; recheck serum potassium in 2 h

Desired fall in glucose at rate of 50–100 mg/dL/h until glucose less than 250; q 1 h glucose checks

Once glucose under 250 mg/dL, change to D5 ½ NS at 200–250 mL/h until DKA resolves

If serum potassium 3.4–5.5 mEq/L, give 20 to 30 mEq of potassium in each liter of IV fluid to keep serum potassium level 4–5 mEq/L; check Chem 7, Phos q 2–4 h

Adjust drip to maintain glucose 150–200 mg/dL until DKA resolves

Saline lock when DKA has resolved and taking adequate orals

Phosphorus: replace with K-phos when serum phosphorus is less than 1mg/dL

For low blood sugars, consider adding glucose and not stopping insulin within the first 48 h of DKA diagnosis

Transition to SQ insulin when anion gap normal, bicarbonate greater than 18 mEq/L and tolerating diet well

Clinical Presentation of DKA
- Symptoms: polyuria, polydipsia, nausea, vomiting, and abdominal pain
- Signs: tachycardia, dry mucous membranes, "fruity breath," Kussmaul respirations, ileus, lethargy, or somnolence

Factors Contributing to Morbidity and Mortality in DKA
1. The underlying cause of the DKA—rule out infection, abscesses, bacteremia, substance abuse, myocardial infarction, etc.
2. Electrolyte disturbances
   a. Hypokalemia
   b. Hyperkalemia (due to severe acidosis and K + H + anteport)
   c. Hypophosphatemia
3. Severe acidemia
   a. Consider IV bicarbonate for pH less than 7 or for symptomatic hyperkalemia
4. Cerebral edema
   a. More common with hypotonic fluids, more common in children
   b. Beware of obtundation; give Mannitol while waiting for your head CT
5. Hypoglycemia (check glucose q 1 h while on the drip)
6. Return to ketoacidosis: patients with DKA are ketogenic and remain so for 24–48 after their DKA resolves; should the patient go hypoglycemic, give them more sugar; DO NOT stop their insulin completely if possible.

Potential Transition Regimens
1. In morning, NPH x 1–2 h prior to stopping drip; stop drip when eating a meal; give lispro after meal with carb counting/correction dosing; transition to insulin glargine at bedtime
2. In evening, insulin glargine 2 h prior to stopping drip; stop drip when eating meal; give lispro after meal with carb counting/correction dosing

FIGURE 14.1. Management of Diabetic Ketoacidosis (DKA)

Source: Courtesy of Mark Lepore M.D. Information from *Postgrad Med J* 2007; 83(976): 79–86, *Diab Care* 2003; 26(Suppl 1): S109–17, *Endocrinol Metab Clin N Am* 2006; 35(4): 725–51, AFP 1999; 60(2): 455–64 and *Diab Care*, 2006; 29(12): 2739–48.

6. **TREATMENT OF DIABETES NOT IN DKA**

Basal Insulin: Long-Acting Insulins

- Start with 50% of total daily insulin (TDI; see **Table 14.1**) or 0.2–0.3 units/kg/day SQ given at the same time each day

TABLE 14.1. Estimating Total Daily Insulin (TDI) Needs in Type 2 DM Based on BMI

Insulin Resistance	BMI	Total Daily Insulin (units)
Normal	Less than 25	Weight (kg) × 0.4 = # of units
High	25–30	Weight (kg) × 0.5 = # of units
Markedly high	Higher than 30	Weight (kg) × 0.6 = # of units

Source: Adapted from *Diabetes Care*, 2008; 31(3): 512–3.

- Increase dose 10–20% daily until fasting glucose is less than 140 mg/dL

Prandial Insulin: Rapid-Acting Insulins

- See **Table 14.2**
- Option 1: start with 50% of TDI divided by 3 or 1 unit per 15 g carbohydrates consumed
- Option 2: insulin to carbohydrate ratio is 500/TDI to determine the grams of carbohydrate covered by 1 unit insulin (e.g., if TDI = 100 units, 1 unit insulin covers 5 g carbohydrates)
- Option 3: fixed-dose regimen with 0.05–0.1 unit/kg/meal or 4–10 units/meal rapid-acting insulin
- Increase dose 10% until 2-h postprandial glucose is less than 180 mg/dL

Correction Dose Insulin: Rapid-Acting Insulins

- See Table 14.2
- Used with preprandial insulin to achieve better glycemic control

Correction dose (CD) of rapid-acting insulin $= \dfrac{\text{(actual glucose} - \text{target glucose)}}{\text{correction factor (CF)}}$

$CF = \dfrac{1500}{TDI}$

If glc = 200, goal = 100, and TDI = 30 units: CD = (200 − 100)/(1500/30)= 100/50= 2 units

TABLE 14.2. Insulins

Insulin	Onset (minutes)	Peak (hours)	Duration (hours)
Rapid-Acting Insulins			
Lispro (Humalog)	5–15	0.5–1.5	4–6
Aspart (NovoLog)	5–15	0.5–1.5	4–6
Glulisine (Apidra)	5–15	0.5–1.5	4–6
Short-acting insulins			
Regular (Humulin R)	30–60	2–3	6–10
Regular (Novolin R)	30–60	2–3	6–10
Intermediate-Acting Insulins			
Lente (Humulin L)	60–180	6–14	16–24
NPH (Humulin N)	120–240	4–10	12–18
Long-Acting Insulins			
Glargine (Lantus)	120–240	None	24
Detemir (Levemir)	120–240	6–14	16–20

Glycemic Goals in the Hospital
- Target glucose levels 120–180 mg/dL with insulin in the ICU
- Glycemic goals for medical or surgical inpatients on the general wards
  - Fasting and preprandial glucose are 90–140 mg/dL and postprandial glucose is less than 180 mg/dL
- Diabetes in pregnancy: Fasting level is less than 95 mg/dL and 1-hour postprandial level is less than or equal to 130 mg/dL

Medical Conditions or Medication Therapy Requiring Insulin Adjustments
- TPN: add 1 unit of insulin per 10 g carbohydrate in TPN
- Corticosteroids: add 10 units of basal insulin for prednisone 20–60 mg/day or equivalent
- Decrease insulin when patients are NPO, have AKI, decompensated CHF, or hepatic failure

Transitioning from Parenteral to Subcutaneous Insulin
- Determine the total daily IV insulin (TDI) requirement during the last 8 h of insulin used
  - Less desirable alternative is to estimate TDI using Table 14.1
- Use 80% of TDI to determine estimate for total daily subcutaneous insulin
  - Administer 50% as long-acting basal insulin (e.g., insulin glargine or detemir)
    - Discontinue insulin drip 2 hours after SQ injection of insulin glargine or detemir
  - Administer 50% as prandial insulin (a rapid-acting insulin) divided by 3 with meals

Management of Hypoglycemia
- If patient can take PO (15–15 rule): 15 g carbohydrate PO for glucose that is less than 70 mg/dL and recheck blood glucose in 15 minutes; repeat if necessary
- If patient unable to take PO: 1 amp D50W IV or glucagon 1 mg IM/SC

Limitations of Oral Diabetic Agents for Inpatient Glycemic Control
- Sulfonylureas have a long half-life and cause hypoglycemia with erratic food intake
- Avoid metformin with IV contrast, CrCl that is less than 50 mL/min, or decompensated CHF
- Thiazolidinediones increase the risk of fluid retention and CHF
- No data for the use of GLP-1 receptor agonists (e.g., exenatide), amylin analogues (e.g., pramlintide), DPP-4 inhibitors (e.g., sitagliptin), or meglitinides in the hospital

Medical Nutrition Therapy
- Diet is a modified carbohydrate diet with each meal containing 60 g of carbohydrates
- Calorie prescription: fat 30% or less; saturated fat less than 7%, and protein 15–20%

General Treatment Guidelines for Adult Diabetic Patients
- Exercise: 30 minutes of moderate exercise at least 5 days/week
- Smoking cessation
- ASA 75–162 mg/day if the 10-year risk of CAD is greater than 10% based on Framingham Risk Score
- Statin indicated for: secondary prevention of CAD, age older than 40 years and one additional CV risk factor, LDL is higher than 100 mg/dL despite diet and exercise, LDL is higher than 70 mg/dL despite diet and exercise and patient has another CAD risk equivalent
- Desire BP to be less than 130/80 mmHg; ACEI is first choice
- Immunizations: influenza vaccine annually; pneumococcal vaccine × 1 and repeat × 1 if patient 65 yo or older and patient immunized when younger than 65 yo more than 5 years previously; hepatitis B vaccine for unvaccinated patients 19 yo and older

Perioperative Management of the Diabetic Patient
- Minor surgery in Type 2 DM patients controlled with oral agents
  - Hold oral agents the night prior and on day of surgery
  - Cover glucose is greater than 180 mg/dL with controlled-dose insulin
- Minor surgery in Type 2 DM patients controlled with insulin
  - Use 80–100% insulin glargine the night prior or ½ dose NPH insulin the morning of surgery
  - Restart the normal insulin regimen once patient is eating well after surgery

- Major surgery in Type 2 DM patients
  - Hold oral agents the night prior to and morning of surgery
  - Use 80–100% insulin glargine the night prior or ½ dose NPH insulin the morning of surgery
  - Start continuous insulin infusion prior to surgery and continue perioperatively
- Surgery in Type 1 DM patients
  - Start 5% dextrose fluids at 100–125 mL/h the morning of surgery
  - Control glucose with a continuous insulin infusion perioperatively

Postoperative Diabetic Management

- Target glucose levels 100–150 mg/dL using an insulin infusion after major surgery
  - Fewer infectious complications and lower mortality if glucose is less than 220 mg/dL
- Transition to subcutaneous insulin once patient is tolerating oral intake

7. PROGNOSIS

- Mortality rate of DKA is approximately 2%
- DKA is responsible for 16% of all diabetes-related deaths

8. COMPLICATIONS

- Cerebral edema is typically seen 12–24 hours after treatment initiation of DKA; primarily seen in patients younger than 20 years of age; mortality rate is 20–40% from brain herniation
- ARDS
- Hypertriglyceridemia (typically improves with insulin therapy)
- GI bleed
- Hyperamylasemia and hyperlipasemia
- Acute MI
- Electrolyte abnormalities: hyperkalemia, hypokalemia, hypophosphatemia
- Hypoglycemia from over-aggressive correction of DKA

REFERENCES

N Engl J Med, 2006;355(18):1903–11; *Diabetes Care*, 2004;27(2):553–91; *Diabetes Care*, 2006;29(8):1955–62; *Ann Intern Med*, 2006;145(2):125–34; *JAMA*, 2008;300(8):933–44; *Diabetes Care*, 2008;31(3):511–3; *Diabetes Care*, 2004;27(2):553–91; *N Engl J Med*, 2006;355(18):1903–11; Diabetes Care, 2012;35(Suppl 1):S11.

CHAPTER 15

HYPERTHYROIDISM AND THYROID STORM

1. **EPIDEMIOLOGY**
   - Thyrotoxicosis: Graves' disease accounts for 60–80% of cases, typically around 20–50 yo
     * 50–75% of patients have ophthalmopathy within 1 year prior to or after diagnosis is made
     * Thyroid dermopathy (pretibial myxedema) occurs in less than 5% of patients
     * 10–30% mortality if thyroid storm is untreated
     * 15% of treated patients will develop hypothyroidism 10–15 years later due to the destructive autoimmune process
   - Other causes of thyrotoxicosis: toxic nodule, toxic multinodular goiter, subacute thyroiditis, lymphocytic or postpartum thyroiditis, factitious disorder, exogenous iodide excess (Jod-Basedow phenomenon), TSH-secreting pituitary tumor, trophoblastic disease, Struma ovarii

2. **PATHOPHYSIOLOGY**
   - Primary hyperthyroidism: increased fT_4 from thyroid leads to decreased TSH
   - Secondary hyperthyroidism: increased TSH from pituitary leads to increased fT_4
   - Graves' disease
     * Genetic factors and environmental modifiers (e.g., sudden increase in iodine intake)
     * May also have antithyroid peroxidase antibodies (nonspecific marker of autoimmunity)
     * Autoimmune: thyroid-stimulating immunoglobulins synthesized by thyroid, bone marrow, and lymph nodes stimulate TSH receptors, which leads to increased fT_4
     * Graves ophthalmopathy: activated T-cells infiltrate extraocular muscles (possibly due to expression of TSH receptor in orbit) and release cytokines that induce synthesis of glycosaminoglycans, leading to edema, fibrosis and, ultimately, exophthalmos
   - Thyroid storm precipitated by stress (CVA, infection, trauma, surgery, DKA, radioiodine treatment)

3. **CLINICAL PRESENTATION**
   - Symptoms: nervousness, palpitations, tremor, heat intolerance, sweating, pruritus, increased appetite, hyperdefecation, sleep disturbance, fatigue, dyspnea
   - Signs
     * Tachycardia [LR+ 4.5, LR– 0.2]
     * Skin warm and moist [LR+ 6.8, LR– 0.7]
     * Palpable thyroid [LR+ 2.3, LR– 0.1]
     * Lid retraction [LR+ 33.2, LR– 0.7]
     * Eyelid lag [LR+ 18.6, LR– 0.8]
     * Fine tremor [LR+ 11.5, LR– 0.3]
     * Weight loss
     * Graves': 50–75% have infiltrating ophthalmopathy (exophthalmos), large gland with or without thyroid bruit
     * Toxic multinodular goiter: long-standing large gland with multiple nodules, sometimes tender
     * Thyroiditis: preceding viral illness, tender normal-sized gland
     * Toxic adenoma: single nodule, normal gland size
   - Thyroid storm: delirium, severe tachycardia, fever, vomiting, diarrhea, dehydration

4. **DIAGNOSIS OF HYPERTHYROIDISM**

- See **Figure 15-1**

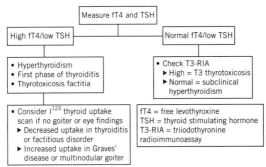

FIGURE 15.1. An Approach to Patients with Suspected Hyperthyroidism

5. **DIFFERENTIAL DIAGNOSIS**

- Sympathomimetic intoxication (cocaine or amphetamines)
- Anxiety attack
- Nonhyperthyroid atrial fibrillation

6. **WORKUP OF HYPERTHYROIDISM**

- Labs: TSH, fT4, total T3 by RIA, CBC, BMP
- Consider thyroid-stimulating immunoglobulin (TSI), anti-TPO (thyroid peroxidase antibody)
- ECG for tachycardia to rule out Afib
- Echocardiogram only if Afib or CHF is present
- Radioioxdide uptake scan if clinical presentation is not diagnostic of Graves' Disease (GD)
  - Increased uptake in GD and toxic multinodular goiter
  - Decreased uptake in thyroiditis and factitious hyperthyroidism
    - Thyroiditis will have elevated thyroglobulin and factitious hyperthyroidism will have low thyroglobulin levels

7. **TREATMENT**

Treatment Options for Hyperthyroidism

- If thyroid gland less than or equal to 2 × normal and soft, mild–moderate hyperthyroidism, children, or pregnant or lactating women, recommend using antithyroid drugs (ATDs)
  - Induction dose: methimazole 15 mg PO q 12 h or propylthiouracil 100 mg PO q 8 h
  - Check CBCD and LFTs for pharyngitis, pruritic rash, jaundice, abdominal pain, nausea, dark urine, acholic stools, or metallic taste (ATD can induce agranulocytosis, hepatotoxicity, or rash)
  - Optimal duration of ATDs is 12–18 months
  - Consider measuring TSI levels prior to stopping ATDs
- Radioiodine ablation indications: thyroid is more than 2 × normal or hard, multinodular goiter, high TSI titer, young man, relapse after ATD therapy, women planning pregnancy 6 months or more in the future, CI to ATD therapy, or high surgical risk
  - Radioiodine ablation or surgery are options for *refractory* atrial fibrillation
  - Pretreat with methimazole if pt is symptomatic or has an initial fT4 is more than 2 × normal
    - Stop methimazole 3–5 days prior to I[131] therapy
  - Stabilize comorbid cardiopulmonary conditions prior to I[131] therapy

- Total thyroidectomy for: pregnant patients with thyroid storm, severe exophthalmos intolerant of or refractory to ATDs, large goiter with compressive symptoms, a suspicious thyroid nodule, desire pregnancy in less than 6 months, noncompliance, or relapse after ATDs and refusing I[131] therapy
  - ATD therapy until euthyroid, then SSKI × 10 days before surgery
  - Follow Ca and iPTH postthyroidectomy
  - Start levothyroxine 1.7 mcg/kg/day immediately postop
- Propranolol is an adjunctive agent for tachycardia, tremors, and nervousness

Treatment of Graves' Ophthalmopathy (GO)

- Smoking cessation
- Orbital radiotherapy
- Oral steroids are indicated for mild active GO; unclear benefit for moderate–severe active GO

Subclinical Hyperthyroidism

- Young, asymptomatic patient and nonnodular thyroid disease; clinically follow
- Consider low-dose ATDs to normalize TSH if: symptomatic with osteoporosis, osteopenia, or atrial fibrillation; nodular thyroid disease; or older than 65 years with TSH less than 0.1 mU/L
- If symptoms resolve with therapy, can consider I[131] radioiodine ablation

Management of Hyperthyroidism in Pregnancy

- Use lowest effective dose of propylthiouracil
- Check TSI titers during third trimester of maternal Graves' disease to assess risk of neonatal Graves' disease
- If thyroidectomy is necessary, perform during the second trimester

Management of Thyroid Storm

- Supportive care: fluid resuscitation with D5NS, thiamine, and a multivitamin daily
- Find and treat precipitating cause (infection, MI, stroke, DVT, PE, or substance abuse)
- Antithyroid drugs: propylthiouracil 500 mg load, then 200–300 mg PO q 4 h or methimazole 20–30 mg PO q 6 h
  - Consider an initial load of propylthiouracil 600 mg PO (especially during pregnancy)
- SSKI 5 gtts PO q 6 h or Lugol's solution 4–8 gtts PO q 6–8 h; start at least 1 hour after ATDs
- Propranolol 40–80 mg PO q 4 h or esmolol 50–100 mcg/kg/min IV
- Acetaminophen as needed for fever; avoid salicylates as they can aggravate thyrotoxicosis
- Hydrocortisone 100 mg IV q 8 h or dexamethasone 2 mg IV q 6 h × 4 doses, especially if hypotensive

8. **COMPLICATIONS**

- HEENT: corneal ulceration leads to optic neuropathy, which leads to blindness and extraocular muscle dysfunction, then diplopia, periorbital, or conjunctival edema
- CV: congestive heart failure, atrial fibrillation, elevated total cholesterol, and decreased HDL
- Endo: glucose intolerance, oligomenorrhea, amenorrhea, anovulatory infertility, gynecomastia, reduced libido, erectile dysfunction, and decreased spermatogenesis
- Pulm: hypercapnia, hypoxemia, and increased pulmonary artery systolic pressure
- GI: diarrhea
- Heme: normochromic, normocytic anemia
- Renal: osteoporosis and fractures
- Derm: warm, hyperpigmentation, pruritus, alopecia, vitiligo, pretibial myxedema
- Psych: anxiety, restlessness, insomnia, emotional lability, and in severe cases, psychosis, agitation, and depression
- Thyroid storm
  - Hypotension, cardiac arrhythmia, cardiovascular collapse, hyperpyrexia (up to 104–106°F), psychosis, delirium, stupor, coma, liver failure
  - See **Table 15.1**

TABLE 15.1.   Diagnostic Criteria for Thyroid Storm

Criteria	Points	Criteria	Points
Temperature (°F)		*GI-Hepatic Dysfunction*	
99–99.9	5	Absent	0
100–100.9	10	Diarrhea, vomiting, abdominal pain	10
101–101.9	15	Marked, unexplained jaundice	20
102–102.9	20	*Tachycardia*	
103–103.9	25	90–109	5
104 or higher	30	110–119	10
CNS Effects		120–129	15
Absent	0	130–139	20
Mild agitation	10	140 or higher	25
Delirium, psychosis, or signicantly increased lethargy	20	*Congestive Heart Failure*	
Seizures or coma	30	Absent	0
Atrial Fibrillation		Mild	5
Absent	0	Moderate	10
Present	10	Severe	15
Precipitating event absent	0	*Precipitating event present*	10

A total score of 45 or higher is highly suggestive, 25–44 is possible, and less than 25 is unlikely to be thyroid storm

Source: Adapted from *Endocrinol Metab Clin N Amer,* 1993; 22: 263–277.

REFERENCES

Endocrinol Metab Clin North Am, 2006;35(4):663–86; *J Clin Endocrinol Metab,* 2007;92(1):3–9; *Obstet Gynecol Surv,* 2007;62(10):680–8; *Lancet,* 2003;362(9382):459–68.

McGee S. Thyroid and its disorders. In: McGee S. *Evidence Based Physical Diagnosis*, 3rd ed. Philadelphia, PA: Saunders-Elsevier; 2012:192–209.

CHAPTER 16

HYPOTHYROIDISM AND MYXEDEMA COMA

1. **EPIDEMIOLOGY**
   - Worldwide most common cause is iodine deficiency
   - In iodine-sufficient areas, Hashimoto's thyroiditis is the primary cause
   - Congenital hypothyroidism: affects 1 in 4000 newborns; 80–85% of cases due to thyroid dysgenesis, 10–15% due to inborn errors of hormone synthesis
   - Incidence of subclinical hypothyroidism is 6–8% in women and 3% in men

2. **PATHOPHYSIOLOGY**
   - Primary hypothyroidism: increased fT_4 in thyroid leads to increased TSH
   - Secondary hypothyroidism: decreased TSH from pituitary leads to decreased fT_4
   - Hashimoto's thyroiditis: lymphocytic autoimmune inflammatory response results in fibrosis and ultimately follicular atrophy, which decreases fT_4
     - Genetic component: HLA-DR polymorphisms
     - Cytotoxic CD8+ T-cells cause destruction of thyroid cells
   - Antithyroid peroxidase and antithyroglobulin antibodies are not directly pathogenic, but rather are markers of autoimmunity; may have thyroid-blocking TSH receptor antibodies
   - Myxedema coma: usually precipitated by hypoventilation (medications, pneumonia, CHF, MI, GI bleeding, CVA); associated with impaired conversion of T_4 to T_3 and adrenal insufficiency

3. **CLINICAL PRESENTATION**
   - Symptoms: weakness, lethargy, cold sensation, decreased sweating, thick tongue, forgetfulness, constipation
   - Signs
     - Cool/dry skin [LR+ 4.7, LR− 0.9]
     - Coarse skin [LR+ 3.4, LR− 0.7]
     - Delayed reflexes [LR+ 3.4, LR− 0.6]
     - Periorbital edema [LR+ 1, LR− 0.6]
     - Coarse hair
   - "Hypothyroid speech": slow rate and rhythm, deep and low-pitched, sometimes slurring
   - Myxedema coma
     - Myxedematous face: puffy, macroglossia, ptosis, periorbital edema, coarse sparse hair
     - Altered mental status, alopecia, bladder distention, delayed reflex relaxation, dry cool skin, decreased GI motility, hyperventilation, hypothermia, nonpitting edema, bradycardia, anorexia, nausea, abdominal pain, ileus, urinary retention, constipation, pericardial effusion, acute kidney injury, and potentially hypotension
     - Lab findings: hyponatremia, anemia, elevated lactic acid and CK, and hyperlipidemia

4. **DIAGNOSIS**
   - See **Figure 16.1**

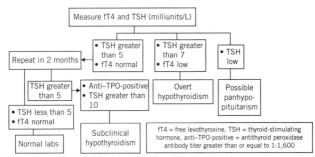

FIGURE 16.1.   An Approach to the Patient with Suspected Hypothyroidism

5. DIFFERENTIAL DIAGNOSIS

- Depression
- Sepsis
- Adrenal insufficiency
- See **Table 16.1**

TABLE 16.1.   Thyroiditis Syndromes

Category	Hashimoto's Thyroiditis	Painless Postpartum Thyroiditis	Painful Subacute Thyroiditis	Painless Sporadic Thyroiditis	Painful Suppurative Thyroiditis
Onset	Usually 30–50 years	Within 4 months postpartum	20–60 years	Usually 30–40 years	Children + 20–40 years
Anti-TPO antibodies	High titers in 90%	High titers	Low titer or absent	High titers	Absent
ESR	Normal	Normal	High	Normal	High
24 h–RAI ^{123} I uptake	Variable*	Less than 5%	Less than 5%	Less than 5%	Normal or low

anti-TPO = antithyroid peroxidase antibody, ESR = erythrocyte sedimentation rate, RAI ^{123} I = radioactive iodine-123 uptake scan
* Uptake is high in rare cases of hashitoxicosis, but usually is low
Source: Adapted from *NEJM*, 2003; 348(26): 2646–55.

6. WORKUP OF HYPOTHYROIDISM

- Labs: TSH, fT4, antithyroid peroxidase antibody, CBC, CMP, fasting lipid panel, ESR, and CK
- ECG
- Echocardiogram for any clinical suspicion of a pericardial effusion
- Consider a I^{123} radioiodine uptake scan if suppurative thyroiditis or Hashitoxicosis is a possibility

7. INITIAL TREATMENT OF HYPOTHYROIDISM

- Start full replacement dose of levothyroxine 1.6–1.7 mcg/kg/day for young, healthy adults
- Consider starting 1.3 mcg/kg/day levothyroxine in elderly patients or those with CAD

Management of Subclinical Hypothyroidism

- Levothyroxine for: TSH higher than 10, α-TPO antibody-positive, infertility, or pregnancy
  - Titrate levothyroxine dose to achieve TSH levels 1–2.5 milliunits/L

Management of Myxedema Coma

- Evaluate/treat precipitants (infection, CHF, stroke, trauma, MI, or hypothermia)
- Intubation for inability to protect airway or ventilatory failure
- Passive rewarming with Bair Hugger, warm IV fluids, and heat lamps
- Volume resuscitation with D_5NS
- Levothyroxine 300–500 mcg (5–8 mcg/kg) IV load, then 100 mcg IV daily, then 1.7 mcg/kg PO daily
- Hydrocortisone 100 mg IV q 8 h × 2–3 days, then gradually taper over 5–7 days

8. **COMPLICATIONS**

- Myxedema coma (coma, hypothermia, hyponatremia, hypercapnia)
- Carpal tunnel syndrome
- Peripheral neuropathy
- Depression
- HEENT: treatment-induced hypothyroidism leads to persistent proptosis, goiter, dysphagia
- Heme: normocytic, normochromic anemia; pernicious anemia
- CV: dyspnea on exertion/reduced exercise capacity, pericardial effusion, elevated blood pressure, heart failure
- Pulm: fatigue, dyspnea on exertion, hypoventilation, macroglossia, obstructive sleep apnea
- GI: constipation/ileus
- Endo: hypercholesterolemia, hyperprolactinemia results in amenorrhea and galactorrhea, hyponatremia, obesity
- Gyn: oligo/amenorrhea or menorrhagia, decreased fertility, increased incidence of spontaneous abortion; decreased libido/erectile dysfunction/delayed ejaculation
- Skin: nonpitting edema (myxedema)

REFERENCES

Endocrinol Metab Clin North Am, 2007:36(3):595–615; *Endocrinol Metab Clin North Am,* 2006;35(4):687–98; *J Intensive Care Med,* 2007;22(4):224–31; *N Engl J Med,* 2001;345(4):260–265; *Am Fam Physician,* 2001;64(10):1717–24; *Am Fam Physician,* 2000;62(11):2485–90.

McGee S. Thyroid and its disorders. In: McGee S. *Evidence Based Physical Diagnosis,* 3rd ed. Philadelphia, PA: Saunders-Elsevier; 2012:192–209.

CHAPTER 17

ADRENAL INSUFFICIENCY

1. EPIDEMIOLOGY

- Most common cause is iatrogenic by rapid withdrawal of glucocorticoid treatment with a 0.5–2% prevalence in developed countries
- Most common cause of primary adrenal insufficiency is autoimmune adrenalitis

2. PATHOPHYSIOLOGY

- Regulation of adrenal steroid production by the hypothalamic-pituitary-adrenal axis
- Stress induces CRH release from hypothalamus; anterior pituitary releases pro-opiomelanocortin, which is cleaved to ACTH; circulating ACTH binds to nuclear receptors, leading to cortisol secretion from adrenal glands
- Other cleavage products of pro-opiomelanocortin stimulate melanocytes, which leads to hyperpigmentation in states of ACTH excess (Addison's disease)
- Renin-angiotensin-aldosterone system
  - Decreased renal perfusion pressure induces renin release from juxtaglomerular cells, activating angiotensin I, angiotensin II, and ultimately aldosterone; aldosterone promotes Na reabsorption and increases K secretion by kidneys

3. CLINICAL PRESENTATION

- Fatigue/malaise, generalized weakness, anorexia, weight loss, nausea/vomiting
- Hypotension
- Hyponatremia, hyperkalemia with mild hyperchloremic acidosis, hypoglycemia
- Hyperpigmentation if primary adrenal insufficiency (ACTH stimulates melanocytes)
- See **Tables 17.1** and **17.2**

TABLE 17.1. Etiologies of Adrenal Insufficiency

Primary Adrenal Insufficiency	Secondary Adrenal Insufficiency
• Metastatic carcinoma of lung, breast, kidney, stomach, colon, or lymphoma • Tuberculosis (TB) or fungal infection • Adrenoleukodystrophy • AIDS-associated infections* • Waterhouse-Friderichsen syndrome • Autoimmune adrenalitis • Adrenal hemorrhage/infarct • Antiphospholipid syndrome • Meds: etomidate, fludrocortisone, ketoconazole, megestrol acetate, phenobarbital, phenytoin, high-dose progestins, or rifampin	• Systemic glucocorticoid therapy more than 3 consecutive wks within the last year • Pituitary or hypothalamic tumors or postirradiation or postsurgery • Lymphocytic hypophysitis • Postpartum pituitary necrosis (Sheehan's syndrome) • Pituitary TB, sarcoidosis, cryptococcosis, or histoplasmosis

* Most commonly HIV, cytomegalovirus infections, histoplasmosis, or mycobacterial infections
Source: Adapted from *Endo Met Clin N Amer,* 2006; 35(4): 767–75.

TABLE 17.2. Signs and Typical Labs in Adrenal Insufficiency (AI)

Both Types of AI	Primary AI	Secondary AI
• Unexplained fever • Hypotension or orthostatic hypotension • Hyponatremia • Hypoglycemia • Mild hypercalcemia • Normocytic anemia • Eosinophilia	• Hyperpigmentation of palmar creases, extensor surfaces, and buccal mucosa • Hyperkalemia • Nonanion gap acidosis • Possible vitiligo	Pituitary lesions may exhibit: • Amenorrhea • Secondary hypothyroidism • Diabetes insipidus • Sexual dysfunction

Source: Adapted from *NEJM*, 2003; 348(8): 727–34.

4. DIAGNOSIS OF ADRENAL INSUFFICIENCY IN MILD ILLNESS

- Overt adrenal insufficiency very likely if early morning cortisol level is less than 3 mcg/dL, possible if it is less than 10 mcg/dL and unlikely if cortisol is 18 mcg/dL or higher
- A 250-mcg cosyntropin stimulation test can assess for adrenal insufficiency if random cortisol equivocal
  - Poststimulation cortisol level of 18 mcg/dL or higher excludes primary adrenal insufficiency and most cases of secondary adrenal insufficiency
  - Poststimulation cortisol less than 18 mcg/dL diagnoses primary or secondary adrenal insufficiency

Diagnosis of Relative Adrenal Insufficiency (RAI) in Critical Illness

- Avoid checking an ACTH-stimulation test in the setting of septic shock
- Random cortisol of less than 10 mcg/dL diagnoses RAI and levels that are greater than 34 exclude RAI
- 250-mcg ACTH stimulation test if random cortisol levels are between 10 and 34 mcg/dL
  - RAI highly likely if cortisol rise is less than 9 mcg/dL; an increase of 16.8 mcg/dL or more excludes RAI

5. DIFFERENTIAL DIAGNOSIS

- Sepsis
- Hypothyroidism
- Etomidate use
- Occult malignancy
- Hemochromatosis

6. TREATMENT OF PRESUMED ADRENAL CRISIS

- 5% dextrose in isotonic saline infusion until normotensive
- Administer dexamethasone 4 mg IV and perform a cosyntropin stimulation test
- Hydrocortisone 100 mg IV q 8 h until results of cosyntropin stimulation test known

Maintenance Therapy of Adrenal Insufficiency

- Maintenance oral dose: prednisone 5–7.5 mg/day, hydrocortisone 20–25 mg/day, or dexamethasone 0.25–0.75 mg/day
  - Increase maintenance dose 2–3-fold during moderate illness or minor surgery
  - Hydrocortisone 100 mg IV q 8 h during severe illness or for major surgery
- Consider adding fludrocortisone 0.1 mg PO q morning in primary AI or orthostatic symptoms
- Add DHEA 25–50 mg PO q morning for women with fatigue, low libido, or dysthymia
- *Patients should have a Medic Alert bracelet and medical identification card*

7. COMPLICATIONS

- Adrenal crisis
- Psychosis
- Depression
- Cognitive impairment

- Electrolyte abnormalities: hypoglycemia, hyponatremia (88%), hypercalcemia (rare: 6–33%), hyperkalemia (64%, concomitant mild hyperchloremic acidosis)
- Auricular cartilage calcification: possible complication of chronic AI, rare in females, no improvement with treatment of AI

REFERENCES

N Engl J Med, 2003;348(8):727–34; *Ann Intern Med,* 2003;139(3):194–204; *Crit Care Med,* 2008;36(6):1937–49; *Am J Respir Crit Care Med,* 2006;174(12):1319–26; *Curr Opin Crit Care,* 2007;13(4):363–9; *Endocrinol Metab Clin North Am,* 2006;35(4):767–75.

CHAPTER 18

CALCIUM DISORDERS

HYPERCALCEMIA

1. **EPIDEMIOLOGY**
   - 99% of body's 1–2 kg of calcium resides in skeleton
   - 50% of total blood calcium is ionized; the rest is ionically bound to albumin and immunoglobulins
   - Acute illness and acidosis dissociate calcium from protein so they make levels of total calcium misleading; ionized calcium is more accurate in acute illness (4.2–5.2 mg/dL)
   - 90% from hyperparathyroidism or malignancy
   - 20% of cancer patients have hypercalcemia

2. **PATHOPHYSIOLOGY**
   - Abnormal PTH axis
     - Increased PTH: parathyroid adenoma or hyperplasia
     - Altered Ca-sensing receptor in parathyroid gland: familial hypocalciuric hypercalcemia (nonpathologic)
     - Secretion of PTH-related peptide: humoral hypercalcemia of malignancy
   - Bony abnormalities
     - Bone destruction: metastatic breast CA, myeloma
     - Increased bone resorption: hyperthyroidism, immobilization
   - Increased 25-(OH) Vitamin D: granulomatous diseases, lymphoma, Vitamin D toxicity
   - Positive Ca balance
     - Increased Ca intake: milk-alkali syndrome, TPN
     - Decreased Ca excretion: thiazides

3. **CLINICAL PRESENTATION**
   - See **Table 18.1**
   - "Stones, bones, (abdominal) moans, psychiatric groans, and irregular heart tones"
     - Stones: nephrolithiasis, nephrogenic DI, dehydration
     - Bones: bone pain, arthritis, osteoporosis, osteitis fibrosa cystica (if secondary to hyperparathyroidism)
     - Moans: nausea, vomiting, anorexia, constipation, abdominal pain, pancreatitis, peptic ulcer disease
     - Groans: impaired concentration, confusion, lethargy, muscle weakness
     - Tones: hypertension, shortened QT, arrhythmias, vascular calcifications

TABLE 18.1. Clinical Presentation of Hypercalcemia

• Bone pain • Renal stones	• Diffuse abdominal pain, anorexia, nausea, and constipation • Lethargy, fatigue, depression, confusion, and cognitive impairment

4. **WORKUP**
   - Discontinue culprit medications: Vitamin D or Vitamin A excess; thiazide diuretics, lithium, estrogens, androgens, theophylline, ganciclovir, or foscarnet
   - Labs: Ca, Phos, albumin, 25-(OH) Vitamin D, iPTH, BMP, SPEP
   - Optional labs based on clinical probability: TSH, PTHRP, PPD, ANCA, ACTH-stimulation test
   - ECG
   - Chest X-ray

5. <u>**TREATMENT OPTIONS FOR ASYMPTOMATIC PRIMARY HYPERPARATHYROIDISM**</u>

- Daily PO intake of elemental calcium 1000–1200 mg and Vitamin D 400–600 IU
- Parathyroid surgery indicated for any of the following: serum calcium is higher than 11.2 mg/dL, nephrolithiasis, osteitis fibrosa cystic, CrCl is less than 60 mL/min, bone density scan reveals a T-score less than or equal to –2.5 at any site, age younger than 50 yo, OR medical surveillance is not desirable or possible
  - Surgery indicated for all patients with symptomatic primary hyperparathyroidism

Treatment of Hypercalcemic Crises (serum calcium Is Greater Than 13.5–14 mg/dL)

- Aggressive isotonic saline hydration 2–4 L/day
- Hypercalcemia of malignancy: treat CA with surgery, chemotherapy, or radiation
  - Bisphosphonates: zoledronic acid 4 mg IV or pamidronate 90 mg IV over 4 h
  - Calcitonin 4 units/kg SC q 12 h if severe (avoid if creatinine is greater than or equal to 4.5 mg/dL)
  - Refractory cases: gallium nitrate 200 mg/m^2 IV daily × 5 days (avoid if creatinine is greater than or equal 2.5 mg/dL)
- Granulomatous disease: treat disease and add hydrocortisone 100 mg IV q 8 h × 3–5 days then taper

6. <u>**COMPLICATIONS**</u>

- Neuro: altered mental status, somnolence, coma, death
- Cardiovascular: dysrhythmias, hypertension, CAD (long-term)
- Renal: nephrogenic DI, renal insufficiency, nephrocalcinosis
- GI: peptic ulcer, pancreatitis

HYPOCALCEMIA

1. <u>**PATHOPHYSIOLOGY**</u>

- PTH is primary protection against hypocalcemia: PTH disorders can cause life-threatening hypocalcemia, parathyroid agenesis, surgery, radiation, autoimmune destruction, mutations to Ca-sensing receptor, PTH receptor mutations, pseudohypoparathyroidism
- Vitamin D disorders cause less severe hypocalcemia due to partial compensation by PTH: Vitamin D deficiency, Vitamin D resistance, altered Vitamin D metabolism
- Hyperphosphatemia: burns, rhabdomyolysis, tumor lysis syndrome, pancreatitis
- Increased consumption: hungry bone syndrome
- See **Table 18.2**

TABLE 18.2. Hypocalcemia Etiologies

• Chronic renal failure • Hypoparathyroidism • Tumor lysis • Postthyroidectomy • Alcohol abuse • Loop diuretics, phenytoin, phenobarbital, glucocorticoids, rifampin, aminoglycosides, cisplatin, amphotericin B, Cinacalcet, foscarnet, EDTA, carbamazepine, isoniazid, theophylline, PPI, H2-blockers, and Strontium-89	• Rhabdomyolysis • Respiratory alkalosis • Acute pancreatitis • Neck radiation • Postparathyroidectomy from hungry bone syndrome	• Severe hypomagnesemia • Massive transfusions • Vitamin D deficiency

2. <u>**CLINICAL PRESENTATION**</u>

- Tetany (neuromuscular irritability)
  - Mild: perioral numbness, paresthesias of hands/feet, muscle cramps
  - Severe: carpopedal spasm, laryngospasm, seizures
    - Trousseau's sign: inflate BP cuff above SBP for 3 minutes; causes carpopedal spasm (adduction of thumb, flexion of MCPs, extension of interphalangeals, flexion of wrist)
    - Chvostek's sign: tap facial nerve just anterior to ear, causes contraction of ipsilateral facial muscles (present in 10% of normocalcemic people)

3. <u>WORKUP OF HYPOCALCEMIA</u>

- Calcium (corrected) (g/dL) = calcium + (0.8 × [4 − serum albumin in g/dL])
- If hypocalcemia etiology unclear, check intact PTH and 25-hydroxyvitamin D levels

4. <u>TREATMENT OF HYPOCALCEMIA</u>

- 1.5–2 g elemental calcium orally with meals daily divided bid–tid
- Add calcitriol 0.25 mcg PO daily–tid or ergocalciferol 50,000 units PO weekly for 8 weeks for hypoparathyroidism or Vitamin D deficiency
- Calcium gluconate 1–2 g IV over 20 min for severe, symptomatic hypocalcemia
- Must correct hypomagnesemia for effective PTH activity

5. <u>COMPLICATIONS</u>

- Ophthal: cataracts
- Neuro: seizures, tetany, basal ganglia calcification, movement disorder (parkinsonism, hemiballismus, choreoathetosis)
- Cardiovascular: refractory hypotension and refractory heart failure, dysrhythmias (i.e., Torsades de Pointes, heart block)
- GI: pancreatitis
- Musculoskeletal: osteopenia/osteoporosis, laryngospasm

REFERENCES

J Clin Endocrinol Metab, 2009;94(2):2335–9; *N Engl J Med,* 2004;350(17):1746–51; *Crit Care Med,* 2004; 32(4 Suppl):S146–54; *Am J Med Sci,* 2007;334(5):381–5; *Am Fam Physician,* 2004;69(2):333–339; *Am Fam Physician* 2003; 67(9):1959–66, 2003:1959–66; *Ann Intern Med,* 2008;149(4):259–63.

CHAPTER 19

SODIUM DISORDERS

HYPONATREMIA

1. PATHOPHYSIOLOGY

- Hypovolemic: decreased total body H_2O but severely decreased total body Na
  - Renal loss of Na: hypoaldosteronism, salt-wasting nephropathy, diuretics, osmotic diuresis
  - Extrarenal loss of Na: GI (diarrhea, vomiting, pancreatitis), insensible losses (burns, trauma)
- Euvolemic: increased total body H_2O with constant total body Na
  - Increased ADH results in increased H_2O reabsorption via vasopressin receptors: SIADH, glucocorticoids, hypothyroidism, stress
- Hypervolemic: increased total body Na but relatively greater increase in total body H_2O
  - Renal loss of Na: renal failure
  - Edematous states (increased total body Na but decreased effective circulating volume): nephrotic syndrome, cirrhosis, CHF

2. CLINICAL PRESENTATION

- Often asymptomatic
- Nonspecific symptoms when Na is less than 120: headache, lethargy, nausea
- A cause of falls in the elderly
- Severe hyponatremia: seizures and coma
- See **Figure 19.1**

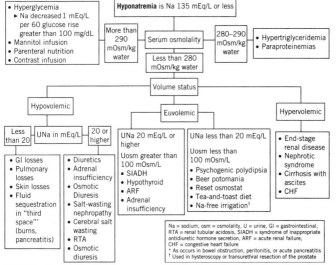

FIGURE 19.1. Workup of Hyponatremia

3. **GENERAL GUIDELINES FOR THE TREATMENT OF HYPONATREMIA**

- Hypovolemic, hypotonic hyponatremia
  - Use isotonic saline until euvolemic
- Hypervolemic or hypotonic, euvolemic hyponatremia
  - Free water restriction to 500–800 mL daily in severe cases and 1000–1500 mL daily in mild to moderate cases
  - Conivaptan 20 mg IV load, then 20–40 mg IV infusion over 24 h × 1–4 days
    - Alternatives: tolvaptan 15–60 mg PO daily; lixivaptan 50–100 mg PO bid
- Treat severe, symptomatic hyponatremia (lethargy, delirium, seizures, or coma) from any cause until Na is at least 120 mEq/L
  - 3% NS
  - Furosemide IV plus NS at a rate to match 50% hourly urine volume
  - Stop when symptoms resolve or 10 mmol/L increase in first 24 hours
  - For *acute* severe symptomatic hyponatremia with neurological symptoms (e.g., exercise-induced hyponatremia): 100 mL bolus 3% NS and may repeat × 1 until severe neurological symptoms resolve
- IV fluid rate approximated by the following equation for the correction of hyponatremia or hypernatremia:

$$\text{Change in serum Na} \atop \text{(after 1 L infusate)} = \frac{[(\text{infusate Na} + \text{infusate K}) - \text{serum Na}]}{\text{Total body water (L)} + 1}$$

Total body water (L) = 0.6 × weight (kg) for young males and 0.5 × weight (kg) for females or elderly males

- Maximum correction of chronic hyponatremia for longer than 48 h is 1 mEq/L/h, 10 mEq/L in 24 h, and less than 18 MEq/L in 48 h
  - More rapid correction can lead to osmotic demyelination syndrome

Treatment of SIADH

- Remove offending meds, treat underlying condition, and restrict fluids
- Infusions of isotonic saline alone usually worsens the hyponatremia of SIADH
- Consider demeclocycline 300–600 mg PO bid for treatment of chronic SIADH

Reset Osmostat (or "Sick Cell Syndrome")

- Occurs with severe malnutrition, Tb, AIDS, alcoholics, terminal CA, and pregnancy
- Patients appropriately regulate serum osmolality around a reduced set point

4. **PROGNOSIS**

- Decreased life expectancy when Na is less than 125 mEq/L in chronic CHF or cirrhosis with ascites

5. **COMPLICATIONS**

- Neuro: tentorial herniation due to cerebral edema results in compressed brain stem and respiratory arrest/death
- Osmotic demyelination syndrome with too rapid correction of chronic hyponatremia

HYPERNATREMIA

1. **PATHOPHYSIOLOGY**

- Loss of H_2O is greater than loss of Na
  - Renal loss of H_2O
  - Osmotic diuresis: hyperglycemia, postobstructive, mannitol
  - H_2O diuresis: diabetes insipidus
    - Nephrogenic (renal resistance to ADH): genetic, hypercalcemia, hypokalemia, lithium
    - Central (failure to secrete ADH)
- Extrarenal loss of H_2O: insensible losses, GI losses (osmotic diarrhea)
- Na intake is greater than H_2O intake
- Hypertonic saline (iatrogenic)

2. <u>**CLINICAL PRESENTATION**</u>

- Irritability
- Restlessness
- Lethargy
- Muscle twitches
- Hyperreflexia

3. <u>**TREATMENT OF HYPERNATREMIA**</u>

- Step 1: NS 10–20 mL/kg over 1 hour if significant hypovolemia
- Step 2: correct free H_2O deficit over 48–72 hours
  - May have a rate of correction of 1 mEq/L/h for severe symptomatic hypernatremia until symptoms resolved
  - Maximum correction is 10 mEq/L in first 24 hours
  - Monitor sodium q 4 h

4. <u>**COMPLICATIONS**</u>

- Most complications occur in setting of acute hypernatremia
- Pediatric mortality 20% in acute hypernatremia and 10% in chronic hypernatremia
- Neuro: may include seizures, cerebral hemorrhage, paralysis, encephalopathy, spasticity/hypertonicity in children (incidence 15%)
- Renal: acute renal failure
- Heme: DIC

REFERENCES

N Engl J Med, 2007;356(20):2064–72; *South Med J,* 2006;99(4):353–62; *JAMA,* 2004;291(16):1963–71; *Am Fam Physician,* 2004;69(10):2387–94; *Am J Med,* 2007;120(11 Suppl 1):S1–21; *Int J Clin Pract,* 2009;63(10):1494–508; *Am Fam Physician,* 2000;61(12):3623–30.

CHAPTER 20

POTASSIUM DISORDERS

HYPOKALEMIA

1. ### PATHOPHYSIOLOGY
   - Transcellular shifts: metabolic acidosis, insulin, β-agonists, TPN, hypokalemic periodic paralysis
   - Increased loss of K
     - Renal: diuretics, salt-wasting nephropathies, hyperaldosteronism, Liddle's syndrome, vomiting, nasogastric suctioning, type 2 RTA, Mg deficiency
     - Extrarenal: diarrhea, sweating

2. ### CLINICAL PRESENTATION
   - Muscle weakness, cramps, rhabdomyolysis (symptoms start approximately when K is less than 2.5 mEq/L)
   - Respiratory muscle weakness can be fatal
   - Cardiac arrhythmias: PAC, PVC, sinus bradycardia, PAT, junctional rhythms, AV block, VTach, VFib
   - EKG changes: ST depression, decrease in T wave amplitude, U waves (especially in V4–V6)

3. ### TREATMENT OF HYPOKALEMIA
   - Estimate potassium repletion using **Table 20.1**
   - IV KCl for ventricular arrhythmias, digoxin toxicity, paralysis, or severe myopathy
     - Maximum rate is 10 mEq/L/h through PIV or 20 mEq/L/h through central line
   - PO KCl in divided doses for all other causes except:
     - Hypokalemic periodic paralysis requires no more than 40 mEq PO KCl
     - Renal tubular acidosis is treated with K-citrate or K-bicarbonate
   - Must correct hypomagnesemia to effectively correct hypokalemia

TABLE 20.1.   Estimated Total Body Potassium Deficit

Serum (K+) Concentration	Estimated (K+) Deficit
3.0 mEq/L	120–200 mmol
2.5 mEq/L	200–333 mmol
2.0 mEq/L	300–500 mmol
1.5 mEq/L	400–666 mmol

4. ### COMPLICATIONS
   - Cardiovascular: arrhythmias
   - GI: ileus, hepatic encephalopathy in cirrhotic patients
   - Musculoskeletal: weakness, hypokalemic periodic paralysis, flaccid paralysis

HYPERKALEMIA

1. ### PATHOPHYSIOLOGY

   - Transcellular shifts: metabolic acidosis, hyperosmolality, β-blockers, digoxin, succinylcholine, trauma, tumor lysis, rhabdomyolysis
   - Decreased renal excretion: ACEIs, ARBs, aldosterone antagonists, K-sparing diuretics, CHF, hypovolemia, NSAIDs, CKD, adrenal insufficiency

2. ### CLINICAL PRESENTATION

   - Muscle weakness, flaccid paralysis, ileus
   - EKG changes: tall, peaked T wave, then loss of P wave then widened QRS
   - See **Figure 20.1**

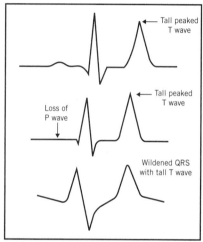

FIGURE 20.1.   ECG Changes of Hyperkalemia

3. ### TREATMENT OF HYPERKALEMIA (MNEMONIC CBIGKDROP)

   - **C**: calcium (1 ampule calcium gluconate IV over 5 min for QRS widening from hyperkalemia)
   - **B**: bicarbonate (1 ampule sodium bicarbonate IV over 5 min; most helpful if acidosis present)
     - β₂-agonist: albuterol 10–20 mg nebulized over 1 hour
   - **I**: insulin (10 units regular insulin IV)
   - **G**: glucose (1 ampule of 50% dextrose unless patient already hyperglycemic)
   - **K**: kayexalate (30–60 g PO or 30–50 g in 100 mL enema PR)
   - **D**: (drop) dialysis

Electrocardiogram Changes with Hypokalemia and Hyperkalemia
- Hypokalemia: ST depression, then U waves
- Hyperkalemia: peaked T waves result in PR prolongation which leads to QRS widening, and P waves disappear leading to sinusoidal pattern

4. **COMPLICATIONS**
- Cardiovascular: arrhythmias (sinus bradycardia, sinus arrest, slow idioventricular rhythm, ventricular tachycardia/fibrillation, asystole); conduction abnormalities (RBBB, LBBB, bifascicular block, atrioventricular block)
- Neuro: muscle weakness (ascending, flaccid); hyperkalemic periodic paralysis

REFERENCES

N Engl J Med, 1998;339(7):451–8; *Crit Care Clin*, 2002;18(2):273–88; *Arch Intern Med*, 2004;164(14):1561–6.

CHAPTER 21

PANHYPOPITUITARISM

1. **PATHOPHYSIOLOGY**
   - Anatomy
     - Posterior pituitary releases vasopressin (ADH) and oxytocin
     - Hypothalamic neurons directly innervate posterior pituitary
     - Anterior pituitary releases prolactin, growth hormone, ACTH, LH, FSH, and TSH
     - Pituitary portal plexus transmits releasing factors from hypothalamus to anterior pituitary
   - Causes of pituitary insufficiency
     - Developmental: dysplasia, Kallmann syndrome, Prader-Willi syndrome, etc
     - Trauma: postoperative, postradiation, head injuries
     - Neoplastic: adenomas, parasellar masses, craniopharyngioma, metastases, meningioma
     - Infiltrative/inflammatory: lymphocytic hypophysitis, hemochromatosis, sarcoidosis, histiocytosis X
     - Inflammatory: Tb, histoplasmosis, toxoplasmosis, tertiary syphilis
     - Vascular: pituitary apoplexy (postpartum = Sheehan's syndrome)
   - See **Table 21.1**

TABLE 21.1.   Causes of Adult-onset Hypopituitarism

Pituitary tumors	Pituitary apoplexy	Peripituitary lesions: meningioma, glioma, craniopharyngioma, brain metastases
Pituitary surgery	Sheehan's syndrome	
Pituitary radiotherapy	Head trauma	Pituitary infections: syphilis, TB, or fungal
Subarachnoid hemorrhage	Infiltrative disorders: sarcoidosis, histiocytosis X, hemochromatosis, or lymphocytic hypophysitis	

Source: Adapted from *Pituitary,* 2005; 8(3–4): 183–91.

2. **CLINICAL PRESENTATION**
   - ACTH: adrenal insufficiency
   - TSH: hypothyroidism
   - LH/FSH
     - Men: decreased libido, ED, eventually diminished facial hair, gynecomastia, soft testes
     - Women: menstrual irregularities, hot flashes, decreased libido, vaginal dryness
   - GH: decreased exercise tolerance
   - See **Table 21.2**

TABLE 21.2.   Symptoms of Adult-onset Hypopituitarism

Deficiency Syndrome	Clinical Presentation
Corticotrophs	Fatigue, weakness, dizziness, nausea, vomiting, anorexia , weight loss, hypoglycemia, and shock (in severe cases)
Thyrotropin	Tiredness, cold intolerance, constipation, weight gain, hair loss, dry, coarse skin, bradycardia, hoarseness, slow cognition, hypothermia
Gonadotropin	Women: amenorrhea, infertility, loss of libido, and osteoporosis Men: decreased libido, erectile dysfunction, hair loss, and decreased muscle/bone mass
Growth hormone	Decreased muscle mass, central obesity, fatigue, weakness, premature atherosclerosis, and decreased quality of life

Source: Adapted from *Pituitary,* 2005; 8(3–4): 183–91.

3.   WORKUP OF SUSPECTED HYPOPITUITARISM

- Corticotroph deficiency: morning cortisol less than 3.5 mcg/dL or poststimulation cortisol less than 18 mcg/dL after 250 mcg cosyntropin challenge, and ACTH level low/low–normal
- Thyrotrope deficiency: TSH levels low or low–normal and fT4 levels low
- Gonadotroph deficiency: LH and FSH levels low; females—estradiol low; males—testosterone low
- Somatotrope deficiency: GH and IGF-1 levels low or inappropriately normal
- Lactotroph deficiency: prolactin levels high if stalk compression or prolactinoma
- Visual field testing as a sign of optic chiasm compression
- MRI of pituitary in all patients with confirmed hypopituitarism
- DEXA-bone mineral densitometry at baseline and every 2 years

Replacement Dosing for Hypopituitarism

- Glucocorticoids: hydrocortisone 15 mg q morning and 10 mg q evening, or prednisone 5–7.5 mg/day
- Thyroid: levothyroxine 1.6–1.7 mcg/kg PO daily and titrate to normalize fT4 levels
  - *Do not follow TSH levels (they will always be low)*
- Hypogonadism in premenopausal women: 35 mcg ethinyl estradiol oral contraceptive pills
- Hypogonadism in men: injectable or transdermal testosterone replacement
- Growth hormone deficiency: treatment only after consultation with an endocrinologist
- Central DI: DDAVP 10–20 mcg intranasally bid, or vasopressin 0.1–1.2 mg/day PO divided bid to tid
- *All patients with panhypopituitarism should have a Medic Alert bracelet*

4. COMPLICATIONS

- Adrenocorticotropin deficiency
  - Most serious complication due to development of adrenal crisis
- Growth hormone deficiency
  - Reduced bone mineral density
  - In adults, can cause insulin resistance, hyperlipidemia, and central obesity all of which combine to cause two-fold increase in cardiovascular mortality
- Gonadotropin deficiency
  - Adults: skin thinning and wrinkle formation, reduced exercise capacity and muscle mass, reduced bone mineral density, reduced libido
  - Men: azoospermia/infertility, erectile dysfunction
  - Women: oligo or amenorrhea, hot flashes, vaginal dryness, dyspareunia, breast atrophy
- Thyrotropin deficiency: same as complications of hypothyroidism
- Prolactin deficiency: postpartum failure of lactation
- Vasopressin (ADH) deficiency: diabetes insipidus (i.e., polyuria, polydipsia, hypernatremia)

REFERENCES

Postgrad Med J, 2006;82(966):259–66; *Pituitary*, 2005;8(3–4):183–91.

SECTION 3

GASTROENTEROLOGY

CHAPTER 22

EVALUATION OF ACUTE ABDOMINAL PAIN

1. **PATHOPHYSIOLOGY**
   - Inflammation of parietal peritoneum causes somatic pain directly over inflamed tissue
     - Stomach acid and pancreatic enzymes are particularly irritating
   - Abdominal wall muscle spasm leads to guarding
   - Obstruction of hollow organ causes visceral pain that is poorly localized and achy in quality
   - Contraction of smooth muscle results in intermittent "colicky" pain
   - Referred pain: convergence of visceral afferents with somatic afferents leads to pain referred to corresponding dermatome (convergence-projection hypothesis)
   - Other causes of abdominal pain: metabolic (DKA, porphyria), neurogenic (zoster, tumors), functional (IBS), abdominal wall spasm, vascular (SMA thrombosis, AAA rupture), pain referred from thorax

2. **CLINICAL PRESENTATION**
   - Peritoneal signs
     - Rigidity (involuntary) [LR+ 3.7 for peritonitis] matters more than guarding (voluntary) [LR+ 2.2]
     - Rebound tenderness (maintain pressure over an area of tenderness, then withdraw hand abruptly) [LR+ 2.0, LR– 0.4]
   - Special studies for appendicitis
     - McBurney's point tenderness: 2" from the ASIS in the direction of the umbilicus [LR+ 3.4]
     - Rovsing's sign: pushing on the LLQ causes pain in the RLQ [LR+ 2.3]
     - Psoas sign: patient lies on L side, doctor hyperextends the R hip [LR+ 2.0]
     - Obturator sign: flex R hip and knee, internally rotate R hip [LR+ 1]
   - See **Figure 22.1**

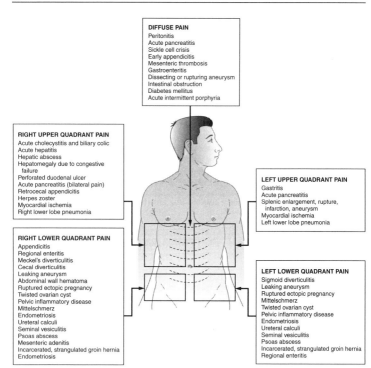

FIGURE 22.1.   Differential Diagnosis of Acute Abdominal Pain

Source: Adapted from Wagner DK. *Curr Topic* 1978; 1 (3).

3. WORKUP OF ABDOMINAL PAIN

- History
  - **O:** onset (duration)
  - **P3:** position, palliating factors, provoking factors
  - **Q:** quality (character of pain)
  - **R:** radiation
  - **S:** severity, associated symptoms (e.g., anorexia, vomiting, diarrhea, constipation, fever)
  - **T:** timing (constant or intermittent, diurnal or nocturnal)
- Labs
  - CBCD, chemistry panel, amylase/lipase, UA with micro, urine pregnancy test in all women of childbearing age
- Radiographic testing
  - Acute abdominal series: free intraperitoneal air (up to 40% false-negative rate for perforating ulcers) or bowel obstruction
    - Sensitivity 69% and specificity 57% for bowel obstruction
    - In one study, results changed management 4% of the time

- Ultrasound: diagnostic procedure of choice for acute cholecystitis, acute cholangitis, and to assess for abdominal aortic aneurysm
  - Sensitivity 88% and specificity 80% for acute cholecystitis
  - Sensitivity 76% and specificity 95% for acute appendicitis
  - Sensitivity 61% and specificity 99% for diverticulitis
  - In two studies, results altered management 22% of the time
- CT scan with oral/IV contrast: diagnostic procedure of choice for acute abdominal pain in nonpregnant adults, except for acute cholecystitis
  - 95% PPV for acute appendicitis: appendix larger than 6 mm and periappendiceal fat stranding
  - Sensitivity 94% and specificity 99% for diverticulitis
  - Sensitivity 94% and specificity 96% for SBO
  - Sensitivity 96% and specificity 93% for LBO
  - Comparable sensitivity to mesenteric angiography for mesenteric ischemia (93% vs 96%), but lower specificity than angiography (79% vs 99%)
  - More sensitive than ultrasound for acute abdominal pain (89% vs 70%, P less than 0.001)
  - Prospective studies demonstrated a change in management 46–60% of the time
- MRI scans in pregnant women
  - Sensitivity 90–100% and specificity 94–98% for acute appendicitis
  - MRI is accurate for nephrolithiasis, bowel wall thickening, intra-abdominal abscesses, fibroid degeneration, adnexal torsion

REFERENCES

McGee S. Abdominal pain and tenderness. In: McGee S. *Evidence Based Physical Diagnosis*, 3rd ed. Philadelphia, PA: Saunders-Elsevier; 2012:441–52.

CHAPTER 23

UPPER GASTROINTESTINAL BLEEDING (UGIB)

1. ## PATHOPHYSIOLOGY
   - Peptic ulcers
     - *Helicobater pylori* infection
     - Bacterial factors: vac A inhibits immune cell function, urease yields ammonia, protease degrades mucous layer, adhesins enable attachment to epithelium
     - Host factors: genetic predisposition?
   - Gastritis
     - Antral-predominant gastritis causes duodenal ulcers
     - Corpus-predominant gastritis cause gastric ulcers and intestinal metaplasia, which lead to carcinoma
     - Nonatrophic pangastritis associated with MALT lymphoma
   - Gastroesophageal varices
   - NSAIDs
     - Inhibit prostaglandin synthesis, leading to decreased mucosal injury
     - Direct topical injury
     - Altered mucous results in reverse diffusion of hydrogen ions plus pepsin
     - Achlorhydria results in increased gastrin
   - Other causes: Mallory-Weiss tear (partial-thickness disruption of GE junction), duodenitis, cancer, aortoenteric fistulas, vascular lesions, Dieulafoy lesion (aberrant vessel in gastric mucosa)

2. ## CLINICAL PRESENTATION
   - May be asymptomatic or present for symptoms of anemia
   - Coffee-ground emesis or hematemesis (present in 56% of patients with bleeds)
   - Stools usually melanotic (70%); brisk bleeds can present as hematochezia

3. ## DIAGNOSIS
   - Definitive diagnosis is with an esophagogastroduodenoscopy

4. ## WORKUP
   - CBC, PT, PTT, BMP, liver panel
     - BUN/crt greater than 36 has a 90–95% sensitivity for predicting UGIB
   - Stool guaiac
   - NGT aspirate if gross blood suggests an active UGIB necessitating a more urgent EGD

   Preendoscopy Clinical Predictors of Poor Outcome with UGIB
   - Age older than 60 yo; cirrhosis; renal failure; cardiopulmonary disease; SBP less than 100 mmHg; concurrent sepsis; APACHE II score of 11 or higher; presence of hematemesis, hematochezia, bright red nasogastric aspirate; or presence of coagulopathy, thrombocytopenia, or Hgb less than or equal to 8 g/dL

   Glasgow-Blatchford Criteria for Low-Risk UGIB Suitable for Outpatient Management
   - BUN less than 18 mg/dL; Hgb greater than or equal to 13 g/dL (men) or greater than or equal to 12 g/dL (women); SBP greater than or equal to 110 mmHg; HR less than 100 bpm; and absence of melena, syncope, current or history of acute/chronic liver disease or heart failure
     - Endoscopic intervention required in 0.5% of these pts and no risk of rebleeding or death
   - See **Tables 23.1** and **23.2**

TABLE 23.1.   Endoscopic Findings as Predictors of Outcome for Peptic Ulcers

Findings	Rebleeding Risk	Surgery Needed	Mortality Risk
Clean base	5%	0.5%	2%
Flat spot	10%	6%	3%
Adherent clot	22%	10%	7%
Visible vessel	43%	34%	11%
Bleeding vessel	55%	35%	11%

Source: Adapted from NEJM, 1994; 331(11): 717–27.

TABLE 23.2.   Rockall Scoring System for Upper Gastrointestinal Bleeds

Score	0	1	2	3
Age (years)	Younger than 60	60–79	80 or older	–
Vitals	HR less than 100 SBP 100 or higher	HR 100 or higher SBP 100 or higher	SBP less than 100	–
Comorbidities	None	–	Chronic heart or lung disease	Renal or liver failure, metastatic cancer
Endoscopic findings	• Mallory-Weiss • No lesion/no SRH	All other diagnoses	Malignant lesion of upper GI tract	–
SRH	Clean base or dark spot on ulcer base	–	Adherent clot, visible or bleeding vessel	–

Rockall Score	Rebleeding	Mortality	Mortality with Rebleeding	Rockall Score	Rebleeding	Mortality	Mortality with Rebleeding
0–2	4.3%	0.1%	–	6	29%	15%	29%
3–4	13%	3%	12%	7	40%	20%	35%
5	17%	8%	21%	8 or higher	48%	40%	53%

HR = heart rate, SBP = systolic blood pressure, GI = gastrointestinal, SRH = stigmata of recent hemorrhage (adherent clot, visible vessel, or bleeding vessel)
Source: Adapted from Lancet, 1996; 347(9009): 1138–40.

5.   INITIAL TREATMENT OF UPPER GI BLEEDS

- Aggressive IV fluid resuscitation if hypovolemic with isotonic saline or PRBC transfusions
- Platelet transfusion for platelet less than 50 K/μL
- Correct coagulopathy with FFP plus or minus Vitamin K (until PTT normalizes in cirrhotic patients)
- Proton pump inhibitors continuous infusion (e.g., pantoprazole or omeprazole 80 mg IVP, then 8 mg/h infusion) preferred over IV bid (esomeprazole, lansoprazole, or pantoprazole)
- EGD within the first 24 hours of admission

Peptic Ulcer Disease

- Endoscopic hemostatic therapy indicated for ulcers with high risk of rebleed: adherent clot, visible vessel, or bleeding vessel
  - Combination of epinephrine injection, bipolar coagulation, and/or hemoclip
  - Clear liquids can be started in 6 hours if patient stable
  - Recommend continuous PPI infusion for 48–72 hours after endoscopic therapy

- Continue PPI PO bid × 4–8 weeks for peptic ulcer disease
- Assess for *H. pylori* infection with gastric biopsies in the setting of gastric ulcers, duodenal ulcers, or duodenitis and treat if present

Duration of Inpatient Observation

- None for Mallory-Weiss tears, gastritis, esophagitis, clean ulcer base, or Rockall score less than 3; 1 day for red spot on ulcer; 1–2 days for adherent clots; 3 days for visible or bleeding vessels treated endoscopically

Gastroesophageal Variceal Bleeds

- Octreotide 50 mcg IV bolus, then infuse at 50–100 mcg/h × 3–5 days for variceal bleeds
- Antibiotic prophylaxis × 7 days: cefotaxime IV or norfloxacin 400 mg PO bid decreases the risk of spontaneous bacterial peritonitis and variceal rebleeding if moderate to large ascites
- Endoscopic variceal ligation (EVL) or sclerotherapy if ligation not possible
  - Serial EVL every 2–3 weeks until varices are obliterated
- β-blockers: propranolol or nadolol titrated to decrease resting heart rate 25%
- Nitrates: isosorbide mononitrate 30 mg PO daily, added to serial EVL and β-blockers
- Transjugular intrahepatic portosystemic shunt (TIPSS) for gastric varices or recurrent esophageal variceal bleeds as a bridge to transplantation
  - Also option for resistant ascites and hepatopulmonary syndrome
  - Contraindications to TIPSS: portosystemic encephalopathy, CHF, pulmonary hypertension, multiple hepatic cysts, active infection, biliary obstruction, hepatic or portal vein thrombosis, central hepatoma, severe thrombocytopenia, or coagulopathy
- Sengstaken-Blakemore balloon tamponade for uncontrollable esophageal variceal bleed as rescue therapy until a TIPSS procedure can be performed
  - The gastric balloon should not remain inflated for more than 48 hours
  - Esophageal balloon should not remain inflated for more than 8 hours at a time
- Patients who are good candidates for transplant should be referred to a liver transplant center for evaluation

6. **PROGNOSIS**

- See Tables 23.1 and 23.2

7. **COMPLICATIONS**

- Overall mortality for UGIB is approximately 10%
- Peptic ulcer disease
  - Hemorrhage/recurrent bleed: increased risk of mortality if older than 60 yo, arterial bleed or visible vessel on ulcer base, presence of shock, coagulopathy, cardiovascular disease
  - Penetrating ulcer: can lead to a fistula (i.e., aortoenteric fistula, choledochoduodenal fistula, gastrocolic fistula)
  - Perforating ulcer (9%): worse outcomes if malnourished or delay in diagnosis
  - Gastric outlet obstruction (3%): highest incidence in pyloric and duodenal ulcers
- Gastric or esophageal varices
- Risk of mortality is 30–50% in each episode of variceal bleeding and risk of rebleeding can be as high as 70%
- Mallory-Weiss tear is rarely associated with Boerhaave's syndrome (esophageal rupture and mediastinal sepsis)

REFERENCES

J Clin Gastroenterol, 2007I;41(6):559–63; *Curr Opin Crit Care*, 2006;12(2):171–7; *Arch Intern Med*, 2007;167(12):1291–6; *Lancet*, 2009;373(9657):42–7; *Gastroenterol Clin North Am*, 2005;34(4):607–21; *N Engl J Med*, 2001;345(9):669–81; *Am Fam Physician*, 2012;85(5):469–76.

CHAPTER 24

LOWER GASTROINTESTINAL BLEEDING (LGIB)

PATHOPHYSIOLOGY

- Colonic diverticula are pseudodiverticula, as they do not involve the entire bowel wall
  - Mucosa protrudes through break in muscularis propria where vasa recti enters
  - Most commonly in sigmoid colon due to elevated luminal pressures generated by stronger contractions in face of constipation
  - Fecal material trapped in pseudodiverticulum forms fecaliths, resulting in inflammation
  - Compression causes perforation
  - Erosion causes bleeding
- Angiodysplasia/vascular ectasias
- Colon cancer erodes into blood vessels
- Inflammatory bowel disease
  - Complex interaction between host and environmental factors results in disordered mucosal immunity, mediated by proinflammatory cytokines (IL-1, IL-6, TNF), causing T-cell activation
- Infectious colitis
- Other causes: hemorrhoids, anal fissures, Meckel's diverticulum, small intestine tumors, postpolypectomy, NSAID colitis, rectal varices, vasculitis, aortocolic fistulas

CLINICAL PRESENTATION

- Melena or hematochezia
- Weakness or fatigue from anemia
- Positive occult blood test

DIAGNOSIS

- Definitive diagnosis is with colonoscopy or flexible sigmoidoscopy
- Alternative modalities include a barium enema or virtual colonography

WORKUP

- See **Figure 24-1**
- CBC, PT, PTT, BMP, liver panel
  - BUN/crt greater than 36 has a 90–95% sensitivity for predicting UGIB
- Stool guaiac

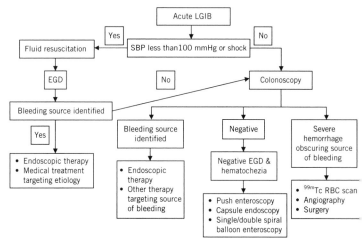

FIGURE 24.1. Suggested Evaluation of Acute Lower Gastrointestinal Bleeding (LGIB)

Source: Adapted from *Best Practice and Research Clin Gastro,* 2008; 22(2): 295–312.

Risk Factors (RFs) of Poor LGIB Outcomes

- SBP less than or equal to 115 mmHg, HR 100 bpm or higher, syncope, nontender abdominal exam, hematochezia during first 4 h of evaluation, history of ASA use, initial Hct 35% or less, and more than 2 active medical comorbidities
- Risk of severe bleeding: low (0 RFs; less than 10%); medium (1–3 RFs; 45%); high (more than 3 RFs; 80%)

5. MANAGEMENT OF LOWER GASTROINTESTINAL BLEEDING

- Bowel rest and aggressive fluid resuscitation with isotonic saline or PRBC transfusions
- FFP for coagulopathy if INR is greater than 1.5 or PTT elevated more than 1.5 × normal
- Platelet transfusion if platelets are less than 50 K/μL
- Treatment of uncontrollable LGIB: angiography with selective embolization versus surgery

Management of Occult GI Bleeding

- Tc⁹⁹m-labeled RBC scan can identify occult GI bleeds if the rate of bleeding is at least 0.1 mL/min
  - Accurate localization 75–95% of time if test is positive within 2 hours of injection
  - Accurate localization 57–67% of time if test is positive after 2 hours of injection
- Angiography can localize the source of LGIB if rate of hemorrhage is at least 0.5 mL/min
  - Sensitivity 30–46% and specificity 100%
  - Allows for selective embolization if bleeding site is found
- Surgery with bowel resection often required for definitive control of bleeding

6. COMPLICATIONS

- Massive hemorrhage
- Shock
- Mortality rate of 10–20% in presence of following risk factors: older than 60 yo, multiorgan system disease, blood transfusion of more than 5 units, bleeding requiring surgical intervention, recent stress (e.g., trauma, sepsis)
- Rebleeding
- Syncope from intravascular volume depletion

REFERENCES

Cleve Clin J Med, 2007;74(6):417–20; *Surg Endosc*, 2007;21(4):514–20; *Eur Radiol*, 2008;18(5):857–67; *Best Pract Res Clin Gastroenterol*, 2008;22(2):295–312; *Am Fam Physician*, 2012;85(5):469–76.

CHAPTER 25

DIARRHEA

ACUTE DIARRHEA

1. ### PATHOPHYSIOLOGY
   - Hypersecretory: voluminous, watery diarrhea with or without vomiting, fever
   - Preformed toxin: *Bacillus cereus, Staphylococcus aureus, Clostridium perfringens*
     - Enterotoxin: *Vibrio cholerae, E. coli, Klebsiella pneumoniae, Aeromonas*
   - Enteroadherence: *E. coli, Giardia, Cryptosporidium*, worms
   - Inflammatory: high fever, severe pain, dysentery (bloody diarrhea)
   - Cytotoxic: *Clostridium difficile, E. coli*
     - Invasive: rotavirus, norovirus, *Salmonella, Campylobacter, Aeromonas, Vibrio parahaemolyticus, Yersinia, Shigella, E. coli, Entamoeba histolytica*
   - Noninfectious: medications, ischemic colitis, diverticulitis, graft-versus-host disease, toxic ingestions, anaphylaxis, initial presentation of IBD

2. ### CLINICAL PRESENTATION
   - Inflammatory: may be watery diarrhea or dysentery (small-volume, mucoid stools with fever, abdominal pain, and tenesmus)
   - Noninflammatory: watery diarrhea, without abdominal pain, without blood or pus in the stool

3. ### WORKUP OF ACUTE DIARRHEA BASED ON CATEGORY OF DIARRHEA
   - No testing if diarrhea lasts less than 3 days, no dehydration, fever under 101.3°F, *and* no blood/pus in stool

   Community-Acquired Diarrhea or Traveler's Diarrhea (TD)
   - Stool for *Clostridium difficile* toxin especially if recent antibiotics, chemotherapy, or institutionalized patient
   - Evaluation of acute bloody diarrhea
     - CBCD, BMP, plus or minus blood cultures
     - Stool culture for *Salmonella, Shigella, Campylobacter*, or *Yersinia*
     - Stool for ova and parasites and giardia antigen if giardia or amebiasis suspected
     - Test for *E. coli* 0157:H7 and shiga toxin (especially if HUS present)
     - CT scan of abdomen if ischemic colitis is likely
   - Stool cultures for vibrio if recent ingestion of shellfish

   Nosocomial Diarrhea (onset after 72 hours of hospitalization)
   - Stool for *Clostridium difficile* toxin
   - Check for *Salmonella, Shigella, Campylobacter*, and/or *E. coli* 0157:H7 if immunocompromised, neutropenic, or suspected systemic enteric infection

   Persistent Diarrhea (More than 7 days)
   - Check all stool studies *prior to* barium/contrast studies (or wait 14 days after)
   - Check stool ova, parasites, and fecal leukocytes (as screen for inflammatory diarrhea)
   - Consider stool studies for giardia (giardia antigen test), *Cryptosporidium, Cyclospora, Isospora*, with or without *Strongyloides*
   - If HIV-positive, add stool for microsporidia, blood cultures for *Mycobacterium avium* complex and consider flexible sigmoidoscopy

4. **GENERAL TREATMENT OF ACUTE INFECTIOUS DIARRHEA**

- IV hydration with isotonic saline or lactated Ringer's solution if patient dehydrated
- Antimotility agents if patients are nontoxic and there is *absence of* fever, blood in stool, no fecal leukocytes, and no traveler's diarrhea; use loperamide or bismuth subsalicylate
  - Avoid narcotics and antimotility agents if bacterial gastroenteritis is suspected
- Insufficient evidence to support use of probiotics (*lactobacilli* or *Saccharomyces*) to prevent antibiotic-associated diarrhea or *Clostridium difficile* infection

Empiric Antibiotics for Bacterial Community-Acquired or Traveler's Diarrhea

- Rifaximin 200 mg PO tid × 3 days is *preferred* for afebrile, nondysenteric TD
  - Oral ciprofloxacin or levofloxacin × 1–3 days an option for TD
- Oral ciprofloxacin or levofloxacin × 5 days for community-acquired diarrhea
- If *E coli* 0157:H7 is a possibility, treat with aggressive hydration but **avoid narcotics and antibiotics** as these can increase the risk of HUS

Empiric Treatment for Severe Nosocomial Diarrhea (presumptive *C. difficile* colitis)

- Discontinue antimicrobials if possible
- Mild–moderate disease: metronidazole 500 mg PO tid × 10 days
- Severe/ongoing disease: vancomycin 125 mg PO qid × 10 days
  - Two of following: temperature above 101°F, age older than 60 yo, albumin less than 2.5 mg/gL, WBC higher than 15K cells/mm^3, or colonic distension on plain films or CT scan of abdomen
- Contact isolation and careful handwashing using soap after contact with patient
- Consider ileal diversion and colonic reperfusion or total colectomy for severe deteriorating disease

Treatment of Persistent Diarrhea

- Treat based on culture results
- If giardia is strongly suspected, empiric therapy with metronidazole or tinidazole

4. **COMPLICATIONS**

- Hypokalemia with nonanion gap hyperchloremic metabolic acidosis
- Dehydration
- Postinfectious irritable bowel syndrome
- Shock
- Recurrent diarrhea can cause malnutrition and growth retardation, particularly in pediatric population

CHRONIC DIARRHEA

1. **PATHOPHYSIOLOGY**

- Secretory: impaired fluid and electrolyte transport cause profuse, watery, painless diarrhea
- Medications, chronic alcoholism, persistent infections, bowel resection, enterocolic fistula, carcinoid, gastrinoma, VIPoma, villous adenoma
- Osmotic: fecal osmotic gap due to nonabsorbed, osmotically active solute leading to output proportional to solute load
- Laxatives, lactose intolerance
- Steatorrhea: fat malabsorption causes malodorous, greasy, floating diarrhea plus weight loss and fat-soluble vitamin deficiencies
  - Pancreatic insufficiency, CF, small intestinal bacterial overgrowth, celiac disease, tropical sprue, Whipple's disease, MAC infection
- Inflammatory: exudative response plus cytokines causes pain, fever, bleeding
  - IBD, microscopic colitis, immunodeficiency, eosinophilic gastroenteritis
  - Dysmotility-related: hyperthyroidism, carcinoid, prokinetic drugs, diabetic diarrhea, IBS
- Factitious: Munchausen syndrome, laxative abuse

2. <u>CLINICAL PRESENTATION</u>

- Physical exam provides clues to etiology
  - Stigmata of chronic disease (episcleritis in IBD, exophthalmos in hyperthyroidism, dermatitis herpetiformis in celiac disease)
  - Scars (surgical causes)
  - Bowel sounds (hypermotility)
  - Tenderness (infection/inflammation)
  - Masses (neoplasia)
  - Rectal exam with occult blood (impaction can cause paradoxical diarrhea)
- See **Table 25.1**

TABLE 25.1. Categories of Chronic Diarrhea

Category	Malabsorption	Inflammatory	Secretory	Osmotic
Stool osmotic gap (mOsm/kg)*	Not applicable	Not applicable	Less than 50 mOsm/kg	Greater than 100–125 mOsm/kg
Fecal leukocytes	Absent	Present	Absent	Absent
Hemoccult	Negative	Positive or negative	Negative	Negative
Nocturnal BMs	No	Possible	Yes	No

*-stool osmotic gap = 290 − 2 x (stool$_{sodium}$ + stool$_{potassium}$), BM = bowel movement

3. <u>WORKUP OF CHRONIC DIARRHEA</u>

- **Dietary history:** after dairy products (lactose intolerance) or "sorbitol-containing" foods
  - Postgastric feeds (especially calorie-dense formulas)
- **Medication-induced:** many antibiotics and antineoplastics, antiretrovirals, acarbose, antacids, colchicine, cyclosporine, digoxin, H$_2$-receptor blockers, misoprostol, metformin, milk of magnesia, NSAIDs, octreotide, olsalazine, orlistat, PPIs, quinidine, theophylline, ticlopidine, and SSRIs
- **Herbs that cause diarrhea:** aloe, buckthorn, cascara sagrada, dandelion root, echinacea, feverfew, ginseng, pokeroot tea, rhubarb root, saw palmetto, and slippery elm
- **Routine labs:** complete blood count, CHEM 7 and thyroid-stimulating hormone, stool osmotic gap, fecal leukocytes, stool ova, and parasites with or without stool giardia antigen and *Clostridium difficile* toxins A/B
- **Malabsorptive diarrhea:** see Table 25.1
  - Typical findings: anemia, decreased serum iron, folate, calcium, magnesium, cholesterol, albumin, and carotene plus or minus Vitamin B$_{12}$
  - 24-hour quantitative stool fat greater than 14 grams diagnostic of steatorrhea
  - Etiologies: pancreatic exocrine insufficiency (screen with bentiromide or pancreolauryl tests), celiac disease (screen with antiendomysial or antitransglutaminase antibodies), lactose intolerance (check lactose tolerance test with 50-gram test dose and measure serum glucose at 0, 60, and 120 minutes), or Whipple's disease (upper endoscopy with small bowel biopsy)
- **Inflammatory diarrhea:** see Table 25.1
  - Stool for ova and parasites × 3 (not valid if barium/contrast study in last 14 days)
  - Stool for *Clostridium difficile* toxin if recent antibiotics, chemotherapy, or hospital exposure, or if residing in a long-term care facility
  - If no infectious cause:
    - Flexible sigmoidoscopy or colonoscopy with biopsy to evaluate for inflammatory bowel disease, collagenous colitis, microscopic colitis, ischemic colitis, radiation colitis, or colon CA
- **Secretory diarrhea:** see Table 25.1
  - Stool for aeromonas, plesiomonas, microsporidia, cryptosporidium, and ova plus parasites
  - Check stool for giardia antigen by enzyme-linked immunoassay test

- Rule out thyrotoxicosis or diabetic enteropathy (nocturnal diarrhea)
- Bile acid diarrhea occurs after extensive ileal resections
- Selective testing for plasma peptides such as gastrin, calcitonin, VIP, somatostatin, or urine 5-hydroxyindole acetic acid if a neuroendocrine tumor syndrome is likely
- **Osmotic diarrhea:** see Table 25.1
  - Stool for laxatives, examine diet, and check meds as indicated earlier
  - D-xylose test positive and stool pH less than 5.6 in carbohydrate malabsorption
- **Irritable bowel syndrome** is a diagnosis of exclusion

INFLAMMATORY BOWEL DISEASE

1. ## PATHOPHYSIOLOGY
   - Complex interaction between host and environmental factors leads to disordered mucosal immunity which then increases proinflammatory cytokines (IL-1, IL-6, TNF), leading to T-cell activation

2. ## CLINICAL PRESENTATION
   - Inflammatory diarrhea
   - Ulcerative colitis: episodic rectal bleeding, diarrhea, pain, tenesmus
   - Crohn's disease: abdominal pain, diarrhea, fever, perianal fistula, heme-positive stools (rarely frank blood)
   - See **Table 25.2**

TABLE 25.2.   Differentiating Ulcerative Colitis from Crohn's Disease

Features	Ulcerative Colitis (UC)	Crohn's Disease (CD)
Passage of mucus or pus	Common	Rare
Rectal bleeding	Common	20–30%
Weight loss and growth failure	Occasionally	Common
Abdominal distension	Only in severe UC	Occasional
Perianal disease and fistulas	Absent	Up to 30%
Abdominal mass	Absent	Sometimes in right lower quadrant
Colorectal involvement	Exclusively	Common
Ileal involvement	Sometimes "backwash ileitis"	Common
Esophagus/duodenum/jejunum	Absent	Infrequent
Bowel obstruction	Rare	Common
Cancer	Common	Occasionally
Extraintestinal manifestations*	Slightly less common	Common
Endoscopic Findings		
Friability and pseudopolyps	Common	Occasionally
Cobblestoning and linear ulcers	Absent	Common
Distribution	Continuous in colon	Segmental distribution
Lab and Pathological Findings		
Elevated CRP/ESR	In severe UC	Common
Anemia	In severe UC	Common
Hypoalbuminemia	In severe UC	Common

(Continued)

Table 25.2 *(Continued)*

Features	Ulcerative Colitis (UC)	Crohn's Disease (CD)
p-ANCA antibodies	60–80% of patients	10–40% (if colitis)
Saccharomyces cerevisiae Ab	1%	50% of patients
Transmural inflammation	No	Yes
Distorted crypt architecture	Yes	Uncommon
Granulomas	No	Yes (15–36% on biopsy)

RLQ = Right Lower Quadrant, CRP = C-reactive protein, ESR = erythrocyte sedimentation rate, p-ANCA = perinuclear antineutrophil cytoplasmic antibodies, Ab = antibodies

* Arthralgias/arthritis, erythema nodosum, pyoderma gangrenosum, oral ulcers, episcleritis, uveitis, keratitis, myocarditis, pericarditis, ankylosing spondylitis, sacroiliitis, primary sclerosing cholangitis, autoimmune hemolytic anemia, myelodysplastic syndrome, interstitial lung disease, myelopathy, peripheral neuropathy, or secondary amyloidosis

Source: Adapted from *Lancet*, 2007; 369(9573): 1641–57, *J Clin Gastroenterol*, 2006; 40(6): 467–75 and *Gastroenterol*, 2007; 133(5): 1670–89.

3. WORKUP OF COLITIS

- Stool culture, ova and parasites, *C. difficile* toxin with or without assay for *E. coli* 0157:H7
- Small bowel follow-through contrast study to rule out strictures consistent with CD

4. MEDICAL TREATMENT OF INFLAMMATORY BOWEL DISEASE (IBD)

- Avoid narcotics, anticholinergics, antimotility agents, and NSAIDs in active colitis
- Rule out infectious colitis (especially *C. difficile* colitis) for any flare of CD or UC
- IBD severity: mild disease is fewer than 4 stools/day and normal ESR; moderate disease with 4–6 stools/day and minimal systemic toxicity; severe disease with more than 6 bloody stools/day and fever, tachycardia, anemia, or an elevated ESR/CRP; fulminant disease with more than 10 bloody stools/day, toxicity, abdominal tenderness and distension, and colonic dilatation on KUB

5-Aminosalicylic Acid Derivatives for Mild–Moderate UC and Maintenance Therapy

- Oral sulfasalazine 1–1.5 g qid or balsalazide 2.25 g tid for colonic involvement
- Mesalamine formulations: oral Asacol or Asacol HD or Pentasa, CANASA suppositories, and Rowasa enemas
  - Asacol 800–1600 mg PO tid for distal ileum and colon
  - Pentasa 500 mg to 1 g PO qid for small bowel and colonic involvement by Crohn's disease
  - Rowasa enemas 1–4 g PR retained for 8 hours at bedtime for distal colon and rectum
  - Canasa suppository 500 mg PR daily or 10% hydrocortisone foam for proctitis
- Maintenance: PO olsalazine 500 mg bid, sulfasalazine 500 mg qid, or mesalamine 1.6 g/day

Treatment of Mild–Moderate CD

- Prednisone 40–60 mg PO daily for moderate CD and UC × 7–14 days until clinical improvement, then wean 5 mg/week until 20 mg/day, then decrease 2.5 mg/week to minimum effective dose
  - Consider budesonide (Entocort) 9 mg/day × 2 wks, then taper to 6 mg/day and then 3 mg/day for ileal or right-sided colonic CD

Corticosteroids for Moderate–Severe CD and UC

- Prednisone 40–60 mg PO daily for moderate CD and UC × 7–14 days until clinical improvement, then wean 5 mg/week until 20 mg/day, then decrease 2.5 mg/week to minimum effective dose
  - Consider budesonide (Entocort) 9 mg/day × 2 wks, then taper to 6 mg/day and then 3 mg/day for ileal or right-sided colonic CD
- Hydrocortisone 100 mg or budesonide 2–8 mg enemas PR daily for proctitis or distal UC
- Methylprednisolone 30 mg IV q12h or 1 mg/kg IV daily for severe CD or UC along with high-dose mesalamine compounds
- Steroids ineffective for perianal fistulas

Immunomodulating Drugs for Refractory Moderate–Severe CD and UC

- Strict bowel rest, IV fluids, and NGT decompression for fulminant colitis or toxic megacolon

- Azathioprine 2–3 mg/kg PO daily or 6-mercaptopurine 1–1.5 mg/kg PO daily for control of steroid-dependent or refractory IBD or as maintenance therapy of fistulizing CD
  - Full effect takes 2–3 months
  - Follow periodic CBCD and liver panel
- Methotrexate 15–25 mg IM weekly for control of moderate, steroid-dependent CD
  - Follow periodic CBCD and liver panel
- Add cyclosporine 2–4 mg/kg/day IV as continuous drip after 7 days of steroids for fulminant colitis or for fistulizing CD
  - Severe sepsis or death can complicate management

Biologic Agents as Alternatives to Steroids for Induction Therapy of Severe IBD
- Infliximab 5–10 mg/kg IV dose at 0, 2, and 6 wks for severe, refractory IBD or fistulizing CD
- Adalimumab 160 mg SQ × 1, then 80 mg at wk 2, then 40 mg at wk 4, then q 2 wks if severe CD

Conditions with Increased Prevalence in IBD
- Thromboembolism, osteoporosis, *C. difficile* colitis, gallstones, primary biliary cirrhosis, nephrolithiasis, and colon CA
- Colon CA screening with colonoscopy after 8–10 years of colitis, then every 1–2 years

Indications for Colectomy
- Fulminant colitis or toxic megacolon refractory to maximum IV therapy × 7–10 days, severe GI hemorrhage, GI perforation, high-grade colonic dysplasia, or suspected carcinoma

PROGNOSIS

- Crohn's disease
  - Severity predictors: age younger than 40 yo, perianal disease, and initial requirement for corticosteroids

COMPLICATIONS

- Crohn's disease
  - Malabsorption
  - Pernicious anemia (Vitamin B_{12} deficiency in severe ileal disease)
  - Osteoporosis and fractures (impaired absorption of Vitamin D/calcium)
  - Formation of sinus tracts and fistulas (enterovesical, enterocutaneous, enterovaginal) or phlegmon/abscess
  - Perianal disease including fissures, fistulas, abscesses
  - Bowel strictures/obstruction/perforation
  - Intestinal carcinoma (risk increased in patients with strictures and perianal disease)
  - Others: thromboembolism, arthritis (including sacroiliitis, ankylosing spondylitis), uveitis, retinal vasculitis/central vein occlusion (rare), primary sclerosing cholangitis, secondary amyloidosis complicated by renal failure, nephrolithiasis
- Ulcerative colitis
  - Massive hemorrhage
  - Toxic megacolon increases risk of intestinal perforation (50% mortality)
  - Bowel stricture/obstruction
  - Colorectal cancer (3–5% incidence: increases with duration and extent of UC)
  - Others: thromboembolism, uveitis/episcleritis, erythema nodosum, pyoderma gangrenosum, arthritis, ankylosing spondylitis, bronchiectasis, AIHA

REFERENCES

Gastroenterology, 1999;116(6):1464–1486; *N Engl J Med*, 1995;332(11):725–9; *Gut*, 2003;52(Suppl 5):v1–15; *Am Fam Physician*, 2011;84(10):1119–26; *N Engl J Med*, 2004;350(1):38–47; *Gastroenterol Clin North Am*, 2003;32(4):1249–67; *Gastroenterology*, 2006;130(5): 1480–91; *J Emerg Med*, 2002;23(2):125–30; *Curr Opin Pharmacol*, 2005;5(6):559–65; *N Engl J Med*, 2008;359(18):1932–40; *Clin Infect Dis*, 2008;46(Suppl1):S32–42; *N Engl J Med*, 2002;347(6):417–29; *Am Fam Physician*, 2003;68(4):707–14; *Gastroenterol Clin North Am*, 2003;33(2):191–208; *Am J Gastroenterol*, 2004;99(7):1371–85; *Gastrointest Endosc*, 2006;63(4):546–57; *Lancet*, 2007;369(9573):1641–57.

CHAPTER 26

ACUTE HEPATITIS

Hepatitis is classified into cholestatic, hepatocellular injury, or infiltrative patterns
- Cholestasis: number of increased alkaline phosphatase is greater than increased liver transaminases
- Hepatocellular injury: number of increased liver transaminases is greater than increased alkaline phosphatase
- Infiltrative diseases of the liver: greatly increased alkaline phosphatase with low bilirubin

1. <u>**EPIDEMIOLOGY**</u>
   - HAV: exclusive fecal–oral transmission; late fall early winter
     - Virtually all recover without sequelae, but 0.05% chance of fulminant hepatitis
     - Vaccine decreased childhood annual incidence by more than 70%
     - 4-week incubation period, replicate in liver, viral shedding in stool, infectivity diminishes rapidly once jaundice is apparent
     - Anti-HAV IgG means immunity
   - HBV: present in all body fluid in infected person
     - 95–99% with acute infection recover without sequelae
     - 5% of cases develop into chronic HepB infection, which is the main reservoir of more than 350–400 millio HBsAg carriers worldwide
     - 25% of these carriers will develop cirrhosis, leading to overall cirrhosis rate of less than 1%; HBeAg positivity correlates with infectivity
     - HBV vaccination has led to a 90% decline in HBV incidence and HCC
   - HCV: blood-borne infection, 5% sexual and perinatal transmission
     - Accidental needle puncture carries a 3% transmission rate
     - Chronic infection prevalence is 85–90%, 60% progress to chronic hepatitis, and 20% develop cirrhosis in 10–20 years
   - HEV: most common form of hepatitis in Asia, Africa, Central America
     - Behaves like HAV

2. <u>**PATHOPHYSIOLOGY**</u>
   - Viral hepatitis
     - Hepatitis viruses are not directly cytotoxic; rather, hepatic injury is due to host immune response to viru
     - Severity and chronicity of infection depends on degree of cytotoxic CD8+ response and production of cytokines
     - Extrahepatic phenomena (glomerulonephritis, polyarteritis nodosa, cryoglobulinemia) in hepatitis B and C due to deposition of immune complexes
   - Toxin-mediated hepatitis
     - Direct toxic effect (acetaminophen, CCl₄, *Amanita phalloides*): dose-dependent, short latency
     - Acetaminophen: hepatotoxic metabolite NAPQI accumulates, depleting glutathione; acetaminophen then binds to hepatocyte proteins, leading to necrosis
     - Idiosyncratic drug reaction (isoniazid, valproate, phenytoin, statins): infrequent, unpredictable, not clearly dose-dependent, depend on host factors such as genetics

3. <u>**CLINICAL PRESENTATION**</u>
   - Often asymptomatic elevation in AST/ALT
   - Symptoms: abdominal pain, fatigue, nausea/vomiting, myalgias
   - Signs: RUQ/epigastric tenderness, jaundice, hepatosplenomegaly
   - See **Table 26.1**

TABLE 26.1.   Causes of Hepatitis

Cholestatic Pattern	Infiltrative Diseases Affecting Liver	Medication-Induced Hepatocellular Injury (cont'd)
• Budd-Chiari syndrome • Gallstones • Hepatocellular carcinoma • Primary biliary cirrhosis • Primary sclerosing cholangitis • Veno-occlusive disease	• CA mets to the liver • Deep fungal infections • Hepatocellular carcinoma • Leukemic infiltrate • Lymphoma • Sarcoidosis • Tuberculosis	• Cyclophosphamide • Dantrolene • Dapsone • Diclofenac • Fluconazole • Fluoxetine • Griseofulvin • Halothane • Heparin • Hydralazine

Medication-Induced Cholestasis		
• Allopurinol • Amoxicillin-clavulanate • Anabolic steroids • Arsenicals • Azathioprine • Benzodiazepines • Carbamazepine • Chlorpromazine • Clindamycin • Clopidogrel • Cyclosporine • Cyproheptadine • Erythromycin • Estrogens • Felbamate • Fluoroquinolones • Fluoxetine • Flutamide • Glucocorticoids • Gold • Histamine$_2$-blockers • Haloperidol • Irbesartan • Mercaptopurine • Methimazole • Methotrexate • Mirtazapine • Naproxen • Niacin • Nitrofurantoin • Oral contraceptives • Penicillamine • Phenothiazines • Propoxyphene • Propylthiouracil • Pyrazinamide • Sulfasalazine • Sulfonylureas • Sulindac • Terbinafine • Tetracycline • Tricyclic antidepressants • Trimethoprim-sulfamethoxazole	**Herbal Hepatotoxins** • Amanita mushrooms • Chaparral leaf • Comfrey • Germander • Gordolobo herbal tea • Greasewood • Jin bu huan • Kava kava • Margosa oil • Mate tea • Mistletoe • Oil of cloves • Pennyroyal (squaw mint) • Skullcap • Valerian root • Yerba herbal tea **Conditions Causing Hepatocellular Injury** • Alcoholic hepatitis • α_1-antitrypsin deficiency • Autoimmune hepatitis • Chronic viral hepatitis • Congestive hepatopathy • Hemochromatosis • Ischemic hepatitis • Nonalcoholic steatohepatitis (diabetes and obesity) • Wilson's disease **Medication-Induced Hepatocellular Injury** • Acarbose • Acetaminophen • Allopurinol • Amiodarone • ACEI • Aspirin/salicylates • Baclofen • Bupropion • Carmustine • Chlorpropamide	• Isoniazid • Ketoconazole • Labetalol • Losartan • MAOI • Methotrexate • Methyldopa • Minocycline • Mithramycin • Nefazodone • Nevirapine • Nifedipine • Nitrofurantoin • NSAIDs • Omeprazole • Paroxetine • Penicillins • Phenobarbital • Phenytoin • Piroxicam • Primidone • Procainamide • Pyrazinamide • Quinidine or quinine • Rifampin • Risperidone • Ritonavir • Sertraline • Statins • Stavudine • Sulfonamides • Tamoxifen • Thiazolidinediones • Trazodone • Valproic acid or divalproate • Venlafaxine • Verapamil • Zidovudine

Source: Information from *NEJM*, 2006; 354(7): 731–9. *Gastroenterology*, 2002; 123(4): 1364–6 and *AFP*, 2005; 71(6): 1105–10.

4. MANAGEMENT OF SEVERE ACUTE ALCOHOLIC HEPATITIS (AAH)

- Severe AAH: Glasgow alcoholic hepatitis score 9 or higher, Maddrey's discriminant score 32 or higher, or MELD score 20 or higher
  - Calculate MELD at www.esot.org/Elita/meldCalculator.aspx
- Possible mortality benefit with glucocorticoids or pentoxifylline for severe AAH
  - PO prednisone 40 mg/day or prednisolone 32 mg/day × 28 days
    - Glucocorticoids contraindicated for acute GI bleed, sepsis, renal failure, or pancreatitis
  - Pentoxifylline 400 mg PO tid is as effective as corticosteroids
- Aggressive nutritional support for 1.2–1.4 times the estimated caloric needs
- Multivitamin, thiamine, folic acid, pyridoxine
- Watch for refeeding syndrome (hypokalemia, hypophosphatemia, hypomagnesemia)
- Consider adding oxandrolone 40 mg PO daily × 30 d for Maddrey score 80 or higher or lack of improvement in Maddrey score or MELD after 10–14 days of therapy

TABLE 26.2. Glasgow Alcoholic Hepatitis Score

Parameters	1 Point	2 Points	3 Points
Age	Younger than 50 yo	50 yo or older	—
WBC (10⁹/L)	Less than 15	15 or higher	—
BUN (mmol/L)	Less than 5	5 or higher	—
INR	Less than 1.5	1.5–2	Greater than 2
Bilirubin (µmol/L)	Less than 125	125–250	Greater than 250

Source: Adapted from *Gut*, 2005; 54(8): 1057–9.

Management of Acute Hepatitis A Virus Infection
- Avoid food handling and unprotected sexual intercourse until immunity develops
- Notifiable disease to public health department
- Hospitalization indicated for severe dehydration related to anorexia, nausea, and vomiting
- Hepatitis A virus vaccine

Management of Acute Hepatitis B Virus Infection
- Nearly all individuals will clear acute infection spontaneously and develop immunity
- Hospitalization is indicated for dehydration related to anorexia, nausea, and vomiting
- Antiviral therapy is generally *not* indicated, except in cases of fulminant hepatic failure with profound jaundice and hepatic encephalopathy when lamivudine may be used
- Avoid unprotected intercourse for 6 months
- HBV vaccine series should be administered to sexual and household contacts of carriers
- HBIG and HBV vaccine are administered to newborns born to HBV-infected mothers

Management of Chronic Hepatitis B Virus Infection
- Indications for HCC screening with ultrasound exam q6–12 months
  - Asian men older than 40, Asian women older than 50, cirrhosis, family history of HCC, Africans older than 20; carrier for more than 40 years with ALT elevation or HBV DNA greater than 2,000 IU/mL
- Options for antiviral therapy when indicated: interferon-α, PEG-interferon-α, lamivudine, adefovir, entecavir, telbivudine, and tenofovir
- Administer HAV vaccine series

Management of Acute Hepatitis C Virus Infection
- Evidence suggests that antiviral treatment is indicated for those patients who do not spontaneously clear infection within 12 weeks
  - Treatment with interferon-α or PEG-interferon-α for 24 weeks is beneficial and cost-effective

Management of Chronic Hepatitis C Virus Infection
- Consider therapy with PEG-interferon-α plus ribavirin $\times$ 14–24 weeks with genotypes 2 or 3; treat for 12 weeks for genotype 1
- Administer HAV and HBV vaccine series

COMPLICATIONS

- Hepatic failure
- Chronic hepatitis
- Cirrhosis
- Hepatocellular carcinoma
- Extrahepatic complications of viral hepatitis (vasculitis, arthritis, glomerulonephritis, myocarditis, optic neuritis, transverse myelitis, thrombocytopenia, aplastic anemia)

FERENCES

Clin Gastro enterol, 2006;40(9):833–41; *Aliment Pharmacol Ther*, 2007;28(9):1166–74.

CHAPTER 27

CIRRHOSIS

1. **EPIDEMIOLOGY**
   - In the United States, 70% is due to EtOH abuse
   - Only 10–30% of alcoholic patients develop cirrhosis
   - Worldwide, viral hepatitis is the most common cause of cirrhosis

2. **PATHOPHYSIOLOGY**
   - Liver fibrosis distorts architecture and induces formation of regenerative nodules that leads to a decl in liver mass and function
   - Spontaneous bacterial peritonitis
     - Translocation of GI flora (usually Gram-negative Enterobacteriaceae) from GI tract to ascites via mesenteric lymph nodes
   - Hepatorenal syndrome
     - Splanchnic vasodilation results in decreased systemic vascular resistance that induces maladaptive renal arterial vasoconstriction, resulting in prerenal azotemia unresponsive to volume resuscitation
   - Hepatopulmonary syndrome
     - Pulmonary vasodilation results in intrapulmonary vascular dilations leading to shunt (worse in upright position), then platypnea and orthodeoxia
   - Gastroesophageal varices
     - Increased intrahepatic resistance plus splanchnic vasodilation increases portal venous pressure, ultimately leading to portocaval anastomoses; in this case, between short gastric veins causing azygous vein
   - Ascites
     - Splanchnic vasodilation increases renin-angiotensin-aldosterone leading to Na retention and increased extracellular volume
     - Constant leak of fluid from vasculature into peritoneum is stimulus for continued Na retention, sinc blood vessels are never fully expanded
     - Decreased liver synthesis of albumin decreases oncotic pressure, worsening leak of fluid from vesse
   - Hepatic hydrothorax
     - Ascites leaks into pleural space (usually R side) through small holes in diaphragm

3. **CLINICAL PRESENTATION**
   - SBP
     - Fevers, chills, diffuse abdominal pain
     - Up to 50% are asymptomatic
     - May have worsening encephalopathy, diarrhea, refractory ascites, worsening renal function, ileus
   - Hepatorenal syndrome
     - Sodium and water retention (Ur Na less than 10 mEq/L, Serum Na less than 130 mEq/L)
     - Decreased urine output (less than 500 mL/24 h)
     - Decreased glomerular filtration rate
       - Type 1: Cr greater than 2.5 mg/dL; usually precipitated by SBP
       - Type 2: Cr greater than 1.5 mg/dL but stable; refractory ascites
   - Hepatopulmonary syndrome
     - Liver disease (portal hypertension with or without cirrhosis)
     - Pulmonary vascular dilation

- Hypoxia
- May have clubbing, cyanosis
- Gastroesophageal varices
  - Asymptomatic until they bleed
  - Suspect varices in any upper gastrointestinal bleed in a cirrhotic
- Ascites
  - Increased abdominal girth, recent weight gain, ankle swelling
  - Underlying disease: heart failure, cirrhosis, nephrotic syndrome, or malignancy
  - Clinical signs include
    - Bulging flanks (hard to differentiate from obesity) [LR+ 1.8, LR− 0.5]
    - Flank dullness: when supine, bowel floats to the top and fluid gathers in the flanks; percuss from umbilicus toward the flank and listen for the transition from tympany to dullness [LR+ 1.7, LR− 0.4]
    - Shifting dullness: roll the patient on his/her side and repeat the percussion; the dependent side should be dull, and the elevated side tympanic [LR+ 2.1, LR− 0.4]
    - Fluid wave: place a hand on one flank and percuss the other—the "fluid wave" should be palpable in your nonpercussing hand [LR+ 5.3, LR− 0.6]
- Hepatic hydrothorax
  - Pleural effusion in setting of cirrhosis without cardiac or pulmonary disease
  - 85% are right-sided
  - May present (rarely) in the absence of ascites

DIAGNOSIS OF CIRRHOSIS

- Gold standard is a percutaneous liver biopsy; presumptive diagnosis by abnormal labs, exam, and imaging (ultrasound or radionuclide liver/spleen scan)
- Ultrasound is 90% sensitive for the diagnosis of cirrhosis
- See **Table 27.1**

ABLE 27.1. Child-Turcotte-Pugh Scoring System for Cirrhosis Classification

Categories	1 Point	2 Points	3 Points
Albumin (g/dL)	Greater than 3.5	2.8–3.5	Less than 2.8
Bilirubin (mg/dL)	Less than 2.0	2.0–3.0	Greater than 3.0
International Normalized Ratio	Less than 1.7	1.7–2.3	Greater than 2.3
Presence of ascites	None	Diuretic controlled	Diuretic resistant
Encephalopathy	None	Grade 1–2 (mild)	Grade 3–4 (severe)
Class A = 5–6 points; Class B = 7–9 points; Class C = 10 or more points			
1- and 2-yr mortality rates: Class A, 0% and 15%; Class B, 20% and 40%; Class C, 55% and 65%			

ource: Adapted from *Crit Care Med,* 2006; 34(Suppl 9): S225–31.

WORKUP OF CIRRHOSIS

- Labs: complete blood count, CHEM 7, liver panel, prothrombin time, and α-fetoprotein
- Labs to consider: hepatitis B and C virus serologies, iron studies, antimitochondrial, antinuclear and antismooth muscle antibodies, serum ceruloplasmin, α_1-antitrypsin level, and blood cultures for any suspicion of SBP
- A percutaneous liver biopsy is indicated if the diagnosis is equivocal
- Imaging studies: abdominal ultrasound with Doppler of portal vein blood flow
- Ascitic fluid analysis: cell count with differential, culture and Gram stain, protein, albumin, and LDH
- Consider screening EGD to assess for esophageal or gastric varices in all patients with newly diagnosed Childs B or C cirrhosis
  - All patients with varices should receive propranolol or nadolol unless contraindicated

6. <u>COMPLICATIONS OF CIRRHOSIS</u>

- Any complication indicates decompensated cirrhosis

9. <u>EVALUATION OF ASCITES</u>

- See **Table 27.2**
- Diagnostic paracentesis for all new-onset ascites, decompensated liver disease, or for an acute upper gastrointestinal bleed and send peritoneal fluid for:
  - Protein, albumin, glucose (glc), cell count, lactate dehydrogenase (LDH) and culture (bedside inoculation of aerobic/anaerobic blood culture bottles gives optimal yield)
  - If SAAG low, consider placing a PPD test and sending fluid for cytology

TABLE 27.2.   Etiologies of Ascites

High SAAG (1.1 g/dL or higher)	Low SAAG (less than 1.1 g/dL)
• Cirrhotic ascites	• Peritoneal carcinomatosis
• Alcoholic hepatitis	• Peritoneal tuberculosis
• Right-sided congestive heart failure	• Pancreatic ascites
• Multiple liver metastases	• Biliary ascites
• Fulminant hepatic failure	• Nephrotic syndrome
• Budd-Chiari syndrome	• Lupus serositis
• Portal vein thrombosis	• Bowel infarction or obstruction
• Veno-occlusive disease	• Postoperative lymphatic leak
• Fatty liver of pregnancy	

SAAG = serum-ascites albumin gradient; SAAG greater than or equal to 1.1 g/dL = portal hypertension (97% accuracy)

Source: Adapted from *Hepatology*, 2004; 39(3): 841–56.

7. <u>GENERAL MANAGEMENT OF CIRRHOTIC ASCITES</u>

- Dietary restriction to 1–2 grams sodium daily is essential for successful control
- Consider fluid restriction up to 1,500 mL/day if serum Na is less than or equal to 125 MEq/L
- Avoid aspirin, NSAIDs, COX-2 inhibitors, aminoglycosides, ACEI, ARB, or α-1 blockers
- Immunize all nonimmune patients with HAV and HBV vaccine series

Management of Moderate-Volume Cirrhotic Ascites

- Spironolactone 100 mg PO q morning or amiloride 10 mg PO daily

Management of Large-Volume Cirrhotic Ascites

- Begin spironolactone 100 mg PO q morning and furosemide 40 mg PO q morning
- Double dosages q 3–5 days until urine Na is higher than urine K and weight loss 1 lb/day or maximal doses of spironolactone 400 mg PO q morning and furosemide 160 mg PO q morning
- Monitor for encephalopathy, renal insufficiency, and hyponatremia and discontinue diuretics for any of these complications

Management of Refractory Ascites (diuretic-resistant ascites)

- Large volume paracentesis q 2–4 weeks with or without infusion of 8–10 g albumin for each liter of ascitic fluid if more than 5 liters of ascitic fluid is removed
- Alternative is a transjugular intrahepatic portosystemic shunt (TIPS procedure)
  - Absolute contraindications to TIPS: portosystemic encephalopathy, CHF, pulmonary hypertension, multiple hepatic cysts, active infection, biliary obstruction, hepatic or portal vein thrombosis, central hepatoma, severe thrombocytopenia, coagulopathy (INR greater than 2, Childs-Pugh score 11 or higher, or total bilirubin greater than 5 mg/dL
  - Relative contraindication is a total bilirubin of 3 mg/dL or higher and age 65 or older
- Recommend referral of patients with ascites for liver transplantation

Spontaneous Bacterial Peritonitis (SBP)

- Clinical features: abdominal pain, fever, encephalopathy, UGIB, nausea, vomiting, or asymptomatic (up to 50%)

- **Diagnosis**: ascitic fluid neutrophils greater than or equal to 250/mm³ and monomicrobial bacterial growth with bedside inoculation of blood culture bottles with ascitic fluid
- SBP variants
  - Neutrocytic ascites: ascitic fluid neutrophils greater than or equal to 250/mm³ and sterile cultures
    - Treated identically to SBP
  - Bacterascites: monomicrobial bacterial growth but ascitic fluid neutrophils less than 250/mm³
    - Repeat paracentesis after 48–72 h of therapy and treat with antibiotics *only* if second set of cultures is positive
- Secondary bacterial peritonitis likely if ascitic fluid white blood count is greater than 10,000/μL, glc is less than 50 mg/dL, LDH is greater than 250 U/L, protein is greater than 1 g/dL, alkaline phosphatase is greater than 240 units/L, carcinoembryonic antigen (CEA) is greater than 5 ng/mL, or polymicrobial Gram stain or culture growth
    - CT scan of abdomen if secondary bacterial peritonitis is a possibility
- **SBP treatment**
  - Cefotaxime 2 g IV q 8 h or ceftriaxone 2 g IV daily × 5–7 days
  - Albumin 1.5 g/kg IV on day 1, then 1 g/kg IV on day 3 has a 19% decrease in absolute mortality and decreases the risk of hepatorenal syndrome
  - Repeat paracentesis after 48 h of treatment and consider change in antibiotics if neutrophil count does not decrease by at least 25%
- **SBP prophylaxis**
  - Trimethoprim-sulfamethoxazole DS 1 tab PO 5 days/week, norfloxacin 400 mg PO daily, or ciprofloxacin 750 mg PO weekly
  - Indicated for prior SBP, if ascitic fluid protein is less than 1 g/dL or Tbili is greater than 2.5 mg/dL
  - Norfloxacin 400 mg PO bid or Ceftriaxone 1 g/day × 7 days for acute variceal bleed; improves survival and decreases risk of SBP or variceal rebleed

Gastroesophageal Variceal Bleed

See page 100

Hepatic Encephalopathy

- Precipitants: GI bleed, medications, high protein intake, infection, or electrolyte disorders
- Treatments: lactulose 30–45 mL PO tid; titrate to 2–4 loose bowel movements daily
- Add neomycin 1–3 g PO qid or rifaximin 550 mg PO bid or 200 mg PO tid for refractory cases

Hepatorenal Syndrome

- Diagnosis of exclusion; serum creatinine (crt) greater than 1.5 mg/dL or CrCl less than 40 mL/min; urinary indices mimic prerenal azotemia (UNa is less than 10 mEq/L); absence of shock; no recent nephrotoxic drugs; absence of parenchymal renal disease, proteinuria, microhematuria, or structural renal disease
- No sustained renal improvement after fluid challenge with albumin 1 g/kg IV and stopping diuretics × 48 hours
- **Therapy options**
  - Midodrine 7.5–12.5 mg PO tid *plus* octreotide 100–200 mcg SQ tid
  - Norepinephrine 0.5–3 mg/h infusion
  - Terlipressin 1 mg IV q 8–12 h
    - Add to all above, albumin 1 g/kg IV on day 1, then 20–40 g IV daily
    - Duration of treatment is 5–15 days until crt is less than 1.5 mg/dL
  - TIPSS is an alternative for refractory HRS as a bridge to transplantation

Hepatopulmonary Syndrome

- Dyspnea and deoxygenation accompanying change from a recumbent to a standing position and usually clubbing is present
- Diagnosis requires an increased alveolar-arterial oxygen gradient and intrapulmonary vascular dilatations

- Diagnosis with ^{99m}-Tc-labeled albumin perfusion lung scan showing more than 6% uptake in the brain, contrast-enhanced echocardiography with bubbles in the left heart after the third heart beat, or pulmonary arteriography to diagnose intrapulmonary vascular dilatations with right-left shunting
- Treatment is with orthotopic liver transplantation and oxygen supplementation

Hepatic Hydrothorax

- Right-sided pleural effusion (85%), left-sided (13%), bilateral (2%)
- Pleural fluid with transudative characteristics, pleural fluid pH greater than 7.4, and serum-pleural fluid albumin gradient greater than 1.1
- 1–2 g/day sodium restriction and diuretics as per large volume ascites
- Transjugular intrahepatic portosystemic shunt for diuretic-resistant effusions
- Therapeutic thoracentesis is acceptable if necessary
- Tube thoracostomy with chemical pleurodesis
- VATS with repair of diaphragmatic defects

Portopulmonary Hypertension

- Pulmonary arterial hypertension that develops in the setting of portal hypertension
- Noninvasive methods to predict pulmonary hypertension
  - CT pulmonary angiogram: the diameter of the main pulmonary arteries is greater than or equal to 29 mm and segmental artery-to-bronchus ratio is greater than 1 in at least 3 pulmonary lobes OR the main pulmonary artery diameter is greater than the aorta diameter
  - 2D-echocardiography can predict pulmonary hypertension
- Gold standard for assessing pulmonary hypertension is a pulmonary artery catheterization
- Perioperative Management of the Cirrhotic Patient
  - Risk factors for surgery in cirrhotic patients
  - Obstructive jaundice: hematocrit greater than 30%, total bilirubin greater than 11 mg/dL, malignancy, creatinine greater than 1.4 mg/dL, albumin less than 3 g/dL, age older than 65 yo, AST greater than 90 IU/L, and BUN greater than 19 mg/dL
    - Acute alcoholic hepatitis: elective surgery is contraindicated
    - Fulminant hepatic failure: consider candidacy for liver transplantation
  - Cirrhosis scoring systems predictive of postoperative complications or death
  - Child-Turcotte-Pugh class and mortality rate for abdominal or cardiac surgery
    - Nonemergent abdominal surgery: Class A = 10%, Class B = 30%, Class C = 82%
    - Emergent abdominal surgery: Class A = 22%, Class B = 38%, Class C = 100%
    - Elective cardiac surgery: Class A = 0%, Class B = 50%, Class C = 100%
  - MELD (Model for End-Stage Liver Disease) score
    - Calculator available at: www.esot.org/Elita/meldCalculator.aspx
    - Minimum lab value is 1.0 and maximum creatinine is 4 mg/dL; max score is 40
    - For elective abdominal operations, 90-day mortality rate is: 10% if MELD score is 8 or lower; 25% if MELD score 9–16; and 50% if MELD score is higher than 16
    - 30-day mortality for nontransplant surgery increases 1% per point for MELD scores between 6 and 20 and 2% per point for scores higher than 20
    - Recommend no nonemergent surgery if MELD score is higher than 15; consider surgery with close monitoring for MELD score 10–15, and proceed with surgery for MELD scores less than 10

Preoperative Management of Decompensated Cirrhosis

- Nutritional recommendations: intake of 1–1.5 g/kg/day of protein and B vitamins
- Coagulopathy: Vitamin K 10 mg PO daily × 3 days helps coagulopathy from malnutrition
  - Prolonged PTT is more predictive of bleeding risk compared with elevated INR
    - Recommend FFP transfusions to normalize PTT before an invasive procedure
- Thrombocytopenia: platelet transfusion if less than 50,000/mm^3 before invasive procedures
- Ascites: aggressive preoperative management minimizes the risk of postoperative pulmonary complications or wound dehiscence

- Hyponatremia: fluid restrict to 1–1.2 liters/day for serum sodium less than 125 mmol/L
- Hepatic encephalopathy: correct all metabolic abnormalities, avoid sedative/narcotics, and use lactulose 20–30 g PO q 6–8 h titrated to 3 loose BMs/day
- Substance abuse: patients should be sober for several months prior to elective surgery

Postoperative Care

- Consider enteral and parenteral nutrition initially after major surgery
- Platelet transfusion if surgical bleeding and counts less than 70,000/mm^3
- Hepatic encephalopathy: lactulose titrated to 3 loose BMs/day, plus or minus neomycin or rifaximin
- Early mobility and ambulation
- DVT prophylaxis with intermittent pneumatic compression stockings

Treatment of Decompensated Cirrhosis

- Orthotopic liver transplant
- MELD calculator is used to assess mortality risk of pts with decompensated cirrhosis; it is available at www.esot.org/Elita/meldCalculator.aspx
- Contraindications to liver transplantation: active substance abuse, noncompliance with medical therapy, severe cardiovascular disease, uncontrolled systemic infection, extrahepatic malignancy, severe psychiatric or neurologic disorders, and absence of a splanchnic venous inflow system

PROGNOSIS

- Those with compensated cirrhosis have a 10-year survival rate of approximately 90%
- The likelihood of turning into decompensated cirrhosis within 10 years is 50%
- Median survival time in patients with decompensated cirrhosis is approximately 2 years
- Four clinical stages of cirrhosis and their prognosis
  - Stage 1: no gastroesophageal varices or ascites—mortality rate 1% per year
  - Stage 2: gastroesophageal varices (but no bleeding) and no ascites—mortality rate 4% per year
  - Stage 3: presence of ascites with or without gastroesophageal varices (but no bleeding)—mortality rate 20% per year
  - Stage 4: patients with GI bleeding due to portal hypertension with or without ascites—57% mortality rate per year
- Spontaneous bacterial peritonitis
  - In hospital mortality rate 10–30%; 70–80% 2-year mortality
- Hepatorenal syndrome
  - Prognosis is poor; type 1 hepatorenal syndrome has a hospital survival of less than 10%, and median survival time is 2 weeks
  - Type 2 hepatorenal syndrome has a median survival time of around 6 months
- Hepatopulmonary syndrome
  - Median survival: 24 months; 5-year survival: 23%; prognosis worse if coexisting medical conditions and older age
- Gastroesophageal varices
  - Patients with esophageal variceal bleeding have a 1-year mortality of 30–40%
  - Those who have esophageal varices without bleeding or ascites (compensated cirrhosis) have a mortality rate of 3.4% per year
  - Early rebleeding is common, and occurs within 5 days of admission in 21% of patients with Child-Pugh grade A, 40% of patients classified as grade B, and 63% of patients classified as grade C

REFERENCES

epatology, 2004;39(1):1; N Engl J Med, 2004;350(16):1646–54; Brit Med J, 2003;326(7392):751–2; Am Fam
'hysician, 2006;74(5):756–62; South Med J, 2006;99(6):600–6; J Clin Gastroenterol, 2004;38(1):52–8;
'in Liver Dis, 2006;10(2):371–85; Crit Care Med, 2004;32(Suppl 4):S106–15; Am J Surg, 2004;188(5):580–3;
rit Care Med, 2006;34(Suppl 9):S225–31; Nat Clin Pract Gastroenterol Hepatol, 2007;4(5):266–76;
Engl J Med, 2008;358(22):2378–87; Hepatology, 2005;41(1):1.

illiams J. Does this patient have ascites? In: Simel DL, Rennie D, eds. The Rational Clinical Examination.
ew York, NY: McGraw-Hill; 2009:65–71.

CHAPTER 28

ACUTE PANCREATITIS

1. **EPIDEMIOLOGY**
   - Annual incidence is 17 in 100,000: 80% are interstitial and mild, 20% are necrotizing and severe
   - Mortality is 3% for interstitial pancreatitis, 17% for necrotizing pancreatitis
   - 45% due to gallstones; 35% due to alcohol; 10% due to other identifiable causes; 10% idiopathic

2. **PATHOPHYSIOLOGY**
   - Local autodigestion (activation of trypsin and other proteolytic enzymes within pancreas instead of intestine) leads to inflammatory response (recruitment and activation of neutrophils and macrophages), then systemic effects of enzymes and cytokines cause vasodilation, edema, SIRS, ARDS, and multiorgan failure

3. **ETIOLOGIES**
   - Gallstones
   - Alcohol
   - Post-ERCP
   - Hypertriglyceridemia
   - Medications
   - Autoimmune
   - Other: apolipoprotein CII deficiency, scorpion bite, trauma

4. **CLINICAL PRESENTATION**
   - Epigastric pain, radiates to the flank and/or back; dull, boring, achy quality; worse when supine; relieved by sitting or fetal position
   - Associated symptoms: nausea and vomiting, fever, tachycardia, jaundice, restlessness
   - Signs: abdominal distention, epigastric pain, LUQ tenderness

5. **DIFFERENTIAL DIAGNOSIS**
   - Perforated duodenal ulcer
   - Acute cholecystitis
   - Intestinal obstruction
   - Mesenteric ischemia
   - Ectopic pregnancy
   - Renal colic
   - Abdominal aortic aneurysm

6. **WORKUP**
   - Serum amylase and lipase (usually elevated more than 3 × upper limit of normal)
   - Labs: CBCD, chemistry panel, LDH, triglycerides, and oximetry (ABG if hypoxic)
     - ALT level more than 3 × normal has a 95% likelihood of gallstone pancreatitis
   - Chest X-ray
   - Abdominal ultrasound indicated if gallstone pancreatitis a possibility
   - Dynamic CT scan of abdomen with IV/PO contrast using 3-phase pancreatic protocol if hemodynamic instability or severe acute pancreatitis with persistent SIRS at 72 h
   - Fine-needle aspirate of necrotic pancreas for fevers lasting more than 72–96 h to rule out infection

7. **TREATMENT**
   - NPO: aggressive IV fluid resuscitation (at least 5 L/day × 2–4 days) to maintain urine output of 0.5 mL/kg/h or more

- Pain control with IV opioids: morphine or dilaudid preferred over meperidine
- Start early enteral feeds in SAP; nasojejunal peptide-based formula feeds probably safer than gastric feeds
- Early ERCP with sphincterotomy within 72 h of symptom onset for gallstone SAP with bilirubin greater than 1.2 mg/dL and common bile duct greater than or equal to 8 mm, or if biliary sepsis present
  - Cholecystectomy once pancreatitis resolved and prior to discharge
- Insulin infusion to keep glucose 80–150 mg/dL
- Close vigilance for the development of acute kidney injury or respiratory failure in first 7 days
- Empiric antibiotics controversial for necrotizing pancreatitis of more than 30% of pancreas
  - The currently available data do not support prophylactic use of antibiotics in necrotizing pancreatitis as they provide no mortality benefit

Managing Complications of Severe Acute Pancreatitis

- Indications for drainage of pancreatic pseudocyst: pain, larger than 6 cm, and duration longer than 6 weeks
  - Discourage percutaneous drainage because of the risk of infection or fistula formation
- Pancreatic abscess: endoscopic ultrasound or CT-guided percutaneous drainage and antibiotics
- Infected pancreatic necrosis: open pancreatic necrosectomy and antibiotics
  - Early surgery for hemodynamic instability; delay surgery for at least 14 days if clinically stable
- Marked pancreatic ascites: may need ERCP with pancreatic duct stenting if duct disrupted
- Pancreatic fistulas: treat with octreotide infusions or somatostatin injections

PROGNOSIS

Indicators of Severe Acute Pancreatitis (SAP)

- SBP is less than 90 mmHg; PaO$_2$ is less than 60 mmHg; creatinine is greater than 2 mg/dL, GI bleed is greater than 500 mL/day, or DIC
- Peripancreatic fluid collection, pancreatic necrosis, pseudocyst, or abscess
- SAP also if APACHE II score on admission is 8 or higher; Ranson's score 3 or higher; or Balthazar's CT severity index 7 or higher.
- Poor prognostic factors: obesity (BMI greater than 30 kg/m^2) and CRP greater than or equal to 15 mg/dL at 48 hours
- See **Tables 28.1** and **28.2**

BLE 28.1.   Ranson's Criteria

Ranson's Criteria		Prognosis	
On Admission*	At 48 hours*	# of criteria	Mortality
Age older than 55 yo (age older than 70 yo)	Hct decrease more than 10% (same)	2 or fewer	Less than 5%
WBC higher than 16,000/mm³ (more than 18 K)	BUN increase greater than 5 mg/dL (greater than 2)	3–4	15–20%
Glucose higher than 200 mg/dL (more than 220)	Base deficit greater than 4 mEq/L (greater than 6)	5–6	40%
AST (SGOT) more than 250 units/L (more than 400)	Calcium less than 8 mEq/L (same)	7 or more	More than 99%
LDH more than 350 units/L (more than 400)	PaO$_2$ less than 60 mmHg (omitted)		
	Fluid sequestration more than 6 L (more than 4 L)		

Criteria for alcoholic (nongallstone) acute pancreatitis listed first; criteria for gallstone pancreatitis in parentheses
Source: Adapted from *Surg Gyn Obstet*, 1974; 139(1): 69–81 and *Ann Surg*, 1979; 189(5): 654–63.

TABLE 28.2.   CT Severity Index

CT Grade	Description	Points	Necrosis	Points	Total Points	Mortality
A	Normal pancreas	0	Less than 30%	2	0–3	3%
B	Enlarged pancreas, no inflammation	1	30–50%	4	4–6	6%
C	Pancreatic or peripancreatic inflammation	2	More than 50%	6	7–10	17%
D	Single peripancreatic fluid collection	3				
E	2 or more peripancreatic fluid collections, or gas in pancreas or retroperitoneum	4				

Source: Adapted from *Radiology*, 1990; 174(2): 331–6.

9. COMPLICATIONS

- Chronic pancreatitis
- Pancreatic pseudocyst or abscess
- Pancreatic or extrapancreatic necrosis
- Malnutrition from chronic diarrhea (decreased pancreatic enzyme)
- Secondary diabetes (destruction of islet cells)
- ARDS
- Renal failure
- Circulatory shock
- Pancreatic cancer
- Sepsis
- Splenic artery aneurysm

REFERENCES

Crit Care Med, 2004;32(12):2524–36; *Gastroenterology*, 2007;132(5):2022–44; *N Engl J Med*, 2006;354(20): 2142–50; *Am Fam Physician*, 2000;62(1):164–74.

CHAPTER 29

ISCHEMIC BOWEL DISEASE

1. **EPIDEMIOLOGY**
   - 70% present in severe abdominal pain
   - 85% mortality rate associated with late diagnosis
   - 5–15% of acute ischemia is due to mesenteric vein occlusion

2. **PATHOPHYSIOLOGY**
   - Splanchnic circulation represents 30% of total cardiac output; extensive collateral circulation
   - Watershed areas (Griffith's point = splenic flexure, Sudeck's point = descending/sigmoid colon junction) particularly vulnerable to ischemia
   - Acute embolism (75% cardiogenic) occurs most commonly just distal to origin of middle colic artery
   - Acute vasoconstriction: secondary to systemic shock
   - Chronic thrombosis of 2 or more vessels causes intestinal angina

3. **ETIOLOGIES**
   - Acute embolic (50%) vs thrombosis (25%) vs low-flow state and nonocclusive state (15%) vs postcoarctectomy syndrome
   - Mesentery emboli most often lodge in the first branch of SMA, left colic/pancreaticoduodenal artery, heart is primary source
   - Hypoperfusion, the vessel are patent but "pruned" at the "watershed" areas

4. **CLINICAL PRESENTATION**
   - Acute onset of abdominal pain (LLQ), fecal urgency, diarrhea, bright red blood per rectum
   - Associated symptoms: anorexia, nausea/vomiting, distention, maroon stools
   - Signs: fever, tachycardia, abdominal tenderness, abdominal distention

5. **DIAGNOSIS**
   - Definitive diagnosis is with a mesenteric angiogram or via laparotomy

6. **DIFFERENTIAL DIAGNOSIS**
   - Perforated duodenal ulcer
   - Intestinal obstruction
   - Abdominal aortic aneurysm
   - Inflammatory bowel disease
   - Acute pancreatitis
   - Acute appendicitis
   - Acute diverticulitis

7. **WORKUP OF SUSPECTED MESENTERIC ISCHEMIA**
   - Lab abnormalities: leukocytosis with or without increased amylase, CK, and LDH; increased lactate is a late finding
   - ECG, cardiac monitoring, and 2D-echocardiogram: evaluate for cardioembolic event
   - Imaging: KUB normal in mild cases; severe cases: bowel distension, ileus, "thumbprinting"
     - CT scan with PO/IV contrast: identifies intestinal distension, bowel wall thickening, and mesenteric vein thrombosis; pneumatosis intestinalis is a late finding
     - CT angiogram: more sensitive than CT scan for mesenteric arterial thrombosis/stenosis

8. TREATMENT OF MESENTERIC ISCHEMIA

- NPO with bowel rest, volume resuscitation, and discontinue any contributing medications
- NGT decompression to low, intermittent suction for severe ileus with abdominal distension
- Antibiotics indicated for signs of intra-abdominal sepsis or bowel infarction
- Acute heparinization if acute mesenteric arterial/venous thrombosis or cardioembolic event
- Options for refractory mesenteric arterial thrombosis or embolism: catheter-directed thrombolysis, surgical embolectomy, or SMA revascularization for SMA thrombosis
- Consider selective mesenteric arteriography with intra-arterial papaverine infusion for nonocclusive mesenteric ischemia
- Indications for surgery: bowel infarction, perforation, or refractory intra-abdominal sepsis

Ischemic Colitis

- Diagnostic Studies
  - Stool for guaiac testing, culture, with or without C. difficile toxin to rule out infectious colitis
  - Abnormal labs: none in mild cases; elevated WBC, LDH, amylase, and lactate (late) in severe cases
  - ECG, cardiac monitoring, and 2D-echocardiogram find source of cardioembolism in up to 40% of cases
  - Imaging: plain X-rays demonstrate bowel distension with or without air-fluid levels
    - CT scan with PO/IV/rectal contrast demonstrates same findings as in mesenteric ischemia
    - CT angiogram is of limited utility as arterial thrombosis or embolism are essentially never seen
  - Colonoscopy diagnostic modality of choice once patient stable locates segmental ischemia

Treatment of Ischemic Colitis

- NPO with bowel rest, aggressive IV hydration, and discontinuation of offending meds
- Broad-spectrum antibiotics for moderate–severe cases
- NGT decompression with low, intermittent suction for severe ileus and distension
- Indications for surgery: peritonitis, persistent intra-abdominal sepsis, symptomatic colonic strictures, persistent symptoms for more than 2–3 weeks, or chronic protein-losing enteropathy

REFERENCES

South Med J, 2005;98(2):217–22.

Hauser SC. Vascular diseases of the gastrointestinal tract. In: Goldman L, Schafer AI, eds. *Cecil Medicine,* 24th ed. Philadelphia, PA: Saunders-Elsevier; Philadelphia 2012. 928–37.

CHAPTER 30

ESOPHAGEAL DISORDERS

1. ## GASTROESOPHAGEAL REFLUX DISEASE (GERD)
   - Definition: a condition in which the reflux of stomach fluid causes symptoms
   - Common symptoms: heartburn, regurgitation, atypical chest pain, or dysphagia
   - Less common symptoms: odynophagia, subxiphoid pain, nausea, chronic cough, hoarseness, laryngitis, poorly controlled asthma, and dental enamel erosions
   - Esophageal disorders: esophagitis, stricture, Barrett's esophagus, and adenocarcinoma
   - Diagnosis: clinical diagnosis if symptoms typical and good response to therapy
     - 24-h esophageal pH probe (off PPI or H_2-blockers × 7 days) if diagnosis is equivocal
     - EGD if odynophagia, dysphagia, GI bleeding, unexplained anemia, unintentional weight loss, and symptoms refractory to medical therapy
   - Treatment
     - Foods to avoid: citrus fruits, tomatoes, onions, carbonated beverages, spicy food, fatty or fried food, caffeinated beverages, chocolate, mint, and all bedtime snacks
     - Lifestyle changes: smoking cessation, weight reduction, alcohol only in moderation, avoid tight garments, and lying down after meals; raise head of bed 6 inches
     - Medications: PPI daily–bid or H_2-blocker bid for symptom control
       - Chronic use increases risk of hip fracture (0.5%), C. difficile colitis, and pneumonia (OR 1.4–2)
     - Nissen fundoplication if symptoms refractory to meds or intolerant of meds
       - Risks: increased dysphagia (6%), increased flatulence, inability to belch, and increased bowel symptoms

2. ## DYSPHAGIA
   - Diagnosis of motility disorders: esophageal manometry
   - Diagnosis of structural disorders: barium swallow or EGD
   - Neuromuscular causes of oropharyngeal dysphagia: stroke, Parkinson's disease, multiple sclerosis, myasthenia gravis, amyotrophic lateral sclerosis, polio, polymyositis, dermatomyositis, or idiopathic upper esophageal sphincter dysfunction
   - Structural causes of oropharyngeal dysphagia: carcinomas, spinal osteophytes, Zenker's diverticula, proximal esophageal webs, or prior surgery/radiation to neck
   - Esophageal motility disorders: achalasia, diffuse esophageal spasm, scleroderma, reflux-associated dysmotility, and idiopathic ineffective esophageal motility syndrome
   - Structural causes of esophageal dysphagia: carcinomas, benign strictures, mid or distal esophageal rings or webs, vascular compression, or eosinophilic esophagitis with or without stricture
   - Medication-induced esophagitis: bisphosphonates, tetracyclines, quinidine, iron, NSAIDs, aspirin, and potassium chloride
   - Treatment of strictures: Botox injections and pneumatic dilations
   - Treatment of achalasia: surgical/endoscopic myotomy and a partial fundoplication for achalasia
   - Hypercontractile disorders: diltiazem and nitrates, add imipramine for atypical CP

3. ## BARRETT'S ESOPHAGUS (BE, DISTAL ESOPHAGEAL METAPLASIA)
   - Treatment: proton-pump inhibitor bid indefinitely
     - Consider Nissen fundoplication: younger patients and if symptoms refractory to meds
     - Antireflux surgery superior to meds for regression of BE, but rate of cancer equal

- Monitoring: EGD q 3 years if no dysplasia; yearly for low-grade dysplasia; q 3 months for focal high-grade dysplasia vs surgery, endoscopic mucosal resection or mucosal ablation; may screen more frequently if long-segment BE (longer than 3 cm)
- Indications for surgery: multifocal high-grade dysplasia or adenocarcinoma

REFERENCES

Gastroenterology, 2008;135(4):1383–91; *N Engl J Med,* 2008;359(16):1700–7; *J Clin Gastroenterol,* 2005;39(5): 357–71; *J Clin Gastroenterol,* 2008;42(5):652–8; *Ann Surg,* 2007;246(1):11–21; *J Fam Pract,* 2006;55(3):243–7; *Drugs,* 2005;65(Suppl 1):75–82.

CHAPTER 31

DIVERTICULITIS

EPIDEMIOLOGY

- Prevalence of sigmoid diverticuli is 35% in general population and 70% if older than 65 yo in North America
- Diverticula form 80% in sigmoid colon

PATHOPHYSIOLOGY

- Colonic diverticula are pseudodiverticula, as they do not involve the entire bowel wall
  - Mucosa protrudes through break in muscularis propria where vasa recti enters
- Most commonly in sigmoid colon due to increased luminal pressures generated by stronger contractions in face of constipation
- Fecal material trapped in pseudodiverticulum forms fecalith, leading to inflammation

CLINICAL PRESENTATION

- Acute or subacute LLQ abdominal pain and fever
- Associated symptoms: nausea/vomiting, constipation *or* diarrhea, and dysuria
- Signs: LLQ tenderness, often with peritoneal signs (may also be right-sided)

DIFFERENTIAL DIAGNOSIS

- Inflammatory bowel disease
- Ischemic colitis
- Colon cancer
- Bowel obstruction
- Ectopic pregnancy
- Pelvic inflammatory disease
- Ovarian torsion
- Degenerating fibroid
- Renal colic

WORKUP

- Abnormal labs: leukocytosis; fecal occult blood positive in 25–30% of cases
- CT scan with PO/IV contrast demonstrates diverticuli and sigmoid wall thickening; complicated cases with free air, pericolic abscess, fistulas, or colonic obstruction
- Flexible sigmoidoscopy or colonoscopy is indicated within 6 weeks after resolution to rule out cancer

TREATMENT

- Mild: clears with ciprofloxacin or trimethoprim-sulfamethoxazole DS AND metronidazole; or amoxicillin-clavulanate; duration of therapy is 7–10 days
- Moderate–severe: NPO with IV hydration; NGT decompression only for severe distension
  - Antibiotics: piperacillin-tazobactam; ciprofloxacin plus metronidazole; or amp/gent/metro
- Management of pericolic abscesses: percutaneous vs open drainage if abscess is larger than 4 cm
- Urgent surgery for: peritonitis, perforation, uncontrolled sepsis, fistula formation, colonic obstruction, or pericolic abscess not amenable to percutaneous drainage
- Indications for delayed colectomy: 2 or more episodes of acute diverticulitis, presence of colon cancer, and potentially after a single severe episode in patients younger than 50 years old

- Prevention of recurrent disease: possible benefit from mesalamine or rifaximin
  - No proven benefit from probiotics
  - No proven benefit from low-residue diet but patients should ingest 25–30 g/day fiber

7   COMPLICATIONS

- Abscess (occurs in 16% of patients)
- Peritonitis (higher risk with perforation)
- Perforation (mortality 20–30%)
- Fistula (colovesical is greater than colovaginal, which is greater than coloenteric and colouterine; contributes to 20% of surgical management of diverticular complications)
- Obstruction (usually incomplete obstruction; must differentiate from colonic mass)

REFERENCES

Am J Gastroenterol, 2008;103(6):1550–6; *Brit Med J,* 2006;332(7536):271–5; *J Gastroenterol Hepatol,* 2007; 22(9):1360–8; *Am Fam Physician,* 2005;72(7):1229–34.

CHAPTER 32

BOWEL OBSTRUCTION

1. EPIDEMIOLOGY

- SBO most common cause: hernia (without surgery), adhesions (prior surgery)
- Large bowel most common cause is cancer!
- Bowel rest cures 80% of partial SBO and 20–40% of complete SBO
- Infection from bacterial overgrowth, fluid from third space into lumen, air from swallowed nitrogen

2. PATHOPHYSIOLOGY

- Major component of bowel gas is nitrogen from swallowed air that is poorly absorbed
- Proximal accumulation fluid from ingestion, secretions, and deranged Na and H_2O flux
- Vomiting, bowel wall edema, decreased splanchnic venous return resulting in fluid and electrolyte loss
- Law of Laplace: increased bowel diameter increases wall tension
- Occlusion of bowel lumen at 2 points results in strangulation of closed loop, then ischemia, leading to bacterial invasion and peritonitis

3. CLINICAL PRESENTATION

- Colicky abdominal pain, nausea and vomiting, abdominal distention, absence of flatus or bowel movements
  - Distal obstructions have more pain and distention
  - Proximal obstructions have more vomiting with less distention
- Signs: distended, tympanitic abdomen; high-pitched (early) or absent (late) bowel sounds
- See **Figure 32.1**

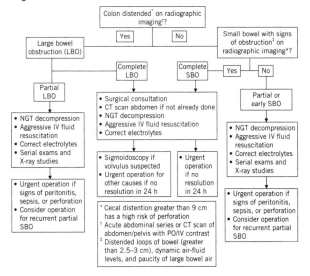

FIGURE 32.1. Evaluation and Management of Bowel Obstruction

4. **DIFFERENTIAL DIAGNOSIS**
   - Inflammatory bowel disease
   - Ischemic colitis
   - Colon cancer
   - Ectopic pregnancy
   - Pelvic inflammatory disease
   - Ovarian torsion
   - Degenerating fibroid

5. **COLONIC PSEUDO-OBSTRUCTION (OGILVIE'S SYNDROME)**
   - Occurs in bedbound, hospitalized elderly patients receiving opiate therapy
   - Treatment: rectal tube or colonoscopic decompression and frequent repositioning
     - Laparotomy and operative decompression if conservative measures unsuccessful or if patient develops worsening abdominal tenderness, fever, or peritonitis

   Toxic Megacolon
   - Complication of inflammatory bowel disease or *C. difficile* colitis
   - Treatment is laparotomy with colectomy and ileostomy or ileal diversion and colonic reperfusion (if secondary to *C. difficile* colitis) and treatment of underlying condition

6. **COMPLICATIONS**
   - Bowel ischemia/necrosis/strangulation from compromised blood flow to distended bowel
   - Bowel perforation of ischemic bowel
   - Intra-abdominal abscess/peritonitis/sepsis from infected and compromised bowel
   - Dehydration from emesis
   - Aspiration

REFERENCES

Am J Surg, 2000;180(1):33–6; *Gut*, 2000;47(Suppl 4):84; *J Am Coll Surg*, 2001;192(3):422–3; *Am Fam Physician*, 2011;83(2):159–65.

CHAPTER 33

BILIARY TRACT DISORDERS

1. **PATHOPHYSIOLOGY**
   Acute Cholecystitis
   - Acute inflammation due to:
     - Mechanical: cystic duct blocked by calculus leading to gallbladder distension, then ischemia
     - Cholesterol stones (80%): supersaturation of bile with cholesterol plus pronucleation chemical milieu and decreased gallbladder motility
       - Risk factors: genetics, obesity, rapid weight loss, estrogen, age, pregnancy
     - Pigment stones (20%): calcium and bilirubin
       - Risk factors: hemolysis, cirrhosis, Gilbert's syndrome, cystic fibrosis, ileal resection, biliary tract infections
     - Chemical: irritation from bile
     - Microbial: *E. coli, Klebsiella, Streptococcus, Clostridium*

   Acute Cholangitis
   - Choledocholith obstructs common bile duct, resulting in static bile infected with bacteria

   Choledocholithiasis
   - Cholesterol stones pass from gallbladder into common bile duct

   Painless Jaundice
   - Bilirubin comes from heme recycling from RBCs; conjugated in liver to solubilize for excretion
   - Overproduction of bilirubin or impaired conjugation leads to indirect hyperbilirubinemia
   - Hemolysis, ineffective erythropoiesis, medications (rifampin), Crigler-Najjar, Gilbert's syndrome, hepatocellular disease (hepatitis, alcohol, acetaminophen, isoniazid, *Amanita phalloides*, Wilson's disease, autoimmune hepatitis)
   - Impaired excretion of bilirubin results in direct hyperbilirubinemia (cholestasis, obstructive jaundice)
   - Dubin-Johnson syndrome, Rotor syndrome, hepatitis, alcohol, primary biliary cirrhosis, primary sclerosing cholangitis, medications (steroids, contraceptives), cholestasis of pregnancy, TPN, veno-occlusive disease, leptospirosis, AIDS cholangiopathy, malignancies (cholangiocarcinoma, pancreatic cancer)

2. **CLINICAL PRESENTATION**
   Acute Cholecystitis
   - RUQ or midepigastric pain, fever, nausea/vomiting
   - Often have a history of biliary colic (RUQ/epigastric pain after fatty meals lasting 4–6 hours)
   - Signs
     - RUQ tenderness [LR+ 1.6, LR− 0.4]
     - Murphy sign: hook fingers underneath the right costal margin and have the patient take a deep breath; sign is positive if they halt the breath because of pain [LR+ 2.8, LR− 0.5]
     - Boas

   Acute Cholangitis
   - Charcot triad: fever and chills, RUQ pain and tenderness, jaundice
   - Reynold's pentad: Charcot triad plus confusion and hypotension; mortality is 70% if all are present

   Choledocholithiasis
   - Afebrile
   - May have jaundice or abnormal liver tests
   - Look for signs of complications (cholangitis, pancreatitis)

Painless Jaundice

- Courvoisier sign: palpable, nontender gallbladder in a jaundiced patient (suggests malignancy)

3. DIFFERENTIAL DIAGNOSIS

- Perforated duodenal ulcer
- Acute appendicitis
- Acute hepatitis
- Right lower lobe pneumonia
- Perforated viscus
- Mesenteric ischemia
- Renal colic
- Fitz-Hugh-Curtis perihepatitis

Acute Cholecystitis

- **Risk factors:** the five Fs are fat, fertile, female, forty (40 yo), and a positive family history
- **Clinical presentation:** persistent, epigastric, or RUQ pain that radiates to the right scapular tip and is associated with nausea and vomiting
  - Serum bilirubin is usually normal, but may increase to 4 mg/dL; jaundice is uncommon
- **Exam:** RUQ tenderness, positive Murphy's sign (arrest of inspiration with gallbladder palpation), and fever
- **Diagnostic studies**
  - Abnormal labs: elevated WBC, alkaline phosphatase, C-reactive protein, and variable rise in liver transaminases and bilirubin
  - Ultrasound detects gallstones (98% sensitivity), gallbladder wall thickening (5 mm or thicker), pericholecystic fluid, and assesses for an ultrasonographic Murphy's sign
  - Hepatobiliary scintigraphy (HIDA scan) with absent gallbladder visualization within 60 minutes suggests acute cystic duct obstruction (90–97% sensitivity)
- See **Tables 33.1** through **33.3**

TABLE 33.1.   Tokyo Guidelines for the Diagnosis of Acute Cholecystitis

Local Symptoms and Signs*	Systemic Signs*	Diagnostic Imaging*
• Murphy's sign present • RUQ pain or tenderness • RUQ mass palpable	• Fever • WBC higher than 12.5K/mm^3 • Elevated C-reactive protein	• Ultrasound or HIDA scan with abnormal findings†

* Acute cholecystitis if 1 or more local symptoms/signs, 1 or more systemic signs, and 1 or more imaging criterion present
† Abnormal ultrasound if gallstones with or without gallbladder wall thickening or pericholecystic fluid; abnormal hepatic scintigraphy (HIDA scan) if gallbladder not visualized within 60 minutes
Source: Adapted from *J Hepatobiliary Pancreat Surg,* 2007; 14(1): 1–121.

TABLE 33.2.   Severity Grading and Treatment for Acute Cholecystitis

Grade	Criteria	Treatment Recommendations
Mild	Mild inflammation, no organ dysfunction	• Laparoscopic cholecystectomy
Moderate	Presence of 1 or more of the following: WBC higher than 18K/mm^3, palpable RUQ mass, duration longer than 72 h, biliary peritonitis, pericholecystic abscess, hepatic abscess, or gangrenous or emphysematous cholecystitis	• Early or delayed cholecystectomy • Antibiotics*
Severe	Presence of 1 or more of the following: septic shock, decreased level of consciousness, acute lung injury, oliguric renal failure, hepatic dysfunction, platelets less than 100K, or DIC	• Percutaneous cholecystostomy • Antibiotics† • Delayed cholecystectomy

* Mild–moderate infections: cefuroxime or ciprofloxacin and metronidazole, ertapenem, cefotetan, or cefoxitin
† Severe infections: piperacillin-tazobactam; imipenem-cilastatin; meropenem; 3rd generation cephalosporin, ciprofloxacin, or aztreonam and metronidazole
Source: Adapted from *J Hepatobiliary Pancreat Surg,* 2007; 14(1): 78–82 and *Clin Infect Dis,* 2003; 37(8): 997–1005.

TABLE 33.3.   Diagnostic Criteria for Acute Cholangitis

Clinical Manifestations	Lab Data	Imaging Findings
History of gallstones	Evidence of inflammatory response*	Biliary dilatation on ultrasound
Fever or chills	Abnormal liver function tests: • Elevated alkaline phosphatase or GGTP • Elevated total bilirubin, AST, and ALT	
Jaundice		
Abdominal pain		

* Elevated heart rate, respiratory rate, WBC, and CRP
Suspected diagnosis: 2 or more clinical manifestations present
Definite diagnosis: Charcot's triad (fever, jaundice, and abdominal pain) or 2 or more clinical manifestations present WITH abnormal lab data and biliary dilatation on ultrasound exam

Source: Adapted from *Curr Gastroenterol Rep,* 2011; 13(2): 166–72.

Acalculous Cholecystitis
- Complicates the course of 1.5% of critically ill patients
- Presents with severe abdominal pain, fever, and minimal abdominal tenderness
- Treatment is with a percutaneous cholecystostomy (or cholecystectomy) and empiric antibiotics

Ascending Cholangitis
- **Clinical presentation:** Charcot's triad of fever, jaundice, and RUQ pain in 50–70% pts
- **Diagnosis:** RUQ ultrasound reveals cholelithiasis; 75% of patients have a dilated common bile duct (CBD) and gallbladder wall thickening
  - Abnormal labs: leukocytosis (90%); elevated alkaline phosphatase, bilirubin, and variable levels of transaminitis
  - ERCP is the gold standard study for the diagnosis and treatment of CBD stones
  - Percutaneous transhepatic cholangiogram (PTHC) and drain placement is an alternative study for diagnosis and treatment if ERCP is unsuccessful or not feasible
- **Treatment:** NPO, IV resuscitation, correct electrolytes, and any coagulopathy
  - Empiric antibiotics: ampicillin plus gentamicin or ciprofloxacin; ceftriaxone or cefepime plus metronidazole; or monotherapy with either piperacillin-tazobactam, ticarcillin-clavulanate, imipenem-cilastatin, tigecycline, or meropenem
  - Duration of antibiotics is 5–7 days
  - Biliary decompression: ERCP with sphincterotomy or PTHC within 24–48 hours
  - Delayed cholecystectomy once clinically stable after biliary decompression

Choledocholithiasis
- **Clinical presentation:** RUQ/epigastric pain, jaundice, nausea and pruritus; up to 50% can present with painless jaundice
- **Diagnostic evaluation:** RUQ ultrasound reveals dilated CBD in 75% of patients
  - Abnormal labs: elevated alkaline phosphatase, bilirubin, and variable transaminitis
  - ERCP with sphincterotomy is the diagnostic and therapeutic modality of choice

4. COMPLICATIONS

Acute Cholecystitis
- Gangrenous gallbladder (most common complication especially in elderly, diabetic, or delayed care)
- Gallbladder perforation
- Pericholecystic abscess/peritonitis/sepsis (especially in perforated)
- Cholecystoenteric fistula (due to chronic pressure necrosis from stone on gallbladder wall)
- Gallstone ileus (commonly at terminal ileum)

Acute Cholangitis

- Development of Raynaud's pentad: confusion, hypotension + triad of Charcot (fever, RUQ pain, jaundice), which leads to severe mortality and morbidity
- Acute pancreatitis
- Hepatic abscess

Choledocholithiasis

- Cholangitis
- Pancreatitis

REFERENCES

Gastrointest Endosc Clin N Am, 2007;17(2):289–306; *Curr Gastroenterol Rep,* 2003;5(4):302–9; *N Engl J Med,* 2008;358(26):2804–11.

Singh VK, Piccini JP, Kalloo AN. Biliary Tract Disease. In: Nilsson KR, Piccini JP *Osler Medical Handbook,* 2nd ed. Johns Hopkins University; 2006 Philadelphia.

Trowbridge R. Does this patient have acute cholecystitis? In: *The Rational Clinical Examination.* McGraw Hill; 2009:137–44.

SECTION 4

HEMATOLOGY

CHAPTER 34

ANEMIA

1. **EPIDEMIOLOGY**
   - 90% due to nutritional deficiency, anemia of chronic disease, and bleeding
   - Iron-deficiency anemia: most common form of anemia with 30% worldwide prevalence (36% in developing countries and 8% in developed countries)
   - Anemia of chronic disease: most common causes are chronic infection, cancer, autoimmune diseases, solid organ transplantation, and CKD

2. **PATHOPHYSIOLOGY**
   - Hemolytic anemia
     - Decreased red cell survival results in hypoxia which upregulates hypoxia-inducible factor, stimulating erythropoietin (epo) release from kidney; epo stimulates erythroid marrow; increased RBC breakdown results in polychromatophilic macrocytes, reticulocytes, increased heme breakdown leading to hyperbilirubinemia, and hypersplenism
   - Microcytic
     - Ineffective erythropoiesis due to defective cytoplasmic maturation
       - Fe deficiency
       - Heme synthesis deficits
         - Acquired
         - Sideroblastic anemia (iron taken up into mitochondrial rings but not incorporated into heme)
         - Inherited
         - Defective hemoglobin structure: sickle cell disease
         - Defective globin synthesis: thalassemias
   - Normocytic
     - Hypoproliferative marrow due to:
       - Inflammation: anemia of chronic disease associated with increased IL-6 (decreases epo production) and increased hepcidin (decreases Fe absorption and release)
       - Decreased erythropoietin: anemia of chronic kidney disease
   - Macrocytic
     - Ineffective erythropoiesis due to defective nuclear maturation (failure of DNA synthesis) results in megaloblasts
     - Conversion of dUMP to dTMP (precursor for thymine nucleotides) requires folate
     - Conversion of homocysteine to methionine requires folate, B_{12}, and B_6
     - Conversion of methylmalonyl-CoA to succinyl-CoA requires B_{12} only

3. **CLINICAL PRESENTATION**
   - Symptoms of all anemia: fatigue, generalized weakness, exertional dyspnea/lightheadedness and headache
   - Signs of anemia: pallor, glossitis (iron, folate, B_{12} deficiency), koilonychia or angular cheilitis (iron deficiency), peripheral neuropathy, paresthesias, ataxia, decreased proprioception and vibratory sensation (B_{12} deficiency), jaundice (hemolysis), splenomegaly (CA, thalassemia, hemolysis), dark urine (hemolysis)

   Peripheral Blood Smear Findings in Different Causes of Anemia
   - Basophilic stippling: thalassemias, sideroblastic anemia, and lead poisoning
   - Heinz bodies: G6PD deficiency, unstable hemoglobins, and thalassemia major
   - Howell-Jolly bodies: sickle cell anemia, and functional or anatomic asplenia

- Hypersegmented neutrophils: megaloblastic anemia (Vitamin B_{12} or folate deficiency), or drugs (azathioprine, hydroxyurea, methotrexate, or zidovudine)
- Nucleated RBCs: chronic hemolysis and any cause of extramedullary hematopoiesis
- Rouleaux formation: monoclonal gammopathies (e.g., multiple myeloma)
- Schistocytes: microangiopathic hemolytic anemia (DIC, TTP/HUS, HELLP syndrome)
- Spherocytes: hereditary spherocytosis, or autoimmune hemolytic anemia
- Spur cells: end-stage cirrhosis
- Stomatocytes: alcoholism and chronic liver disease
- Target cells: chronic liver disease, hemoglobinopathies (especially thalassemia), or postsplenectomy
- Tear drop cells: myelofibrosis, myelophthisic process (cancer or granulomatous infection in the bone marrow), and megaloblastic anemia
- Toxic granules: sepsis or severe inflammatory states
- See **Figure 34.1** and **Table 34.1**

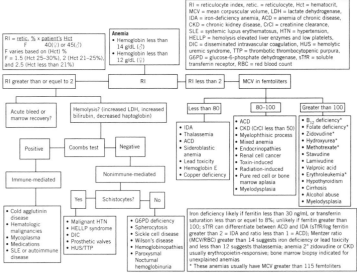

FIGURE 34.1.   Evaluation of Anemia

TABLE 34.1. Evaluation of Microcytic Anemias in Hospitalized Patients

Studies	Iron-Deficiency Anemia (IDA)*	Anemia of Chronic Disease (ACD)†	Thalassemia	Sideroblastic Anemia
Iron (mcg/dL)	Less than 30–50	Less than 30–50	50 or greater	50 or greater
TIBC (mcg/dL)	250–400 or greater	Less than 250	Normal	Normal
Ferritin (mcg/L)	50 or less‡	Greater than 100	Greater than 100	Greater than 100
Transferrin saturation (Fe/TIBC)	Less than 15%	Greater than 15%	20% or greater	20% or greater
MCV/RBC	14 or greater	–	13 or less	–
RDW	Elevated	Normal	Normal	Normal
PBS findings	Hypochromic	–	Basophilic stippling; target cells	Basophilic stippling
sTfR(mg/L)/ log[ferritin(mcg/L)]	Greater than 2	Less than 1	–	–
Zinc protoporphyrin (mcg/dL)	Greater than 1.24	Less than 1.24	–	–
Hgb electrophoresis	Normal	Normal	Abnormal	Normal
Bone marrow findings	Low iron stores	May be abnormal (infection or CA)	–	Ringed sideroblasts

TIBC = total iron binding capacity, MCV = mean corpuscular volume, RBC = red blood count, RDW = RBC distribution width, PBS = peripheral blood smear, sTfR = soluble transferrin receptor, Hgb = hemoglobin, CA = cancer

* Cases of iron-refractory, iron-deficiency anemia frequently from elevated hepcidin levels, which blocks enteral iron absorption

† Can be from cancer, autoimmune diseases, chronic infections, or chronic inflammatory states

‡ Ferritin less than 50 mcg/L for pts with chronic inflammation, liver disease, or acute illness makes IDA highly likely; ferritin is an acute phase reactant so pts can have IDA with level greater than 100 mcg/L

Source: Information from *Crit Care,* 2004; 8(Suppl 2): S37–41, *AFP,* 2000; 62(7): 1565–72, *NEJM,* 1999; 341(26): 1986–95, *NEJM,* 2005; 353(11): 1135–46, and *NEJM,* 2005; 352(10): 1011–23.

4. EVALUATION OF NORMOCYTIC ANEMIAS

- Labs: reticulocyte count, serum iron, TIBC, ferritin, B_{12} and homocysteine levels, BUN, creatinine, and an erythropoietin level
  - Homocysteine elevated in B_{12} or folate deficiency
  - Methylmalonic acid elevated in B_{12} deficiency; test if high suspicion and low normal B_{12} level (200–400 pg/mL)
- Other tests: urinalysis, chest X-ray, and SPEP with serum immunofixation (for myeloma)
- Exam: for signs of occult malignancy (lymphadenopathy, splenomegaly, and stool guaiac test)
- Anemia of chronic kidney disease: begins if CrCl is less than 50 mL/min; especially if CrCl 30 or lower
- Treatment of folate/B_{12} deficiency: folate 1 mg PO daily, cyanocobalamin 2 mg PO daily
  - Initial therapy of B_{12} deficiency should be IM B_{12} due to poor absorption of B_{12} by megaloblastic epithelium of GI tract

Indications for Bone Marrow Biopsy

- Normocytic or macrocytic anemia of unclear etiology; definitive diagnosis of IDA, sideroblastic anemia, or multiple myeloma; staging/cytogenetic analysis for various cancers

Erythropoietic Agents for Anemia Treatment

- FDA indications: anemia associated with incurable cancer patients on chemotherapy, HIV infection, and CKD
- Off-label uses: myelodysplasia or ACD due to infection, cancer, or autoimmune diseases
- Supplemental iron indicated if transferrin saturation is less than 20% and serum ferritin is less than 100 mcg/L

- In ACD, iron dextran 100 mg slow IVP with epoetin alfa significantly improves Hgb response compared with oral iron supplementation; continue oral iron after Hgb is greater than 10 g/dL
- Target Hgb is 12 g/dL or less; risk of arterial/venous thrombosis, MI/CVA, or tumor progression if Hgb is greater than 12 g/dL
- Dose: epoetin alfa 50–100 units/kg SQ 3 × weekly for CKD; 100–300 units/kg IV/SQ 3 × weekly if zidovudine-induced anemia; 40,000 units SQ weekly for chemotherapy-induced anemia
  - Darbepoetin 0.45 mcg/kg IV/SQ every 1–2 weeks for CKD; 2.25 mcg/kg SQ weekly or 200 mcg SQ every 2 weeks for chemotherapy-induced anemia

Autoimmune Hemolytic Anemias (AIHA)

- 90% of cases are from extravascular hemolysis in the reticuloendothelial system
- Intravascular hemolysis (10% of cases): markedly elevated LDH, decreased haptoglobin, indirect hyperbilirubinemia, hemoglobinemia, hemoglobinuria, positive urine hemosiderin stain, and reticulocyte index higher than 2
  - ABO-incompatible transfusion reaction or paroxysmal nocturnal hemoglobinuria
- Warm-antibody (IgG): direct Coombs-positive; idiopathic; lymphoproliferative disorders (e.g., CLL); SLE, RA, and other autoimmune diseases; HIV; HCV; EBV; and meds
  - Meds: cephalosporins (60% of all cases in the United States), chlordiazepoxide, cladribine, fenfluramine, fludarabine, interleukin-2, levodopa, mefenamic acid, methyldopa, methysergide, NSAIDs, penicillins, penicillamine, phenothiazines, phenazopyridine, procainamide, quinidine, rifampin, sulfa drugs, thiazides, and tricyclics
    - Medication-induced AIHA will have **no** pure red blood cell antibodies present
    - Indirect Coombs test will be **negative** in medication-induced AIHA
- Warm AIHA treatment
  - First-line: prednisolone 1 mg/kg/day and once stable taper to 20 mg/day over 2 weeks, then decrease 5 mg/day every 2 weeks
  - Second-line: IVIG or rituximab
  - Third-line: splenectomy for refractory cases
    - Avoid RBC transfusion if possible
- Cold-antibody (IgM): idiopathic, monoclonal gammopathies (Waldenström's macroglobulinemia), CLL, lymphomas, mycoplasma, and infectious mononucleosis
  - Tertiary syphilis and paroxysmal cold hemoglobinuria (IgG-mediated hemolysis)
  - Treatment of cold AIHA
    - Avoidance of cold and consider rituximab or fludarabine
    - Steroids and splenectomy are both ineffective for cold AIHA

Nonimmune-Mediated Hemolytic Anemias

- Microangiopathic hemolytic anemias: DIC, HELLP syndrome, TTP/HUS, prosthetic heart valves, and malignant hypertension
  - Treat underlying disease including prompt delivery in HELLP syndrome
  - Urgent plasma exchange for TTP (medical emergency)
- G6PD deficiency: hemolysis is precipitated by drugs (aspirin, chloroquine, chloramphenicol, dapsone, doxorubicin, metformin, methylene blue, nitrofurantoin, primaquine, phenazopyridine, quinidine, sulfacetamide, sulfamethoxazole, or Vitamin C), infection, diabetic ketoacidosis (DKA), or fava beans
- Hemoglobinopathies: sickle cell anemia or thalassemias
- RBC membrane disorders: hereditary spherocytosis (HS) or paroxysmal nocturnal hemoglobinuria (PNH has an increased risk of venous thromboembolism and aplastic anemia)
  - HS therapy: folate and consider splenectomy for moderate–severe disease
  - PNH diagnosed by peripheral blood flow cytometry (absent CD55 and CD59)
  - Hematology consult: treat with eculizumab therapy or if marrow failure possible stem cell transplant

- Infection/toxins: malaria, babesiosis, *Bartonella*, clostridia, or snake/spider envenomations
- Hemolytic transfusion reactions: acute or delayed

5. COMPLICATIONS

- Cognitive impairment
- Hemolytic anemia
  - Thromboembolism (i.e., venous thrombosis, pulmonary thrombosis, stroke) due to hypercoagulable state from increased platelet activation, thrombin and fibrin generation, and tissue factor activity; risk of thromboembolism increased with splenectomy
  - Splenomegaly resulting from increased red cell destruction (i.e., sickle cell disease, hereditary spherocytosis), which increases risk of rupture in trauma
  - Jaundice
- Vitamin B_{12} deficiency
  - Neurologic problems such as paresthesias and ataxia with loss of vibration and position sense, spasticity, incontinence from dysfunctional myelin formation

REFERENCES

N Engl J Med, 1999;340(6):438–47; *JAMA*, 2003;289(8):959–62; *Transfusion*, 2002;42(8):975–9; *Lancet*, 2003;361(9352):161–9; *N Engl J Med*, 2005;353(11):1135–46; *N Engl J Med*, 2005;352(10):1011–23; *Blood*, 2004;103(8):2925–8; *Lancet*, 2007;369(9572):1502–4; *Eur J Haematol*, 2004;72(2):79–88; *Am Fam Physician*, 2004;69(11):2599–606; *Am Fam Physician*, 2010;82(11):1381–8; *Am Fam Physician*, 2009;79(3):203–8.

CHAPTER 35

SICKLE CELL ANEMIA

1. ## EPIDEMIOLOGY
   - Prevalence at birth is about 1 in 600 births
   - There are about 2 million carriers, nearly all are of African ancestry; more than 70,000 have actual disease
   - Identification of children by age 2 yo with transcranial Doppler to assess risk and treatment of stroke can decrease risk by 90%

2. ## PATHOPHYSIOLOGY
   - Mutated β-globin gene: glutamate to valine substitution at 6th amino acid position
     - Homozygotes: sickle cell disease
     - Heterozygotes: sickle cell trait (generally asymptomatic)
   - Fetal hemoglobin (HbF) replaced by HbS (instead of normal HbA) at 3–9 months old
   - Deoxygenated HbS polymerizes, forming stiff, sticky RBCs
     - Microvascular occlusion results in tissue ischemia and infarction (spleen, CNS, bones, joints, liver, kidney, lungs)
     - Splenic destruction causes hemolytic anemia

3. ## DIAGNOSIS
   - Peripheral blood smear exam is suggestive; hemoglobin electrophoresis is definitive

4. ## MANAGEMENT OF COMPLICATIONS
   - **Vaso-occlusive crises** (bony crises)
     - Aggressive hydration (3–4 liters/day), oxygen, opioids, and NSAIDs
     - Morphine 4–6 mg IV load, then 2–4 mg IV q 5–10 min or hydromorphone 1–2 mg IV load, then 0.5–1 mg IV q 5–10 min until pain controlled, then initiate an opiate PCA
     - NSAIDs (unless renal disease): ibuprofen 600 mg PO q 6 h or ketorolac 30 mg IV q 6 h (max 5 days)
   - **Acute chest syndrome:** acute onset of cough, fever, tachypnea, hypoxia, and alveolar infiltrates; life-threatening complication of sickle cell disease
     - Treatment: IV hydration (but avoid overhydration), oxygen, antibiotics (e.g., ceftriaxone and azithromycin OR moxifloxacin), exchange transfusion, pain control, bronchodilators, folic acid, and frequently necessitates mechanical ventilation
     - Frequently occurs as a postoperative complication after general anesthesia
   - **Stroke:** in adults, hemorrhagic strokes (especially subarachnoid hemorrhage) occur more than ischemic strokes
     - Treatment: exchange transfusion followed by maintenance transfusions to keep HbS under 30%, which minimizes recurrences
   - **Avascular necrosis:** commonly affects the femoral head, humeral head, or the acetabulum
     - Treatment: tissue decompression procedures, or joint replacement
   - **Osteomyelitis:** focal pain and fever; occurs at sites of bone necrosis; *Salmonella* more common than *S. aureus*
     - Treatment: 4–6 weeks of IV antibiotics targeting organism identified by bone cultures
   - **Skin ulcers:** typically, overlying the lateral malleolus or anterior shins
     - Local wound care with wet then dry dressings, hydrocolloid dressings, or Unna boots
   - **Proliferative retinopathy:** screen annually; laser photocoagulation for neovascularization
   - **Renal dysfunction:** hyposthenuria; papillary necrosis presents as painless hematuria
     - Treatment of papillary necrosis: IV hydration and urinary alkalinization

- **Cholelithiasis:** present in most adults
- **Medullary carcinoma of kidney:** increased risk in sickle cell trait or anemia and carries a poor prognosis

Sickle Cell Disease in Pregnancy

- Preterm delivery: 25% risk in SS and 15% risk in SC disease
- Preeclampsia: 20% risk SS and 9% risk in SC disease
- Increased frequency of vaso-occlusive pain crises
    - Encourage increased hydration during pregnancy
- No proven benefit of prophylactic exchange transfusions to alter rate of complications
- Preconception interventions: stop hydroxyurea if prescribed; start folic acid 1–4 mg/day and MVI

Preventative Care

- Immunizations: pneumococcus, haemophilus influenza type b, influenza, and hepatitis B virus
- OCPs, barrier methods, and depo-medroxyprogesterone acetate are safe contraceptive methods
- Preoperative care: prophylactic transfusion to Hgb 10 g/dL, generous hydration, supplemental oxygen, and prevent hypothermia prior to general anesthesia
- Consider hydroxyurea 15–35 mg/kg PO daily for 3 or more vaso-occlusive crises/year or a history of acute chest syndrome
    - Avoid for severe hypoplastic anemia, leukopenia, thrombocytopenia, or during pregnancy

5. PROGNOSIS

- Without bone marrow transplant, age at death is 42 years for men and 48 years for women in patients with sickle cell anemia
- For hemoglobin SC disease, life expectancy is 60 years for men and 68 years for women

REFERENCES

J Emer Med, 2007;32:239. *Anesthesiol,* 2004;101:766. *N Engl J Med,* 2008;359:2254. *Mayo Clin Proc,* 2008;83:320. *J Emerg Med,* 2007;32(3):239–43; *Anesthesiology,* 2004;101(3):766–85; *N Engl J Med,* 2008;359(21):2254–65; *Mayo Clin Proc,* 2008;83(3):320–3; *N Engl J Med,* 1999;340(13):1021–30; *N Engl J Med,* 2008;358(13):1362–9.

CHAPTER 36

BLEEDING DISORDERS

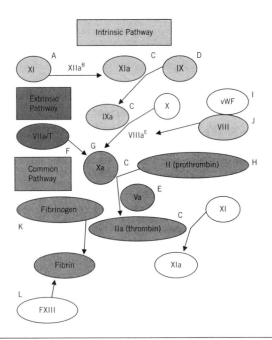

A = FXI deficiency, B = FXII deficiency, C = Antithrombin III action, D = FIX deficiency (Hemophilia B or Christmas disease), E = Proteins C & S action, F = Tissue factor (TF) or extrinsic pathway, G = TF pathway inhibitor, H = Prothrombin deficiency, I = vWF (von Willebrand factor) binds to FVIII to decreased FVIII concentration and activity, J = FVIII deficiency or (hemophilia A), K = fibrinogen deficiency or dysfibrinogenemia, L = fibrin stabilizing factor

FIGURE 36.1. Bleeding Disorders and the Clotting Cascade

Source: Adapted from *Cell,* 1988;53(4):505–18.

TABLE 36.1.   Coagulation Studies for Various Bleeding Diatheses

Disorder	PTT	PTT with Mixing Study	PT	Other Tests
vWD	Increased	NL	NL	RCA + RIPA decreased and low vWD antigen
Hemophilia A	Increased	NL	NL	RCA NL and FVIII decreased
Hemophilia B	Increased	NL	NL	Decreased FIX
Inhibitors to fibrinogen, II, V, or X; or lupus anticoagulant	Increased	Increased	Increased	Direct inhibitor and lupus anticoagulant testing
Inhibitors to VIII, IX, XI, or XII	Increased	Increased	NL	Direct inhibitor testing
FV, FVII, or FX deficiency*	Increased	NL	Increased	Decreased factor levels
FVIII, FIX, FXI, FXII deficiency*	Increased	NL	NL	Decreased factor levels
Prothrombin deficiency	Increased	NL	Increased	Decreased prothrombin
Dysfibrinogenemia	Increased	NL	Increased	Decreased fibrinogen, increased TCT
Vitamin K deficiency	Increased	NL	Increased	Normal TCT
DIC	Increased	NL	Increased	Decreased PLT, increased TCT, decreased fibrinogen, increased D-Dimer
Severe liver disease	NL or increased	NL	Increased	Abnormal liver panel

Roman numerals refer to specific clotting factors; PTT = partial thromboplastin time, PT = prothrombin time, vWD = von Willebrand disease, NL = normal, RCA = ristocetin cofactor activity, RIPA = ristocetin-induced platelet aggregation, TCT = thrombin clotting time, DIC = disseminated intravascular coagulation, PLT = platelet

* Single factor levels usually have to decrease to less than 30% of normal before elevation in PT or PTT is seen

Source: Information from *Haemophilia*, 2006;12(Suppl 3):68–75 and *Med Clin North Am*, 2001;85(5):1277–310.

TABLE 36.2   Coagulation Abnormalities That Can Occur in Advanced Liver Disease

Clinical Syndromes	PT	aPTT	Thrombin time	Fibrinogen	Platelets	D-Dimer	Fibrinolysis*
Factor VII deficiency	↑	NL	NL	NL	NL	NL	NL
Fibrinolysis	NL	NL	NL/↑	NL	NL	NL/↑	↑↑
Deficiency of Factors II, V, and VII	↑↑	NL/↑	NL	NL	NL	NL	NL
DIC	↑	↑	↑	↓↓	↓	↑↑	NL/↑
Hypofibrinogenemia	NL/↑	NL/↑	↑	↓↓	NL	NL	NL/↑
Dysfibrinogenemia	↑	NL/↑	↑	NL	NL	NL	NL/↑

* Extensive fibrinolysis can be assessed by clot lysis time, euglobulin lysis time, D-dimer assay, fibrinogen degradation assay, or thromboelastogram clot lysis index

↑ signifies an elevated level, ↑↑ signifies a very elevated level, ↓ signifies a decreased level, ↓↓ signifies a very decreased level

Note: Significant bleeding with invasive procedures or operations typically does not occur if INR is 2 or less AND PTT normal; lumbar puncture or regional neuraxial anesthesia is safe if INR is 1.7 or less AND PTT normal; elevated PTT and bleeding history are the 2 biggest risk factors for bleeding tendency in a patient with cirrhosis

Source: Adapted from *Advances in Medical Sciences*, 2010; 55 (1): 16–21.

CHAPTER 37

PANCYTOPENIA

1. ## ETIOLOGIES

   - **Drug-induced or chemical-induced**: acetazolamide, alcohol, allopurinol, antithyroid drugs, arsenic poisoning, aspirin, benzene, captopril, carbamazepine, systemic chemotherapy, chloramphenicol, chloroquine, chlorpromazine, colchicine, corticosteroids, dapsone, felbamate, furosemide, gold, insecticides, interferon-alfa, lisinopril, lithium, mebendazole, nizatidine, NSAIDs (butazones, diclofenac, indomethacin, and piroxicam), penicillamine, pentoxifylline, phenobarbital, phenylbutazone, phenothiazines, phenytoin, quinidine, sulfonamides, sulindac, ticlopidine, tolbutamide, thiazides, and toluene
   - **Gamma radiation-induced**
   - **Bone marrow replacement by cancer**: hematologic or metastatic solid organ malignancies
   - **Infections:** bacterial septic shock; tuberculosis; invasive fungal, brucellosis, babesiosis, leishmaniasis; HIV, HCV, HBV, non-A, B, or C hepatitis virus; CMV, EBV, or parvovirus B19 infections
   - **Autoimmune disorders**: systemic lupus erythematosus and Sjögren's syndrome
   - **Hematologic disorders**: aplastic anemia, paroxysmal nocturnal hemoglobinuria, osteopetrosis, myelodysplastic syndromes, agnogenic myeloid metaplasia with myelofibrosis, multiple myeloma, hairy cell leukemia, or copper deficiency
   - **Megaloblastic syndromes**: Vitamin B_{12} or folate deficiency
   - **Miscellaneous**: Gaucher's or lipid storage diseases, sarcoidosis, copper deficiency, heavy metal poisoning, or Niemann-Pick disease
   - **Hypersplenism**

2. ## EVALUATION OF PANCYTOPENIA

   - History of recent chemotherapy, radiation therapy, or culprit medication/chemical exposure
   - Exam for occult malignancy, infection, or autoimmune disorder
   - Labs: CBCD; chemistry panel; LDH; B_{12} and homocysteine levels; HIV, HCV, and HBV serologies, with or without ANA
   - Bone marrow biopsy for unexplained pancytopenia for routine studies, flow cytometry, and cultures for bacteria, acid-fast bacilli, and fungus

3. ## COMPLICATIONS

   - Neutropenia increases risk of infection (typically bacterial), septic shock
   - Thrombocytopenia results in bleeding

REFERENCES

Lancet, 2005;365(9471):1647–56; *Ann Intern Med,* 2002;136:534–46; *N Engl J Med,* 2004;350(6):552–9.

CHAPTER 38

THROMBOCYTOPENIA

1. ## DEFINITION
   - Platelet count less than 150K cells/μL

2. ## WORKUP
   - History and exam: assess for splenomegaly or lymphadenopathy and check medication list
   - Check peripheral blood smear: platelet clumping, platelet size and morphology, presence of schistocytes or spherocytes, and assess other cell lines
   - Labs: complete blood count with differential and coagulation studies
     - If schistocytes, confirm hemolysis with significantly increased LDH and indirect hyperbilirubinemia and reticulocyte count; check direct Coombs test
     - If direct Coombs-negative, check DIC panel (positive = DIC, negative = TTP/HUS)
   - Consider bone marrow biopsy if etiology unclear, multiple cell lines abnormal or older than 60 yo

3. ## RISKS OF COMPLICATIONS AT DIFFERENT PLATELET COUNTS
   - Greater than 50K: major surgery safe (except surgery of the brain, spinal cord, or eye: need more than 100K)
   - 20–50K: risk of major bleeding low
   - 10–20K: risk of mild–moderate bleeding (low risk for spontaneous hemorrhage)
   - Less than 10K: high risk for spontaneous hemorrhage (especially if less than 5K)
   - Consider platelet transfusion if platelets are less than 10K; less than 20K with active bleeding, infection, or qualitative platelet dysfunction; less than 50K prior to an invasive procedure or surgery; less than 100K prior to neurologic or ophthalmologic surgery or if intracranial hemorrhage; or if intracranial or life-threatening hemorrhage and patient on antiplatelet therapy (especially clopidogrel)
     - Avoid platelet transfusion in HUS/TTP, antiphospholipid antibody syndrome, HIT, DIC, HELLP syndrome, or severe ITP unless the patient has a CNS bleed
     - 1 unit random donor platelets usually increases platelet count about 10K
     - 1 unit single donor platelets usually increases platelet count about 50K

4. ## ETIOLOGIES
   ### Pseudothrombocytopenia
   - Platelet clumping in 0.1% of all blood draws; EDTA-mediated
   ### Decreased Platelet Production
   - Congenital causes (May-Hegglin anomaly, Bernard-Soulier syndrome, thrombocytopenia with absent radius and Wiskott-Aldrich syndromes, and Fanconi syndrome)
   - Storage diseases
   - Myelodysplasia (older than 60 yo), lymphoproliferative disorders, aplastic anemia, or marrow infiltration by tumor
   - Meds/toxins: alcohol*, thiazides, estrogens, ganciclovir and chemotherapy*, or radiation*
   - Vitamin deficiencies: B_{12} or folate
   - Infection: sepsis, tuberculosis, measles, HIV, rubella, mumps, parvovirus, varicella virus, hepatitis B virus, hepatitis C virus, and Epstein-Barr virus
   ### Immune-Mediated Platelet Destruction (most common mechanism)
   - Idiopathic thrombocytopenic purpura (ITP): diagnosis of exclusion with **isolated** thrombocytopenia, normal peripheral blood smear, and spleen size
     - Test for *H. pylori* infection and treat for *H. pylori* if present
     - Antiplatelet antibody panel **usually not** useful for diagnosing routine or classic ITP

* Medications commonly associated with thrombocytopenia

- Treatment usually reserved for platelet counts less than 30K; initial treatment corticosteroids
  - Prednisone 1–1.5 mg/k/d × 2–3 weeks
    - Alternative is dexamethasone 40 mg PO daily × 4 days
  - 2nd-line agents: IVIG 1 g/k/day × 2 days if PLT less than 5K, major bleeding, or extensive purpura
    - $Rh_o(D)$ immune globulin if Rh-positive patient
  - Thrombopoietic agents for refractory ITP: romiplostim or eltrombopag
  - Splenectomy if refractory to thrombopoietic agents
  - Consider rituximab therapy for recalcitrant cases
- Pregnant patients with ITP can receive either steroids or IVIG
  - If necessary splenectomy can be done during the 2nd trimester
  - Avoid vacuum- or forceps-assisted deliveries
- Evan syndrome: hemolysis, spherocytosis, and positive direct Coombs test
- Meds (common): abciximab, amiodarone, amphotericin B, carbamazepine, cimetidine, clopidogrel, digoxin, fluconazole, heparin, interferon-alpha, linezolid, penicillins, phenytoin, quinidine, quinine, ranitidine, trimethoprim-sulfamethoxazole, valproic acid, and vancomycin
- Meds (less likely): acetaminophen, acyclovir, albendazole, allopurinol, aminosalicylic acid, aspirin, atorvastatin, captopril, cephalosporins, chlorpromazine, chlorpropamide, ciprofloxacin, clarithromycin, colchicine, danazol, deferoxamine, diazepam, eptifibatide, ethambutol, felbamate, furosemide, haloperidol, hydroxychloroquine, inamrinone, indinavir, isoniazid, isotretinoin, itraconazole, levamisole, lithium, mesalamine, minoxidil, nitroglycerin, NSAIDs, octreotide, penicillamine, pentoxifylline, primidone, procainamide, pyrazinamide, rifampin, sirolimus, spironolactone, sulfasalazine, tamoxifen, thiothixene, tirofiban, and ticlopidine
- Infection: cytomegalovirus, toxoplasmosis, HIV, Epstein-Barr virus, and *H. pylori*
- Miscellaneous: SLE, antiphospholipid antibody syndrome, myelodysplasia, posttransfusion purpura, Type IIB (platelet-type) von Willebrand disease, or IgA deficiency

HEPARIN-INDUCED THROMBOCYTOPENIA

1. <u>DIAGNOSIS</u>

- Calculate "4 Ts score" (see **Table 38.1**); a score under 4 makes HIT very unlikely
  - Send heparin-platelet 4 antibody for scores 4 or higher
  - If heparin-platelet 4 antibody is elevated, perform a functional assay (serotonin release assay or a heparin-induced platelet activation assay) to confirm the diagnosis of HIT
  - Negative heparin-platelet factor 4 antibody excludes HIT with 95% accuracy

TABLE 38.1.   Pretest Probability of Heparin-induced Thrombocytopenia (the 4 "T's")

Category	2 Points	1 Point	0 Points
Thrombocytopenia	More than 50% platelet decrease to level 20 K or higher	30–50% decrease, nadir 10–19 K, or more than 50% decrease postop	Less than 30% decrease, or nadir less than 10 K
Timing of platelet decrease	5–10 days; within 1 day if heparin exposure in past 30 days	More than 10 days, or within 1 day if heparin exposure 31–100 days ago	Less than 4 days and no recent heparin exposure
Thrombosis or skin abnormalities	New thrombosis, skin necrosis, or acute systemic reaction with IV heparin bolus	Progressive or recurrent thrombosis, erythematous skin lesions, or suspected (not proven) thrombosis	None
Other etiologies present	None	Possible	Definite

First day of heparin is day 0; high probability = score 7–8, intermediate = 4–6, low = score 0–3
Note: Absence of heparin-platelet factor 4 antibodies excludes HIT more than 95% of the time

Source: Adapted from *Circulation,* 2004;110(18):e454–8.

2. TREATMENT OF HEPARIN-INDUCED THROMBOCYTOPENIA

- Discontinue heparin/LMWH and start argatroban, lepirudin, danaparoid, or bivalirudin until PLT are greater than 150K
- Start warfarin when PLT are greater than 100K and then bridge with nonheparin anticoagulant for at least 5 days and until INR 2–3 × 48 h for treatment of thrombosis
  - Continue warfarin for 3–6 months
- Fondaparinux is safe for DVT prophylaxis in patients with HIT and platelets greater than 100K
- Recommend repeating a functional assay prior to elective surgery for a history of HIT
  - Heparin use is safe if functional assay is negative

Non–immune-mediated platelet destruction (direct Coombs-negative)

- Presence of microangiopathic hemolytic anemia: DIC, HUS/TTP, HELLP syndrome, or malignant hypertension
- DIC is associated with sepsis, cancer, trauma, severe pancreatitis, envenomations, hepatic failure, abruption placentae, or amniotic fluid emboli
  - Treat underlying condition and provide supportive therapy
  - Use cryoprecipitate for bleeding with fibrinogen levels less than 100 mg/dL
  - Heparin therapy is not beneficial in acute DIC
- Other causes: vasculitis or shearing of platelets on prosthetic heart valves
- See **Table 38.2**

TABLE 38.2.   DIC Scoring System*

Factors	0 points	1 point	2 points	3 points
Platelet count	Greater than 100,000	50–100,000	Less than 50,000	–
D-dimer (ng/mL)	1000 or less	–	1000–5000	Greater than 5000
Fibrinogen (mg/dL)	Greater than 100	Less than 100	–	–
Prothrombin time prolongation	Less than 0–3 seconds	3–6 seconds	More than 6 seconds	–

* Overt DIC if score is 5 or higher

Source: Adapted from *Crit Care Med*, 2006;34(2):314–20.

- **TTP:** severe deficiency (less than 5%) of ADAMTS 13 enzyme activity supports idiopathic TTP
  - Emergent plasmapheresis and glucocorticoids for idiopathic TTP until PLT are above 150K
  - Recurrent TTP or refractory disease: consider corticosteroids, rituximab, or splenectomy
- **Splenic sequestration** (platelets usually over 40K)
  - Portal hypertension, Gaucher's disease, lymphoma/leukemias, myelofibrosis, or CHF
- **Gestational** (5% of all pregnancies in late 3rd trimester; platelets usually above 70K)
- **Dilutional:** after massive blood transfusions (10 or more units packed red blood cells)
- See **Table 38.3**

TABLE 38.3.   Causes of Thrombocytopenia in the ICU

Condition	Relative Incidence
Sepsis	52.4%
DIC	25.3%
Drug-induced thrombocytopenia	9.5%
Massive blood loss	7.5%
Immune thrombocytopenia	3.4%
HIT	1.2%
Thrombotic microangiopathy	0.7%

Source: Adapted from *Crit Care Clin,* 2011; 27: 281–297.

REFERENCES

Mayo Clin Proc, 2004;79:504. *N Engl J Med,* 2006;355:809. *N Engl J Med,* 2006;354:1927, *N Engl J Med,* 2007;357:580. *N Engl J Med,* 2006; 354:1927. *South Med J,* 2006;99:490.

CHAPTER 39

VENOUS THROMBOEMBOLISM

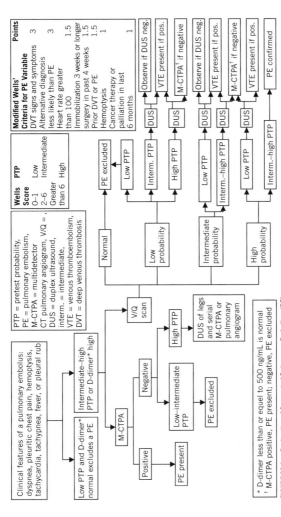

FIGURE 39.1. Evaluation of Suspected Pulmonary Embolism (PE)

* D-dimer less than or equel to 500 ng/mL is normal

† M-CTPA positive, PE present; negative, PE excluded

Modified Wells' Criteria for PE Variable	Points
DVT signs and symptoms	3
Alternative diagnosis less likely than PE	3
Heart rate greater than 100	1.5
Immobilization 3 weeks or longer surgery in past 4 weeks	1.5
Prior DVT or PE	1.5
Hemoptysis	1
Cancer therapy or palliation in last 6 months	1

Wells Score	PTP
0–1	Low
2–6	Intermediate
Greater than 6	High

PTP = pretest probability,
PE = pulmonary embolism,
M-CTPA = multidetector
CT pulmonary angiogram, V/Q = ,
DUS = duplex ultrasound,
interm. = intermediate,
VTE = venous thromboembolism,
DVT = deep venous thrombosis

Clinical features of a pulmonary embolus:
dyspnea, pleuritic chest pain, hemoptysis,
tachycardia, tachypnea, fever, or pleural rub

Low PTP and D-dimer*
normal excludes a PE

Intermediate–high
PTP or D-dimer* high

M-CTPA

Positive → PE present

Negative → Low–intermediate PTP → PE excluded

High PTP → DUS of legs and serial M-CTPA or pulmonary angiogram

V/Q scan

Normal → PE excluded

Low probability → Low PTP / Interm. PTP → DUS / High PTP → DUS

Intermediate probability → Low PTP → DUS / Interm.–high PTP → DUS

High probability → Low PTP → DUS / Interm.–high PTP → PE confirmed

Observe if DUS neg.
VTE present if pos.
M-CTPA† if negative

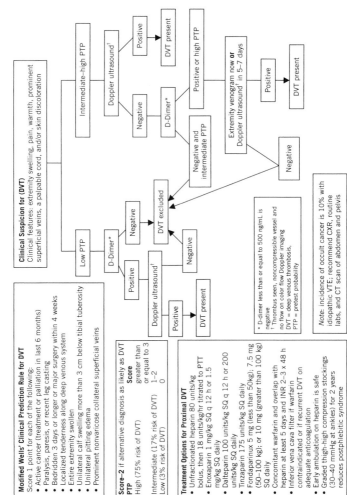

Clinical Suspicion for (DVT)
Clinical features: extremity swelling, pain, warmth, prominent superficial veins, a palpable cord, and/or skin discoloration

Modified Wells' Clinical Prediction Rule for DVT
Score 1 point for each of the following:
- Active cancer (treatment or palliation in last 6 months)
- Paralysis, paresis, or recent leg casting
- Bedridden 3 days or longer or major surgery within 4 weeks
- Localized tenderness along deep venous system
- Entire extremity swollen
- Unilateral calf swelling more than 3 cm below tibial tuberosity
- Unilateral pitting edema
- Prominent nonvaricose collateral superficial veins

Score -2 if alternative diagnosis as likely as DVT

PTP	Score
High (75% risk of DVT)	greater than or equal to 3
Intermediate (17% risk of DVT)	1–2
Low (3% risk of DVT)	0

Treatment Options for Proximal DVT
- Unfractionated heparin 80 units/kg bolus, then 18 units/kg/hr titrated to PTT
- Enoxaparin 1 mg/kg SQ q 12 h or 1.5 mg/kg SQ daily
- Dalteparin 100 units/kg q 12 h or 200 units/kg SQ daily
- Tinzaparin 175 units/kg SQ daily
- Fondaparinux 5 mg (less than 50kg); 7.5 mg (50–100 kg); or 10 mg (greater than 100 kg) SQ daily
- Concomitant warfarin and overlap with heparin at least 5 days and INR 2–3 x 48 h
- Inferior vena cava filter if warfarin contraindicated or if recurrent DVT on adequate anticoagulation
- Early ambulation on heparin is safe
- Graded thigh-high compression stockings (30–40 mmHg at ankles) for 2 years reduces postphlebitic syndrome

* D-dimer less than or equal to 500 ng/mL is negative
† Thrombus seen, noncompressible vessel and no flow on color flow Doppler imaging
DVT = deep venous thrombosis,
PTP = pretest probability

Note: incidence of occult cancer is 10% with idiopathic VTE; recommend CXR, routine labs, and CT scan of abdomen and pelvis

FIGURE 39.2.   Evaluation of Suspected Deep Venous Thrombosis

1. **CLINICAL PRESENTATION**
   - Pulmonary embolism
     - Dyspnea (sudden onset), pleuritic chest pain, hemoptysis, syncope, hypotension
   - Deep venous thrombosis
     - Acute calf pain/tenderness and swelling
     - Signs: ankle/calf swelling [LR+ 1.2, LR− 0.7], asymmetrical by more than 2 cm [LR+ 2.1, LR− 0.5]
     - Classic signs (without diagnostic utility: LR+ 1, LR− 1)
       - Palpable cord
       - Dilated superficial veins
       - Homan's sign: discomfort behind the knee on forced dorsiflexion of the foot
       - Skin erythema
       - Altered skin temperature

2. **DIFFERENTIAL DIAGNOSIS**

   DVT
   - Cellulitis
   - Lymphedema
   - Heart failure
   - Nephrotic syndrome
   - Cor pulmonale

   PE
   - Pneumonia
   - Pleurisy
   - Pleural effusion
   - Pneumothorax
   - Acute MI
   - Pericarditis

3. **TREATMENT OPTIONS FOR DEEP VENOUS THROMBOSIS OR PULMONARY EMBOLI**
   - Unfractionated heparin 80 units/kg bolus, then 18 units/kg/h titrated to PTT 1.5–2.5 × upper limit of normal
   - Enoxaparin 1 mg/kg SQ q 12 h or 1.5 mg/kg SQ daily (avoid if CrCl is less than 15 mL/min)
     - Dose adjustment required for CrCl 15–30 mL/min
     - Follow anti-FXa levels to adjust dosing for patient weight greater than 150 kg or less than 45–50 kg
     - For VTE with cancer, use LMWH for at least 6 months and indefinitely if cancer is still active
   - Dalteparin 100 units/kg SQ q 12 h or 200 units/kg SQ daily
   - Tinzaparin 175 units/kg SQ daily
   - Fondaparinux 5 mg (wt less than 50 kg), 7.5 mg (50–100 kg), or 10 mg (more than 100 kg) SQ daily
   - Start anticoagulation if VTE is suspected while workup is in progress
   - Overlap warfarin and heparin/LMWH/fondaparinux for at least 5 days and until INR 2–3 for 24 hours
   - Early ambulation is recommended for patients with DVT on anticoagulation
   - Inferior vena cava filter if anticoagulation is contraindicated or if recurrent pulmonary embolus on therapeutic doses of anticoagulation
   - Consider catheter-directed thrombolysis for a massive, limb-threatening ileofemoral DVT with symptoms less than 14 days (e.g., phlegmasia cerulean dolens or phlegmasia cerulean alba), good functional status, and life expectancy 1 year or longer for those who have a low risk of bleeding
   - Consider IV tPA100 mg IV over 2 h in a hemodynamically unstable patient with a massive PE or a submassive PE with RV strain (RV hypokinesis, estimated RV systolic pressure greater than 40 mmHg, elevated TnI, BNP greater than 100 pg/mL, or NT-pro BNP greater than 900 pg/mL)

- Absolute contraindications for thrombolytics: prior ICH, history of intracerebral AVM or malignancy, ischemic stroke in last 3 months, suspected aortic dissection, active bleeding or bleeding diathesis, recent spine or brain surgery, recent head or facial trauma
- Relative contraindications: age older than 75 yo, current anticoagulation, pregnancy, noncompressible vascular punctures, CPR for more than 10 minutes, internal bleeding in last 4 weeks, BP greater than 180/110 mmHg, dementia, and major surgery within 3 weeks
- Pulmonary embolectomy is an option for patients at high risk of bleeding
- Chronic thromboembolic pulmonary hypertension
  - Refer for consideration of pulmonary endarterectomy
  - Chronic, life-long anticoagulation
- Knee-high graduated compression stockings 30–40 mmHg at the ankle for at least 2 years after leg DVT

4. COMPLICATIONS OF VENOUS THROMBOEMBOLISM

Deep Venous Thrombosis

- Pulmonary embolism
- Phlegmasia cerulea dolens: uncommon type of DVT involving massive proximal venous thrombosis of lower extremities complicated by venous gangrene, compartment syndrome, and shock
- Venous valvular insufficiency leads to chronic lower extremity edema
- Postphlebitic syndrome (edema, pain, and skin discoloration of affected limb)

Pulmonary Embolism

- Acute right ventricular failure/cor pulmonale leads to hypotension, shock/sudden cardiac death
- Pulmonary hypertension, dyspnea at rest/exercise intolerance
- Pulmonary parenchymal infarction from occluded pulmonary artery
- Arrhythmias/PEA
- Pleural effusion
- Severe hypoxemia
- See **Tables 39.1** and **39.2**

TABLE 39.1.   Risk Factors for Venous Thromboembolic Events (VTE)

Advanced age older than 50 yo	Recent prolonged travel longer than 2 hours
Prolonged immobilization	Major surgery in last 4 weeks
Recent trauma	Inflammatory bowel disease
Previous VTE	Central venous catheter
Medical conditions: severe burns, active cancer, stroke with paresis, inherited thrombophilia, polycythemia, myeloproliferative disorder, obesity, CHF, nephrotic syndrome, inflammatory bowel disease, acute MI, acute respiratory failure, sickle cell disease, paroxysmal nocturnal hemoglobinuria, pregnancy, and collagen vascular disease	
Medications: tamoxifen, raloxifene, thalidomide, lenalidomide, darbepoetin, epoetin alfa, bevacizumab, hormone replacement therapy, or systemic chemotherapy	

Source: Information from *Arch Intern Med*, 2002; 162(11): 1245–8 and *NEJM*, 2001; 344(16): 1222–31.

TABLE 39.2.   Duration of Anticoagulation for Venous Thromboembolic Events

Underlying Condition or Risk Factor(s)	Duration
First episode of LE DVT or PE with reversible risk factors*; any UE DVT	3 months†
First episode of idiopathic VTE or VTE with protein C or S deficiency, elevated FVIII levels, prothrombin gene mutation, hyperhomocysteinemia, or heterozygous Factor V Leiden	6 months†
First episode† of VTE with: active cancer, antiphospholipid syndrome, AT III deficiency, homozygous Factor V Leiden, 2 or more thrombophilic conditions **or** for recurrent, idiopathic VTE **or** life-threatening VTE	Indefinite
VTE in pregnancy: anticoagulate until 6 weeks postpartum (avoid warfarin).	
Unprovoked symptomatic distal DVT	3 months
Symptomatic saphenous or basilic vein thrombosis	4 weeks
Infusional superficial thrombophlebitis treated with PO or topical diclofenac	

* Trauma, immobilization, estrogen use, pregnancy, or recent surgery
† Reevaluate patients after course of anticoagulation with a D-dimer test; recommend continuation of anticoagulation if D-dimer remains elevated 5.4% absolute risk increase of recurrent VTE versus patients with normal D-dimer levels)
LE = lower extremity, DVT = deep venous thromboembolism, PE = pulmonary embolism, UE = upper extremity, VTE = venous thromboembolism, AT III = antithrombin III, PO = per oral
Source: Chest, 2008; 133 (supp): 71–109 and 454, *Circulation*, 2001; 103: 2453–60, *NEJM*, 2006; 355: 1780.

HYPERCOAGULABLE STATES

Testing Recommendations for Thrombophilia in Venous Thrombosis

- **Strongly thrombophilic states**: idiopathic VTE in pts younger than 50 yo, recurrent VTE, or first-degree relative with VTE younger than 50 yo; a cerebral or visceral vein thrombosis, one fetal demise after 10 gestational weeks, or three or more unexplained spontaneous abortions occurring at less than 10 weeks' gestation
- **Weakly thrombophilic states**: idiopathic VTE 50 yo or older or occurring during pregnancy, the early postpartum period, or with estrogen therapy and no family history of thrombophilia
- **Timing for testing of hypercoagulable states:** check all of the lab tests after anticoagulation has been completed and the patient has been off of warfarin for at least 2 weeks
- See **Table 39.3**

TABLE 39.3.   Evaluation of Various Thrombophilic States

Clinical Conditions	Tests to Consider Checking
Strong thrombophilic states	APC resistance*, prothrombin gene mutation, anticardiolipin antibody, lupus anticoagulant, and levels of plasma homocysteine, antithrombin III, protein C, FVIII activity and protein S, anti-B$_2$ glycoprotein 1
Weak thrombophilic states	APC resistance, prothrombin gene mutation by PCR, Factor VIII activity, and levels of protein C and protein S
DVT in an unusual site (cerebral, mesenteric, portal, or hepatic veins)	Levels of proteins C and S and antithrombin III, and evaluate for a myeloproliferative disorder (including test for the JAK2 mutation) and for paroxysmal nocturnal hemoglobinuria
Recurrent miscarriages/stillbirths	Anticardiolipin antibody and lupus anticoagulant

APC = activated protein C, PCR = polymerase chain reaction
* 95% of these cases will be due to a Factor V Leiden mutation; check with a Factor V Leiden by PCR test
Source: Adapted from NEJM, 2001(16); 344: 1222–31.

Suggested Workup for Acquired Hypercoagulable States After VTE event

- Thorough history (particularly, was clot provoked?) and exam (including breast, pelvic, and rectal exam), fecal occult blood testing, urinalysis, complete blood count with peripheral blood smear, chemistry panel, chest X-ray, mammogram (women older than 40 yo), prostate-specific antigen (men older than 50 yo), and colonoscopy (older than 50 years) to evaluate for malignancy
- Urinalysis and serum albumin to screen for nephrotic syndrome
- Inquire about GI symptoms that may represent inflammatory bowel disease
- Examine the patient for orogenital ulcers, uveitis, and skin lesions (Behcet's disease)
- Any use of hormonal meds, tamoxifen, raloxifene, erythropoietic agents, or megestrol

Conditions Associated with Premature Arterial Thrombosis

- Active cancer or myeloproliferative disorders
- Antiphospholipid syndrome
- Hyperhomocysteinemia
- Elevated lipoprotein(a) levels

Screening Asymptomatic Family Members for Genetic Thrombophilia

- No consensus about screening family members of patients with thrombophilia
- Consider screening family members who are contemplating pregnancy or on treatment with hormonal contraception or hormone replacement therapy
- No role for long-term anticoagulation of asymptomatic patients with inherited thrombophilia and no history of a deep venous thrombosis/pulmonary embolus
  - Avoid screening tests for genetic thrombophilia until after 15 years of age

Indefinite Anticoagulation in High-Risk Patients with Thrombophilia or Unprovoked VTE

- One or two unprovoked venous thromboembolic events
- One spontaneous life-threatening thrombotic event
  - If first VTE event is a PE, it is 3 × more likely that 2nd VTE event will be a PE compared with a patient with a DVT as the first VTE event
- One spontaneous thrombosis at an unusual site
- Unprovoked VTE and CA, antiphospholipid syndrome, or antithrombin III deficiency

REFERENCES

Chest, 2008;133(supp):71–109, 454. *Circulation*, 2001;103:2453-60. *N Engl J Med*, 2006; 355:1780. *Ann Int Med*, 2001; 135:367. *Clin in Chest Med*, 2003;24:153. *Lancet Oncol*, 2005;6:401.

CHAPTER 40

PERIOPERATIVE MANAGEMENT OF ANTICOAGULATION AND ANTITHROMBOTICS

1. **MANAGEMENT OF ANTICOAGULATION FOR LOW-RISK SURGERIES OR PROCEDURES**
   - Warfarin may be continued perioperatively for the following procedures:
     - Eye surgery: cataract excision or trabeculectomies
     - Screening GI endoscopy, ERCP or biliary stent insertion without sphincterotomy
     - Dental procedures: restorations, endodontics, prosthetics, uncomplicated extractions, and dental hygiene treatment
     - Dermatologic procedures: Mohs surgery, simple excisions
     - Orthopedic procedures: joint and soft tissue injections or aspirations
     - Minor podiatry procedures

2. **MANAGEMENT OF ANTICOAGULATION FOR URGENT OPERATIONS**
   - Patients requiring urgent surgery may receive Vitamin K 1–2.5 mg PO if INR 1.8–3 or 2.5–5 mg PO if INR is greater than 3
     - Corrects INR less than or equal to 1.5 within 24 hours

3. **MANAGEMENT OF ANTITHROMBOTICS BEFORE OPERATIONS**
   - Aspirin and clopidogrel should be stopped (if possible) 7 days before an elective operation
   - If clopidogrel use and need for emergent surgery, give single pack single donor platelets on call to the OR
   - For patients who have had placement of a coronary stent, continue both aspirin and clopidogrel in the perioperative period if:
     - Bare metal stent in last 6 weeks or drug-eluting stent in last 12 months
   - See **Tables 40.1** and **40.2**

TABLE 40.1. Perioperative Anticoagulation Based on Risk of Thromboembolism

Perioperative Risk of Thromboembolic Event	Conditions	Management
Low (less than 5%/year)	• Nonvalvular afib with CHADS$_2$ score* 3 or lower • St. Jude valve—aortic position • VTE more than 3 months ago • Nonrecurrent stroke/TIA	• Stop warfarin 5 days prior to surgery • Proceed with surgery if INR is less than 1.5 on day of surgery
Intermediate (5–10%/year)	• VTE 1–3 months ago • History of 2 or more strokes/TIAs • St. Jude valve—mitral position • VTE 3–6 months ago and active CA • History of recurrent VTE • Nonvalvular Afib and CHADS$_2$ score* 4–6	• Stop warfarin 5 days prior to surgery • Start enoxaparin† 1 mg/kg SQ q 12 h 36 h after last warfarin dose • Check PT/INR 1 day preop and give Vitamin K 1 mg PO if INR is 2 or higher • Stop enoxaparin 24h preop • Restart enoxaparin 1 mg/kg SQ q 12 h and warfarin 12–24 h postop • Overlap enoxaparin and warfarin 5 or more days and until INR 2–3 × 24 h
High (higher than 10%/year)	• VTE in last month • Arterial embolus within 3 months • Valvular Afib • Cardioembolism from Afib or a mechanical heart valve • Hypercoagulable state • Acute intracardiac thrombus • Older mechanical valve • Any mitral valve prosthesis • Recent ischemic CVA less than 6 months	

* See Table 5.1

† Use unfractionated heparin for wt greater than 155 kg; dose adjust for CrCl 15–30 and avoid if CrCl is less than 15 mL/min

VTE = venous thromboembolism, TIA = transient ischemic attack, INR = international normalized ration, CA = cancer, Afib = atrial fibrillation, PT = prothrombin test, CVA = cerebrovascular accident

Source: Adapted from *Clev Clin J Med,* 2005;72(2):157–63 and *J Thromb Thrombolysis,* 2009;28(1):16–22.

TABLE 40.2. Regimens for DVT Prophylaxis in Medical and Surgical Patients

Category	Options for DVT Prophylaxis
Low-risk patients • Age younger than 40, minor surgery*, no RFs[†]	• Early ambulation • Leg exercises
Moderate-risk patients • Minor surgery and RFs[†] • Surgery in pts 40–60 yo • Major surgery[‡] and no RFs[†]	• Heparin[§] 5000 U SQ q 8 h started 2 h preop • LMWH[‖] 3400 U or less SQ daily • Fondaparinux[¶] 2.5 mg SQ daily • GCS or IPC
High-risk patients • Surgery, 40–60 yo + RFs[†] • Surgery in pts older than 60 yo • Major surgery[‡] and younger than 40 yo and RFs[†] • High-risk medical patient[†]	• Heparin[§] 5000 U SQ q 8 h started 2 h preop • LMWH[‖] more than 3400 U SQ daily • Fondaparinux[¶] 2.5 mg SQ daily • GCS or IPC
Highest risk patients • Major surgery[‡] older than 40 yo and RFs[†] • THA, TKA, or HFS • Major trauma[#] • Spinal cord injury[#] • Critically ill medical patient	• Heparin[§] 5000 U SQ q 8 h started 2 h preop • LMWH[‖] greater than 3400 U SQ daily • Fondaparinux[¶] 2.5 mg SQ daily • Warfarin titrated to INR 2–3 option for THA or TKA **PLUS IPC**
Moderate–high risk patients at high risk for bleeding	• GCS or IPC until bleeding risk is low • Initiate thromboprophylaxis when bleeding risk low

DVT = deep venous thromboembolism, RF = risk factor, LMWH = low molecular weight heparins, GCS = graduated compression stockings, IPC = intermittent pneumatic compression devices, THA = total hip arthroplasty, TKA = total knee arthroplasty, HFS = hip fracture surgery, INR = international normalized ratio
* Eye, ear, dermatologic, laparoscopic, or arthroscopic operations
† Severe burns, immobility, prior VTE, active cancer, stroke with paresis, inherited thrombophilia, polycythemia, myeloproliferative disorder, obesity, CHF, nephrotic syndrome, inflammatory bowel disease, acute MI, acute respiratory failure, sickle cell disease, paroxysmal nocturnal hemoglobinuria, pregnancy, recent trauma, central venous catheter, mechanical ventilation, severe sepsis, shock, and use of the following meds: tamoxifen, raloxifene, thalidomide, lenalidomide, darbepoetin, epoetin alfa, bevacizumab, hormone replacement therapy, or systemic chemotherapy
‡ Thoracic, intraperitoneal, bariatric, open urologic and gynecologic, cardiac, neurosurgical, and cancer operations
§ Caution starting heparin if initial PLT is less than 50 K and discontinue if PLT count falls by 50% or more or to less than 100 K.
‖ LMWH = low molecular weight heparins: enoxaparin 40 mg SQ daily starting 1–2 h preop or 30 mg SQ q 12 h starting 12–24 h postop; dalteparin 2500 units SQ starting 1–2 h preop and 6–8 h postop, then 5000 units SQ daily (not approved for TKR); tinzaparin 75 units/kg SQ daily starting 10–12 h before THR/TKR; dosage adjustment required for CrCl 15–30 mL/min and adjust dose based on anti-FactorXa levels if weight is greater than 155 kg; avoid if CrCl is less than 15 mL/min; caution if initial platelet less than 50 K, and discontinue if platelets fall by 50% or more or to a level less than 100 K
¶ Give 6–8 h postop; avoid if CrCl less than 30 mL/min, weight less than 50 kg, thrombocytopenia with positive antiplatelet antibodies, epidural infusions, or endocarditis; no antidote if active bleeding develops; $T_{1/2}$ ~18 h
# Thromboprophylaxis can generally be started within 36 h of major trauma or spinal cord injury unless intracranial bleeding, active internal bleeding, perispinal hematoma, or uncorrected coagulopathy present.
Source: Adapted from *Chest*, 2008;133(Suppl 6):381S–453S.

DURATION OF THROMBOPROPHYLAXIS

- Those at moderate–high risk of VTE should receive prophylaxis for entire hospitalization
- Extended thromboprophylaxis (28–35 days) for total hip or total knee arthroplasties, hip fracture surgery, or abdominal/pelvic surgery for cancer

ANTITHROMBOTICS AND ANTIPLATELETS WITH REGIONAL ANESTHESIA OR LUMBAR PUNCTURES

- Wait times before epidural or dural punctures or prior to epidural catheter removal
  - Wait 7 days after clopidogrel use, 8–12 h after SQ heparin, 10–12 h after bid prophylactic dose of LMWH, 18 h after daily prophylactic dose of LMWH, 24 h after therapeutic dose of LMWH, 36 h after fondaparinux
- May perform neuraxial block, LP, or remove epidural catheter if INR is less than 1.5 on warfarin
- Start SQ heparin/LMWH 2 h or longer and fondaparinux 12 h after epidural catheter removed
- Wait times after neuraxial anesthesia before initiation of antithrombotics
  - Wait 6–8 h before daily prophylactic LMWH started, 24 h before bid prophylactic or therapeutic LMWH, 4 h before SQ heparin, and 12 h before fondaparinux started

REFERENCES

Cleve Clin J Med, 2005;72(2):157–63; *Reg Anesth Pain Med*, 2003;28(3):172–97; *Anesth Analg*, 2007;105(6):1540–7; *Chest*, 2008;133(Suppl 6):381S–453S.

SECTION 5

INFECTIOUS DISEASE

CHAPTER 41

EVALUATION OF FEVER IN THE HOSPITALIZED PATIENT

1. **DEFINITION OF NOSOCOMIAL FEVER**
   - Fever higher than 38.3°C (100.9°F)

2. **COMMON INFECTIOUS ETIOLOGIES OF FEVER IN THE HOSPITALIZED PATIENT**
   - Hospital-acquired pneumonia
   - Catheter-related bloodstream infection
   - Urinary tract infections (usually catheter-related)
   - *Clostridium difficile*–associated diarrhea
   - Surgical site infections (especially if more than 4 days postop)
   - Hospital-acquired meningitis (rare in the absence of a neurosurgical procedure)
   - Nosocomial endocarditis (beware of patient with a history of IVDU and a new central line)
   - Infected decubitus ulcers

3. **WORKUP OF A NOSOCOMIAL FEVER**
   - Careful exam for any clinical sources of infection
   - Labs: CBCD, blood culture × 2, urinalysis, and urine culture if greater than or equal to 5 WBC/hpf and CXR
     - Sputum culture and Gram stain for pulmonary infiltrate and cough
   - High concern for catheter-related bloodstream infection
     - Remove line; send tip for semiquantitative culture (greater than 10^5 bacteria inidcates CRBSI)
   - Drain and culture any skin abscesses
   - Three separate stool samples for *Clostridium difficile* toxins A and B or a single stool PCR test if diarrhea is present
   - For new fever and new neurological findings or delirium, rule out CNS infection
     - Noncontrast head CT required prior to lumbar puncture for CSF analysis

4. **NONINFECTIOUS CAUSES OF FEVER**
   - Drug fever (10% of fevers in hospitalized patients) usually antimicrobials (e.g., β-lactam drugs, amphotericin B, erythromycin, sulfonamides, antimalarials, and nitrofurantoin), antiepileptic drugs (e.g., barbiturates and phenytoin), antiarrhythmics (e.g., quinidine and procainamide), contrast media, methyldopa, bleomycin, allopurinol, captopril, cimetidine, heparin, hydralazine, thiazides, isoniazid, meperidine, or nifedipine
     - May take longer than 7 days to resolve after stopping the offending agent
   - Malignant hyperthermia
     - Caused by succinylcholine or inhalational anesthetics (halothane most commonly)
     - Clinically presents with increased muscle spasms, fever, and elevated creatinine kinase
     - Usually immediate reaction; may be delayed up to 24 hours in steroid use
   - See **Table 41.1**

TABLE 41.1.   Medical Conditions That Can Cause Fever in Adults

Acute cholecystitis	Munchausen's syndrome (factitious fever)
Acute myocardial infarction	Organ transplant rejection
Adrenal insufficiency	Pancreatitis
Adult Still's disease	Pheochromocytoma
Alcoholic hepatitis	Pulmonary infarction
Aspiration pneumonitis without infection	Sarcoidosis
Dressler's syndrome (pericardial injury syndrome)	SLE flare
Fat emboli	Stroke
Gout/pseudogout	Substance abuse withdrawal syndromes
Heterotopic ossification	Thyroid storm
Immune reconstitution inflammatory syndrome	Thyrotoxicosis
Inflammatory bowel disease	Transfusion reaction
Intracranial bleed	Tumor lysis syndrome
Ischemic colitis	Vasculitis
Jarisch-Herxheimer reaction	Venous thromboembolism
Malignancy (Hodgkin's disease; non-Hodgkin's lymphoma; leukemia; myeloma; sarcoma; tumors of the liver, brain, kidney, colon, gallbladder, or pancreas; or myelodysplasia)	

Source: Adapted from *Crit Care Med* 2008; 36(4): 1330–49 and *Crit Care Med*, 2009; 37 (7 Suppl): S273–8.

CHAPTER 42

INFECTIVE ENDOCARDITIS

1. EPIDEMIOLOGY

- More than 50% cases affect pts older than 60 yo
- ICE-MD study showed diabetes mellitus as an independent predictor of inpatient mortality for pts with IE; also, IE due to *S. aureus* has a 60% chance of embolic events and a 20% chance of mortality
- ICE-PC Study: incidence of microbe: *S. aureus* 31%, *S. viridans* 17%, Enterococci 11%, coagulase-negative Staph 11%, *Streptococcus bovis* 7%, other Strep 5%, non-HACEK (*H*aemophilus aphrophilus, *A*ctinobacillus actinomycetemcomitans, *C*ardiobacterium hominis, *E*ikenella corrodens, and *K*ingella kingae), Gram-negative bacteria 2%, fungi 2%, HACEK 2%
- 75% of IE patients have preexisting heart valve abnormalities
- Other risk factors: prior IE, IVDU, hemodialysis, diabetes, intravascular devices, receiving vancomycin, MRSA infection, persistent bacteremia

2. PATHOPHYSIOLOGY

- Predisposing endothelial injury (MR, AS, AR, VSD, other congenital heart disease, prosthetic valve) leads to clot-rich fibrin and platelets
- Skin or mucosal injury can result in transient bacteremia by organisms that produce adhesion factors (*Staphylococcus, Streptococcus, Enterococcus*), leading to infection of clot or injured endothelium, then infected vegetation
- *S. aureus* produces virulence factors that enable invasion of intact valves
- Metabolically active bacteria on vegetation surface results in continuous bacteremia
- Metabolically inactive bacteria inside vegetation are resistant to killing by antibiotics
- Vegetation fragments and/or immune complexes result in embolic phenomena

3. CLINICAL PRESENTATION

- Fevers, new murmur, fatigue/weakness, particularly in IVDU or patients with artificial valve, hematuria (urinalysis reveals an active sediment)
- Exam stigmata
  - Conjunctival hemorrhages
  - Splenomegaly
  - Petechiae
  - Splinter hemorrhages: linear red/brown, nonblanching lesions in the nailbed
  - Janeway lesions: painless, small erythematous macules on palms and soles
  - Osler's nodes: tender, erythematous, indurated nodules with pale center, 1–2 mm, usually on pads of fingers or toes
  - Roth spots: flame-shaped retinal hemorrhages with pale centers
- See **Table 42.1** and **Figure 42.1**

TABLE 42.1. Modified Duke Criteria for the Diagnosis of Infective Endocarditis (IE)

Major Criteria	Minor Criteria
Positive blood cultures (and no primary focus) • 2 or more blood cultures positive with typical organisms (*Strep viridans* or *bovis*, HACEK group, *S. aureus*, or *enterococcus*) • Positive blood culture or IgG titer greater than 1:800 for *Coxiella burnetti*	Predisposing heart condition, prior IE, or IVDU
	Temperature higher than 100.4°F (greater than 38°C)
	Vascular phenomena: major arterial emboli, septic pulmonary infarcts, mycotic aneurysm, intracranial hemorrhage, conjunctival hemorrhages, and Janeway lesions
Evidence of endocardial involvement • Echocardiogram with a pedunculated vegetation, abscess, prosthetic valve dehiscence, new valvular regurgitation	Immunologic, glomerulonephritis, Osler's nodes, Roth's spots, rheumatoid factor–positive
	Microbiology: positive blood culture or serologies but does not meet major criteria

Definite IE: 2 major criteria, 1 major and 3 minor criteria, or 5 minor criteria

Possible IE: 1 major and 1 minor criteria, or 3 minor criteria

IE rejected: firm alternative diagnosis, resolution of syndrome with antibiotics for less than 4 days, no pathologic evidence at surgery or autopsy with antibiotics less than 4 days

Source: Adapted from *Circulation*, 2005; 111(23): e394–434.

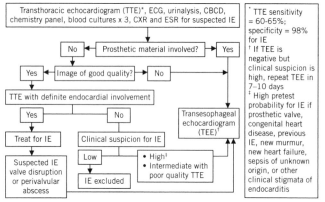

FIGURE 42.1. Algorithm for Evaluation of Suspected Infective Endocarditis (IE)

Source: Adapted from *Eur Heart J*, 2004; 25(3): 267–76 and *Eur Heart J*, 2009; 30(19): 2369–413.

4. EMPIRIC TREATMENT OF SUSPECTED INFECTIVE ENDOCARDITIS

- Native valve endocarditis with risk factors (e.g., hemodialysis, prior MRSA infections, indwelling vascular device, or IVDU): vancomycin plus gentamicin
- Native valve endocarditis without risk factors: nafcillin plus gentamicin
- Prosthetic valve endocarditis: vancomycin plus gentamicin with or without rifampin
- Once a specific organism is identified and sensitivities are known, de-escalate antibiotics based on **Table 42.2**

TABLE 42.2. Antibiotic Therapy for Infective Endocarditis Based on Organism

Organism	Primary Therapy	Alternative Therapy
• *Streptococcus* (penicillin-susceptible*) NVE	• Penicillin G[†] plus gentamicin[‡] 1 mg/kg q 8 h × 2 weeks	• Ceftriaxone 2 g IV q 24 h plus gentamicin[‡] 1 mg/kg q 8 h
• *Streptococcus* (penicillin-intermediate*) NVE or PVE	• Penicillin G[†] plus gentamicin[‡] 1 mg/kg q8 h × 2 weeks	• Ceftriaxone 2 g IV q 24 h plus gentamicin[‡] 1 mg/kg q 8 h
• *Streptococcus* (penicillin-resistant*) NVE or PVE	• Ampicillin-sulbactam[†] plus gentamicin[‡] 1 mg/kg q 8 h	• Vancomycin[§] 30 mg/kg/day plus gentamicin[‡] 1 mg/kg q 8 h
• Methicillin-susceptible *S. Aureus* and NVE[ǁ]	• Nafcillin[†] plus gentamicin[‡] 1 mg/kg q 8 h	• Cefazolin[†] plus gentamicin[‡] 1 mg/kg q 8 h
• Methicillin-resistant *S. Aureus* and NVE[ǁ]	• Vancomycin[§] 30 mg/kg/day plus gentamicin[‡] 1 mg/kg q 8 h	• Daptomycin 8–10 mg/kg IV q 24 h
• *Enterococcus* (penicillin-susceptible*) NVE or PVE	• Ampicillin[†] or penicillin G[†] plus gentamicin[‡] 1 mg/kg q 8 h	• Vancomycin[§] 30 mg/kg/day plus gentamicin[‡] 1 mg/kg q 8 h
• *Enterococcus* (penicillin-resistant*) NVE or PVE	• Ampicillin-sulbactam[†] plus gentamicin[‡] 1 mg/kg q 8 h	• Vancomycin[§] 30 mg/kg/day plus gentamicin[‡] 1 mg/kg q 8 h
• HACEK NVE or PVE	• Ceftriaxone 2 g IV q 24 h	• Ampicillin-sulbactam[†] or ciprofloxacin
• *Brucella* sp.	• PO doxycycline 200 mg/day plus cotrimoxazole 960 mg/q 12 h plus rifampin 300–600 mg/day × 3 months	
• *Coxiella burnetii*	• PO doxycycline 200 mg/day plus hydroxychloroquine 200–600 mg/day × 18 months	• PO doxycycline 200 mg/day plus ofloxacin 400 mg/day × 18 months

* Penicillin susceptible if MIC is less than or equal to 0.12 mcg/mL; intermediate if MIC is greater than 0.12 up to 0.5 mcg/mL; resistant if MIC is greater than 0.5 mcg/mL

† β-lactam dosing guidelines: penicillin G 2–3 million units IV q 4h if MIC is less than or equal to 0.12 mcg/mL or 4 million units IV q 4 h if MIC 0.13–0.5 mcg/mL; nafcillin 2 g IV q 4 h; ampicillin 2 g IV q 4 h; cefazolin 2 g IV q 6 h and ampicillin-sulbactam 3 g IV q 6 h

‡ Synergistic gentamicin × **2 weeks** (maintain gentamicin peak 3–4 mcg/mL); NVE = native valve endocarditis

§ Vancomycin given in divided doses q 8–12 h aiming for a vancomycin trough 15–20 mcg/mL (renal dosing needed)

ǁ For prosthetic valve endocarditis (PVE) add rifampin 300 mg IV q 8 h or 600 mg IV q 12 h to regimen

Note: If possible, avoid systemic anticoagulation during treatment of endocarditis

Source: Adapted from *Circulation*, 2005; 111(23): e394–434 and *Eur Heart J*, 2009; 30(19): 2369–413.

Antibiotic Duration for Native Valve Endocarditis (NVE) and Prosthetic Valve Endocarditis (PVE)

- Duration applies to primary therapeutic antibiotic(s); gentamicin used for 1st 2 weeks only
- NVE: coagulase-negative *Staphylococcus* (4 weeks)
- NVE: *S. aureus* and *Enterococcus* (6 weeks), and HACEK (4 weeks)
- NVE: uncomplicated **penicillin-susceptible** (MIC up to 0.12 mcg/mL) strep NVE (4 weeks)
  - 2 weeks if synergistic gentamicin used
- NVE: **penicillin-intermediate** (MIC greater than 0.12 and up to 0.5 mcg/mL) *Streptococcus* (4 weeks)
- NVE: **penicillin-resistant** (MIC greater than 0.5 mcg/mL) *Streptococcus*, *Abiotrophia defectiva*, *Granulicatella* sp., and *Gemella* sp. (4–6 weeks)
- PVE: *Streptococcus* (6 wks), *S. aureus* and *Enterococcus* (6–8 wks), and HACEK (4 wks)

Indications for Valve Surgery for IE

- Refractory CHF, cardiogenic shock, persistent vegetation after systemic embolization, increase in vegetation size or persistently positive blood cultures despite appropriate antimicrobial therapy for more than 7 days, acute AI or MR with signs of ventricular failure, valve perforation or rupture, valvular dehiscence or rupture, fistula into cardiac chamber or pericardial space, pseudoaneurysm formation, new heart block, perivalvular abscess refractory to antimicrobial therapy, and suspected infection of pacemakers or AICD devices
- See **Tables 42.3** and **42.4**

TABLE 42.3.   Causes of Culture-Negative Infective Endocarditis

Pathogen	Diagnosis
Brucella sp.	Blood cultures, serology, culture, immunohistology, and PCR of surgical material
Coxiella burnetii	Serology (IgG greater than 1:800), tissue culture, immunohistology, and PCR of surgical material
Bartonella sp.	Blood cultures, serology, culture, immunohistology, and PCR of surgical material
Tropheryma whipplei	Histology and PCR of surgical material
Mycoplasma sp.	Serology, culture, immunohistology, and PCR of surgical material
Legionella sp.	Blood cultures, serology, culture, immunohistology, and PCR of surgical material

TABLE 42.4.   Predictors of Poor Outcome in Patients with Infective Endocarditis

Patient Characteristics	IE Complications	Pathogen	Echocardiographic Findings
Age older than 50	CHF	*S. aureus*	Periannular complications
Prosthetic valve	Acute renal failure	Gram-negative bacilli	Severe AI/MR
Insulin-requiring DM	Stroke	Fungi	LVEF less than 0.4
Cardiac disease	Septic shock		Pulmonary hypertension
Chronic renal disease	Periannular complications		Large vegetations (larger than 10 mm)
Chronic lung disease			Severe prosthetic valve dysfunction
Malnourished			Elevated diastolic pressures

Source: Adapted from *Eur Heart J*, 2009; 30(19): 2369–413.

5. COMPLICATIONS

- Cardiac: heart failure (most common cause of death; caused by valvular damage/insufficiency), perivalvular abscess, heart block (from perivalvular abscess extension, most commonly at aortic valve, into proximal ventricular conduction system), acute coronary syndrome (rare; due to extrinsic coronary compression from perivalvular infection), systemic embolization (especially in presence of perivalvular abscess), pericarditis, intracardiac fistulas, aneurysm/pseudoaneurysm, aortic dissection
- Embolization
  - Systemic: usually results from left-sided endocarditis (or rarely, right-sided endocarditis in the presence of a PFO); may cause stroke, blindness, ischemic/gangrenous limbs, splenic/renal infarction, cerebrovascular accident, or spinal cord infarct leading to paralysis
  - Pulmonary emboli/hypoxia due to right-sided endocarditis
- Neurologic: embolic stroke/CVA, encephalopathy, meningitis, meningoencephalitis, brain abscess/cerebritis, seizures
- Mycotic aneurysms
- Vertebral osteomyelitis
- Septic arthritis (especially in presence of *S. aureus, S. viridans*, nongroup A–B hemolytic strep)

REFERENCES

Circulation, 2005;111(23):e394–434; *Eur Heart J*, 2004;25(3):267–76; *Eur Heart J*, 2009;30(19):2369–413; *Circulation*, 2010;121(9):1141–52.

CHAPTER 43

INFECTIONS IN HIV-POSITIVE PATIENTS

1. GENERAL PATHOPHYSIOLOGY

- CD4+ helper T cells are primary target for HIV
- HIV infection of cells requires binding to CD4+ coreceptors (CCR5 or CXCR4)
- Transmission: mucosal breakdown or transport by dendritic cells leads to infection of mucosal CD4+ T cells
- Acute infection: wide dissemination of HIV to CD4+ T cells, especially in gut-associated lymphoid tissue, leads to high-level viremia (acute retroviral syndrome)
- Evasion of immune response: high rate of mutation selects for clones that evade CD8+ T cells
  - Immune activation causes exhaustion of CD8+ T cells
  - Loss of CD4+ helper T-cell function decreases specific humoral and cell-mediated immune response
  - Latent reservoir of resting CD4+ T cells established early in infection
- Viral set point (steady-state level of viremia) directly correlated with speed of progression to AIDS
- CD_4 less than 200 increases susceptibility to opportunistic infections—clinical definition of AIDS
- See **Table 43.1** and **Figure 43.1**

TABLE 43.1. Infectious and Non-infectious Complications of HIV Infection

CD4 Count	Infectious Conditions	Noninfectious Conditions
Greater than 500	• Acute retroviral syndrome • Mucucutaneous candidiasis • Standard bacterial infections	• Generalized lymphadenopathy • Guillain-Barre syndrome • Medication-induced meningitis
200–500	• Bacterial pneumonia • Esophageal candidiasis • Herpes zoster virus infections • Localized herpes simplex virus (HSV)* • Kaposi's sarcoma • Oral hairy leukoplakia • Tuberculosis*	• Anemia • Cervical dysplasia or cancer • Immune thrombocytopenic purpura • Lymphoma (Hodgkin's and NHL) • Mononeuritis multiplex • Seborrheic dermatitis
50–200	• Bacillary angiomatosis (*Bartonella*) • Disseminated coccidioidomycosis • Cryptococcosis • Chronic cryptosporidiosis • Disseminated HSV* • Disseminated histoplasmosis • Microsporidiosis • Miliary tuberculosis* • *Pneumocystis jiroveci* pneumonia* • Progressive multifocal encephalopathy • Toxoplasmosis*	• Cardiomyopathy • Primary CNS lymphoma • HIV-associated dementia • HIV-associated wasting syndrome • Myelopathy • Peripheral neuropathies • Polyradiculopathy • Immunoblastic lymphoma • Immune reconstitution syndrome (IRIS)
Less than 50	• Invasive aspergillosis • Disseminated CMV infections • Disseminated *Mycobacterium avium* complex*	

* Incidence can be decreased with medication prophylaxis

Source: Adapted from *Infect Dis Clin N. Amer,* 2001; 15(2): 433–55.

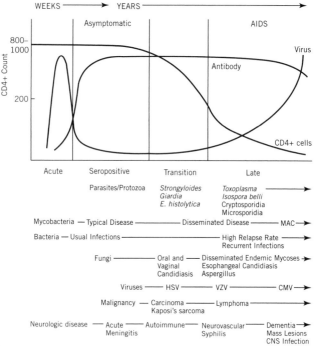

FIGURE 43.1. Time Course of HIV Infection and Opportunistic Infections at Various Stages of HIV Disease

Source: Courtesy of Gail Simpson, M.D., Director of Infectious Disease, Ventura County Medical Center.

MENINGOENCEPHALITIS

1. PATHOPHYSIOLOGY

- Cryptococcal meningitis: inhalation of aerosolized *Cryptococcus neoformans* results in latent infection of lungs; when reactivated, yeast disseminates to CNS; release of capsular polysaccharide results in immune dysfunction
- Progressive multifocal leukoencephalopathy: JC virus infection results in viral inclusions in oligodendrocytes and deformed astrocytes, resulting in multifocal demyelination
- HIV encephalopathy: HIV infection of resident macrophages and astrocytes releases neurotoxins, resulting in white matter disease and neuronal loss

2. CLINICAL PRESENTATION

- Cryptococcal meningitis: headache, fever, confusion, altered mental status, and depressed level of consciousness (CD4 less than 200)
- Viral meningoencephalitis: headache, fever, confusion, delirium, lethargy, focal deficits, seizure
- Cytomegalovirus encephalitis: headache, altered mental status, progressive focal deficits, cauda equina syndrome (CD4 less than 50)
- HSV encephalitis: headache, behavioral, personality, memory changes, and seizures

- VZV encephalitis: vasculitis leading to stroke syndromes
- Neurosyphilis: behavioral/psychological abnormalities, delirium, dementia, focal deficits, stroke syndromes, meningitis, myelitis, uveitis, chorioretinitis, cranial nerve palsies, and rash (CD4 less than 350)

3. MENINGITIS ETIOLOGIES

- Bacterial (including *Listeria monocytogenes*), *Cryptococcus*, viral (HSV, HIV, CMV), *M. tuberculosis*, histoplasmosis, and coccidioidomycosis

4. WORKUP

- Neuroimaging: MRI with/without gadolinium or CT scan of head with contrast
- Routine CSF studies: cell count, glucose, protein, culture and Gram stain, and India ink
- Other CSF studies: cocci titer, VDRL, AFB and/or HSV RNA by PCR, and cytology
- Other studies: PPD; serum crypto antigen, VDRL, and cocci titer; urine histo antigen; blood cultures × 2; CBCD; basic metabolic panel

5. TREATMENT

- Cryptococcal meningitis: treat with amphotericin B 0.7–1 mg/kg/day or liposomal amphotericin B 5–6 mg/kg/day **and** flucytosine 25 mg/kg PO q 6 h × at least 2 wks (watch for cytopenias)
  - Daily lumbar punctures 20–30 mL CSF or lumbar drain to keep CSF closing pressure less than or equal to 20 cmH$_2$O
  - Continue induction phase until CSF fungal cultures are sterile
  - Chronic suppressive phase: fluconazole 800 mg PO daily for lifetime or until immune system is reconstituted
- Neurosyphilis
  - Diagnosis: elevated CSF VDRL titer or serum VDRL/FTA positive and abnormal CSF studies consistent with neurosyphilis
  - Treatment: penicillin G 3–4 million units IV q 4 h or ceftriaxone 2 g IV daily × 14 days
  - Monitoring: desire at least a 4-fold decrease in VDRL titer in 6–12 months
- Bacterial meningitis
  - Empiric therapy with ampicillin, ceftriaxone, vancomycin plus dexamethasone 10 mg IV q 6 h × 96 h
  - Tailor antibiotics based on identification and sensitivities of organism

6. COMPLICATIONS

- Seizures
- Delirium/confusion
- Visual or hearing disturbances
- Dementia
- Abscess formation

CNS MASS LESIONS

1. PATHOPHYSIOLOGY

- Toxoplasmosis: ingestion of *Toxoplasma gondii* cysts releases tachyzoites in GI tract, which go dormant; reactivation of dormant organism results in dissemination to CNS (and other organs), where they cause cell necrosis
- Primary CNS lymphoma: *associated with EBV infection* and increased IL-6 expression by HIV-infected macrophages

2. CLINICAL PRESENTATION

- Focal neurologic deficits, behavioral changes, confusion, occasionally fever, headache; seizure or coma in advanced disease (CD4 less than 50)
- Herniation syndromes
- Cerebral toxoplasmosis typically presents with multiple ring-enhancing lesions at corticomedullary junction and basal ganglia on MRI
- See **Figure 43.2**

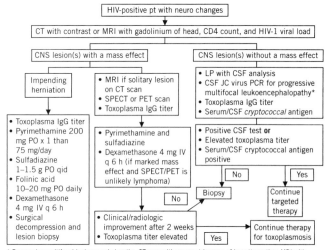

FIGURE 43.2. Management of HIV-Infected Patients with CNS Lesions

Source: Information from *CID*, 2002; 34(1): 103–15, *J Infect*, 2000; 40(3): 274–81 and *Neurology*, 1997(3); 48: 687–94.

PULMONARY INFECTIONS

1. PATHOPHYSIOLOGY OF PNEUMOCYSTIS PNEUMONIA

- *Pneumocystic jiroveci* pneumonia: *Pneumocystis jiroveci* colonization results in ingestion by alveolar macrophages, which then release inflammatory mediators that cause alveolar damage and induce host inflammatory response

2. CLINICAL PRESENTATION OF PNEUMOCYSTIS PNEUMONIA

- Pneumocystis pneumonia: fever, progressive exertional dyspnea, nonproductive cough worsened by breathing deeply

3. WORKUP OF PNEUMONIA DEPENDING OF CXR PATTERN

- See **Table 43.2**
- Focal infiltrate
  - Blood cultures × 2, sputum for culture and Gram stain
  - Consider first morning–induced sputum or BAL for AFB smear and PJP stain × 3
- Diffuse opacities or diffuse nodular infiltrate
  - Blood cultures × 2, sputum for culture and Gram stain and for fungal stain and culture
  - First morning–induced sputum or BAL for AFB smear and PJP stain × 3
  - Serum coccidioidomycosis titers, LDH, and urine histoplasma antigen
- Pneumothorax
  - First morning–induced sputum or BAL for PJP stain × 3
- Mediastinal lymphadenopathy
  - Blood cultures × 2, sputum for culture and Gram stain and for fungal stain and culture
  - First morning–induced sputum or BAL for AFB smear and PJP stain × 3
  - Serum coccidioidomycosis titers, LDH, β_2-microglobulin
  - Urine histoplasma antigen
  - Consider mediastinoscopy and lymph node biopsy if initial blood tests are nonconfirmatory

• See Table 43.2

TABLE 43.2.   Chest Radiographic Patterns of Pneumonia in HIV-Positive Patients

CXR Pattern	Common Pathogens
Focal infiltrate	Bacteria, tuberculosis (TB; especially upper lobes), *P. jiroveci* (uncommon)
Diffuse opacities	*P. jiroveci*, TB, bacteria, fungal*, cytomegalovirus, Kaposi's sarcoma (KS)
Diffuse nodules	Large nodules: KS; Small nodules: tuberculosis, *P. jiroveci*, or fungal*
Pneumothorax	*Pneumocystis jiroveci*
Mediastinal LAD	Tb, nontuberculous mycobacteria, KS, lymphoma, or fungal*
Pleural effusion	Bacteria, TB, KS, lymphoma, fungal*, cardiomyopathy, or hypoalbuminemia
Cavitation	CD4 greater than 200: TB or bacterial; CD4 less than 200: *P. jiroveci*, *Pseudomonas aeruginosa, Rhodococcus equi, Nocardia asteroides*, or fungal*

*Fungal includes coccidioidomycosis, blastomycosis, histoplasmosis, and aspergillosis; LAD = lymphadenopathy
Source: Adapted from *Crit Care Med*, 2006; 34(Suppl 9): S245–50.

TREATMENT OF *PNEUMOCYSTIS JIROVECI* PNEUMONIA

• Trimethoprim-sulfamethoxazole (5 mg/kg trimethoprim component) PO/IV q 6 h
• Trimethoprim 5 mg/kg/day + dapsone 100 mg PO daily
• Atovaquone 750 mg PO bid
• Pentamidine 3–4 mg/kg IV daily
• Add PO prednisone 40 mg bid × 5 days, 40 mg/day × 5 days, 20 mg/day × 11 days if PaO$_2$ is less than 70 mmHg or A-a(O$_2$) gradient is greater than 35 mmHg
• Duration of therapy is 21 days

COMPLICATIONS

• Pneumatocele rupturing to cause a pneumothorax
• Pleural effusion
• ARDS

INFECTIONS

PATHOPHYSIOLOGY

• Candidiasis (oropharyngeal and esophageal): extensive mucocutaneous infection
• CMV esophagitis or colitis: latent infection reactivates in setting of immunosuppression, favored by chronic antigenic stimulation; intranuclear inclusions (seen as "owl's eye" nuclei) induce cellular immune response

CLINICAL PRESENTATION

• Candidal infections of oral cavity: dysphagia or odynophagia
• Candida esophagitis: substernal chest pain (sharp or burning)
• CMV or herpes esophagitis: aphthous ulcers and giant ulcers
• CMV colitis: fever, anorexia, abdominal pain, watery diarrhea with or without blood (CD4 less than 100)
• Cryptosporidium/microsporidium colitis: anorexia, nausea/vomiting, cramps, profuse watery diarrhea, steatorrhea, and severe metabolic disturbances (CD4 less than 100)

WORKUP AND TREATMENT

• Oral infections
  ○ Severe aphthous ulcers: treat with steroids or thalidomide
  ○ Oral candidiasis: treat with nystatin rinses or clotrimazole troches
  ○ HSV ulcers: treat with acyclovir
• Esophagitis/giant ulcers: candida, cytomegalovirus, or herpes simplex virus
  ○ Diagnosis requires EGD with biopsies

- Candida esophagitis therapy: fluconazole
- CMV esophagitis: 2–3 weeks of IV ganciclovir, foscarnet, or cidofovir
- HSV esophagitis therapy: acyclovir
- Evaluation of diarrhea
  - Stool for routine culture including *Salmonella, Shigella,* and *Campylobacter, C. difficile* toxin, ova and parasites × 3, and giardia antigen; special stains for *Cryptosporidium, Isospora, Microsporidia, Cyclospora*; modified acid fast stain, and *E. coli* 0157 (if bloody)
  - Blood cultures for *Mycobacterium avium* complex (if CD4 less than 100)
  - Endoscopy if blood/stool studies unrevealing: small bowel and colon biopsies for MAC, lymphoma, histoplasma, microsporidia, cytomegalovirus, or KS
- Hepatitis: *Mycobacterium avium complex*, HAV, HBV, HCV, fungal or protozoan infection
- HIV cholangiopathy
  - Diagnosis with ERCP
  - Treat with HAART therapy and sphincterotomy; pathogen-directed therapy of no benefit
- Chronic acalculous cholecystitis: CD4 less than 100
  - Diagnosis: HIDA scan with nonvisualization of gallbladder
  - Treatment: cholecystectomy
- Anal warts: treat with podofyllin or 5-fluorouracil
- Proctitis: herpes simplex virus, cytomegalovirus, chlamydia or gonococcal infections, and campylobacte

4. <u>COMPLICATIONS</u>

- Diarrhea: malabsorption/malnutrition, weight loss, electrolyte abnormalities, dyschezia
- Hepatitis: cirrhosis/end-stage liver disease, ascites, SBP, HCV/HIV coinfection increases risk of hepatic steatosis → steatohepatitis → cirrhosis

OCULAR INFECTIONS

1. <u>PATHOPHYSIOLOGY</u>

- CMV retinitis: necrotic inflammation causes perivascular hemorrhage and exudates, which lead to patchy, permanent vision loss

2. <u>CLINICAL PRESENTATION</u>

- Herpes zoster ophthalmicus: shingles involving the ophthalmic distribution of trigeminal nerve
- Kaposi's sarcoma: asymptomatic, mimicking a chalazion or subconjunctival hemorrhage
- Molluscum contagiosum: small, painless umbilicated lesions; may involve the eyelid
- Keratitis: visual loss
- Retinitis: floaters, photopsias, visual-field changes, blurry vision
- Uveitis: syphilis, Tb, or medications (e.g., rifabutin)

3. <u>TREATMENT</u>

- Chorioretinitis: commonly CMV, less likely toxoplasma or syphilis, rarely TB or lymphoma
- CMV retinitis
  - Induction therapy: IV ganciclovir 5 mg/kg bid, foscarnet 90 mg/kg bid or valganciclovir 900 mg PO bid × 14–21 days
  - Maintenance therapy: intravitreal ganciclovir implant or valganciclovir 900 mg PO bid
- Toxoplasma chorioretinitis (rare): treat with pyrimethamine 200 mg PO × 1, then 75 mg/day, sulfadiazine 1–1.5 g PO qid, and folinic acid 20 mg PO 3 × per week
  - Prednisone 1 mg/kg/day tapering over 1-2 weeks for vision-threatening disease

4. <u>COMPLICATIONS</u>

- Inflammatory changes such as keratitis/vasculitis, iritis/uveitis, ischemic papilitis/optic neuritis, retinitis, encephalitis
- Nerve damage such as cranial nerve palsy
- Blindness
- See **Table 43.3**

ABLE 43.3.   Treatment of AIDS-Associated Opportunistic Infections in Adults and Adolescents

Opportunistic Infection	Preferred Therapy, Duration of Therapy, Chronic Maintenance	Alternative Therapy	Other Options/Issues

Pneumocystis pneumonia (PCP)	Preferred treatment for moderate-to-severe PCP
	• Trimethoprim-sulfamethoxazole (TMP-SMX): [15–20 mg TMP and 75–100 mg SMX]/kg/day IV administered q 6 h or q 8 h (AI), may switch to PO after clinical improvement (AI)
	• Duration of therapy: 21 days (AII)
		Alternative therapy for moderate-to-severe PCP
		• Pentamidine 4 mg/kg IV daily infused over greater than or equal to 60 minutes (AI), certain specialists reduce dose to 3 mg/kg IV daily because of toxicities (BI); or
		• Primaquine 15–30 mg (base) PO daily plus clindamycin 600–900 mg IV q 6 h to q 8 h or clindamycin 300–450 mg PO q 6 h to q 8 h (AI)
			Indications for corticosteroids (AI)
			PaO_2 less than 70 mmHg at room air or alveolar-arterial O_2 gradient greater than 35 mmHg
			Prednisone doses (beginning as early as possible and within 72 hours of PCP therapy) (AI):
			  Days 1–5 : 40 mg PO bid
			  Days 6–10 : 40 mg PO daily
			  Days 11–21 : 20 mg PO daily
			IV methylprednisolone can be administered as 75% of prednisone dose
			Benefits of corticosteroid if started after 72 hours of treatment is unknown, but a majority of clinicians will use it in patients with moderate-to-severe PCP (BIII)
			Whenever possible, patients should be tested for G6PD deficiency before use of primaquine

	Preferred treatment for mild-to-moderate PCP • Same daily dose of TMP-SMX as above, administered PO in 3 divided doses (AI); or • TMP-SMX (160 mg/800 mg or DS) 2 tablets tid (AI) • Duration of therapy: 21 days (AII)	Alternative therapy for mild-to-moderate PCP • Dapsone 100 mg PO daily and TMP 15 mg/kg/day PO (3 divided dose) (BI); or • Primaquine 15–30 mg (base) PO daily plus clindamycin 300–450 mg PO q 6–8 h (BI); or • Atovaquone 750 mg PO bid with food (BI)	
	Preferred secondary prophylaxis • TMP-SMX (160 mg/800 mg or DS) tablet PO daily (AI); or • TMP-SMX (80 mg/400 mg or SS) tablet PO daily (AI)	Alternative secondary prophylaxis • TMP-SMX (160 mg/800 mg or DS) PO tiw (BI) • Dapsone 50 mg PO bid or 100 mg PO daily (BI); or • Dapsone 50 mg PO daily plus pyrimethamine 50 mg PO weekly plus leucovorin 25 mg PO weekly (BI); or • Dapsone 200 mg PO plus pyrimethamine 75 mg PO plus leucovorin 25 mg PO weekly (BI); or • Aerosolized pentamidine 300 mg every month via Respirgard II™ nebulizer (BI); or • Atovaquone 1500 mg PO daily (BI); or • Atovaquone 1500 mg + pyrimethamine 25 mg + leucovorin 10 mg PO daily (CIII)	

(Continued)

TABLE 43.3. *(Continued)*

Opportunistic Infection	Preferred Therapy, Duration of Therapy, Chronic Maintenance	Alternative Therapy	Other Options/Issues
Toxoplasma gondii encephalitis (TE)	**Preferred therapy** • Pyrimethamine 200 mg PO x 1, then 50 mg (less than 60 kg) to 75 mg (greater than or equal to 60 kg) PO daily plus sulfadiazine 1000 mg (less than 60 kg) to 1500 mg (greater than or equal to 60 kg) PO q 6 h plus leucovorin 10–25 mg PO daily (can increase 50 mg) (AI) **Duration for acute therapy** • At least 6 weeks (BII); longer duration if clinical or radiologic disease is extensive or response is incomplete at 6 weeks	**Alternative therapy regimens** • Pyrimethamine (leucovorin)* plus clindamycin 600 mg IV or PO q 6 h [AI]; or • TMP-SMX (5 mg/kg TMP and 25 mg/kg SMX) IV or PO bid (BI); or • Atovaquone 1500 mg PO bid with food (or nutritional supplement) plus pyrimethamine (leucovorin)* (BII); or • Atovaquone 1500 mg PO bid with food (or nutritional supplement) plus sulfadiazine 1000–1500 mg PO q 6 h (BII); or • Atovaquone 1500 mg PO bid with food (BII); or • Pyrimethamine (leucovorin)* plus azithromycin 900–1200 mg PO daily (BII)	Adjunctive corticosteroids (e.g., dexamethasone) should be administered only for treatment of mass effect attributed to focal lesions or associated edema (BIII); discontinue as soon as clinically feasible Anticonvulsants should be administered to patients with a history of seizures (AIII) and continued through the acute treatment, but should not be used prophylactically (DIII)
	Preferred chronic maintenance therapy • Pyrimethamine 25–50 mg PO daily plus sulfadiazine 2000–4000 mg PO daily (in two to four divided doses) plus leucovorin 10–25 mg PO daily (AI)	**Alternative chronic maintenance therapy/ secondary prophylaxis** • Clindamycin 600 mg PO every 8 hours plus pyrimethamine 25–50 mg PO daily plus leucovorin 10–25 PO daily (BI) (should add additional agent to prevent PCP [AII]); or • Atovaquone 750 mg PO every 6–12 hours +/- ([pyrimethamine 25 mg PO daily plus leucovorin 10 mg PO daily] or sulfadiazine 2000–4000 mg PO) daily (BII)	
Cryptosporidiosis	**Preferred therapy** • Initiate or optimize ART for immune restoration (AII) • Symptomatic treatment of diarrhea (AIII) • Aggressive oral or IV rehydration and replacement of electrolyte loss (AIII)	**Alternative therapy for cryptosporidiosis** • A trial of nitazoxanide 500–1000 mg PO bid with food for 14 days (CIII) + optimized ART, symptomatic treatment and rehydration and electrolyte replacement	Use of antimotility agents such as loperamide or tincture of opium might palliate symptoms (BIII)

(Continued)

TABLE 43.3. *(Continued)*

Opportunistic Infection	Preferred Therapy, Duration of Therapy, Chronic Maintenance	Alternative Therapy	Other Options/Issues
Microsporidiosis	Initiate or optimize ART; immune restoration to CD4+ count greater than 100 cells/μL is associated with resolution of symptoms of enteric microsporidiosis (AII)		Severe dehydration, malnutrition, and wast-ing should be managed by fluid support and nutritional supplement (AIII) Antimotility agents can be used for diarrhea control if required (BIII)
	Preferred therapy for gastrointestinal infections caused by *Enterocytozoon bienuesi* • Fumagillin 20 mg PO tid (not available in the US) (BII) • TNP-470 (a synthetic analog of fumagillin) might also be effective (not available in the US) (BIII)	Alternative therapy for gastrointestinal infections caused by *E. bienuesi* • Nitazoxanide 1000 mg bid with food for 60 days; effects might be minimal for patients with low CD4+ count (CIII)	
	Preferred therapy for disseminated (not ocular) and intestinal infection attributed to microsporidia other than *E. bienuesi* and *Vittaforma corneae* • Albendazole 400 mg PO bid (AII), continue until CD4+ count greater than 200 cells/μL for greater than 6 months after initiation of ART (BIII)	Alternative therapy for disseminated disease • Itraconazole 400 mg PO daily plus albendazole 400 mg PO bid for disseminated disease attributed to trachipleistophora or anncaliia (CIII)	
	For ocular infection • Topical fumagillin bicylohexylammonium (Fumidil B) 3 mg/mL in saline (fumagillin 70 μg/mL) eye drops: 2 drops every 2 hours for 4 days, then 2 drops qid (investigational use only in the US) (BII) plus albendazole 400 mg PO bid for management of systemic infection (BIII) • Treatment should be continued indefinitely to prevent recurrence or relapse (BIII)		

(Continued)

TABLE 43.3. *(Continued)*

Opportunistic Infection	Preferred Therapy, Duration of Therapy, Chronic Maintenance	Alternative Therapy	Other Options/Issues
Mycobacterium tuberculosis (TB)	Empiric treatment should be initiated and continued in HIV-infected persons in whom TB is suspected until all diagnostic workup is complete (AII)		Directly observed therapy (DOT) is recommended for all HIV patients undergoing treatment for active TB (AII)
—	Treatment of drug-susceptible active TB disease Initial phase (2 months) (AI) Isoniazid (INH)† + [rifampin (RIF) or rifabutin (RFB)] + pyrazinamide (PZA) + ethambutol (EMB); if drug susceptibility report shows sensitivity to INH and RIF and PZA, then EMB may be discontinued before 2 months of treatment are completed (AI) Continuation phase • INH + (RIF or RFB) daily or tiw (AIII) or biw (if CD4+ count greater than 100/μL) (CIII) Duration of therapy Pulmonary TB: 6 months (AI) Pulmonary TB with cavitary lung lesions and (+) culture after 2 months of TB treatment (AII): 9 months Extrapulmonary TB w/ CNS, bone, or joint infections: 9 to 12 months (AII) Extrapulmonary TB in other sites: 6–9 months (AII)	Treatment for drug-resistant active TB Resistant to INH • Discontinue INH (and streptomycin, if used) • (RIF or RFB) + EMB + PZA for 6 months (BII); or • (RIF or RFB) + EMB for 12 months (preferably with PZA during at least the first 2 months) (BII) • A fluoroquinolone may strengthen the regimen for patients with extensive disease (CIII) Resistant to rifamycins • INH + PZA + EMB + a fluoroquinolone for 2 months, followed by 10–16 additional months with INH + EMB + fluoroquinolone (BIII) • Amikacin or capreomycin may be included in the first 2–3 months for patients with rifamycin resistance and severe disease (CIII) Multidrug resistant (MDR, i.e., INH- and RIF-resistant) or extensively drug resistant (XDR: i.e., resistance to INH and RIF, fluoroquinolone and at least 1 injectable agent) TB • Therapy should be individualized based on resistance pattern and with close consultation with experienced specialist (AIII)	Initial phase of TB treatment may also be administered 5 days weekly (40 doses) (AII), or tiw (24 doses) (BII) by DOT For CNS disease, corticosteroid should be initiated as early as possible and continued for 6–8 weeks (AII) RIF is not recommended for patients receiving HIV protease inhibitors (PI) because of its induction of PI metabolism (EII) RFB is a less potent CYP3A4 inducer than RIF and is preferred in patients receiving PIs Rifapentine administered once weekly can result in development of resistance in HIV-infected patients and is not recommended (EI) Therapeutic drug monitoring should be considered in patients receiving rifamycin and interacting ART Paradoxical reaction that is not severe may be treated with nonsteroidal anti-inflammatory drugs (NSAIDs) without a change in anti-TB or anti-HIV therapy (BIII) For severe paradoxical reaction, may consider prednisone or methylprednisolone 1 mg/kg of body weight, gradually reduced after 1–2 weeks (BIII)

(Continued)

BLE 43.3. *(Continued)*

pportunistic fection	Preferred Therapy, Duration of Therapy, Chronic Maintenance	Alternative Therapy	Other Options/Issues
Disseminated *Mycobacterium avium* complex (MAC) disease	Preferred therapy for disseminated MAC At least 2 drugs as initial therapy with • Clarithromycin 500 mg PO bid (AI) + ethambutol 15 mg/kg PO daily (AI) Addition of rifabutin may also be considered • Rifabutin 300 mg PO daily (dosage adjusted may be necessary based on drug–drug interactions) (CI)	Alternative therapy for disseminated MAC (e.g., when drug interactions or intolerance precludes the use of clarithromycin) • Azithromycin 500–600 mg + ethambutol 15 mg/kg PO daily (AII) Addition of a third or fourth drug should be considered for patients with advanced immunosuppression (CD4+ count less than 50 cells/µL), high mycobacterial loads (greater than 2 log CFU/mL of blood), or in the absence of effective ART (CIII) • Amikacin 10–15 mg/kg IV daily; or • Streptomycin 1 g IV or IM daily; or • Ciprofloxacin 500–750 mg PO bid; or • Levofloxacin 500 mg PO daily; or • Moxifloxacin 400 mg PO daily	Testing of susceptibility to clarithromycin and azithromycin is recommended (BIII) In ART-naïve patients, may consider with-holding initiation of ART until after 2 weeks of MAC treatment to lessen drug interactions, reduce pill burden, and potentially lower occurrence of IRIS (CIII) NSAIDs may be used for patients who experience moderate-to-severe symptoms attributed to ART-associated IRIS (CIII) If immune reconstitution inflammatory syndrome (IRIS) symptoms persist, short term (4–8 weeks) of systemic corticosteroid (equivalent to 20–40 mg of prednisone) can be used (CIII)
	Chronic maintenance therapy (secondary prophylaxis) • Same as treatment drugs and regimens Duration: lifelong therapy (AII), unless in patients with sustained immune recovery on ART (BII)		

(Continued)

TABLE 43.3. *(Continued)*

Opportunistic Infection	Preferred Therapy, Duration of Therapy, Chronic Maintenance	Alternative Therapy	Other Options/Issues
Bacterial respiratory diseases	Preferred empiric outpatient therapy (oral) • A β-lactam plus a macrolide (azithromycin or clarithromycin) (AII) *Preferred β-lactams:* • High-dose amoxicillin or amoxicillin/clavulanate *Alternative β-lactams:* • Cefpodoxime or cefuroxime	Alternative empiric outpatient therapy (oral) • A β-lactam plus doxycycline (CIII) *For penicillin-allergic patients or those with β-lactam use in prior 3 months:* • A respiratory fluoroquinolone (levofloxacin 750 mg/day, gemifloxacin, or moxifloxacin) (AII)	Patients receiving macrolide for MAC prophylaxis should not receive macrolide monotherapy for empiric treatment of bacterial pneumonia Fluoroquinolones should be used with caution in patients where TB is suspected but is not being treated Empiric therapy with a macrolide alone is not routinely recommended, because of increasing pneumococcal resistance (DIII) Once the pathogen has been identified by a reliable microbiologic method, antibiotics should be directed at the pathogen (BIII) For patients begun on IV antibiotic therapy, switching to PO should be considered when patient is clinically improved and able to tolerate oral medications Chemoprophylaxis may be considered for patients with frequent recurrences of serious bacterial respiratory infections (CIII) Clinicians should be cautious of using antibiotics to prevent recurrences because of the potential for developing drug resistance and drug toxicities
	Preferred empiric therapy for non-ICU inpatient • A β-lactam (IV) plus a macrolide (AII) *Preferred β-lactams:* • Cefotaxime, ceftriaxone, or ampicillin-sulbactam	Alternative empiric therapy for non-ICU inpatient • A β-lactam (IV) plus doxycycline (CIII) *For penicillin-allergic patients or those with β-lactam use in prior 3 months:* • An IV respiratory fluoroquinolone (levofloxacin 750 mg or moxifloxacin) (AII)	
	Preferred empiric ICU inpatient therapy • A β-lactam (IV) plus azithromycin IV (AII) or an IV respiratory fluoroquinolone (levofloxacin 750 mg or moxifloxacin) (AII) *Preferred β-lactams:* • Cefotaxime, ceftriaxone, or ampicillin-sulbactam	Alternative empiric ICU therapy *For penicillin-allergic patients or those with β-lactam use in prior 3 months:* • Aztreonam IV plus an IV respiratory fluoroquinolone (BIII)	
	Preferred empiric Pseudomonas therapy (if risks present) • An antipneumococcal, antipseudomonal β-lactam plus either ciprofloxacin or levofloxacin 750 mg/day (BIII) *Preferred β-lactams:* • Piperacillin-tazobactam, cefepime, imipenem, or meropenem	Alternative empiric *Pseudomonas* therapy • An antipneumococcal, antipseudomonal β-lactam plus an aminoglycoside plus azithromycin (BIII) • Above β-lactam plus an aminoglycoside plus an antipneumococcal fluoroquinolone* (BIII) *For penicillin-allergic patients or those with β-lactam use in prior 3 months:* • Replace the β-lactam with aztreonam (BIII)	
	Preferred empiric methicillin-resistant *Staphylococcus aureus* (if risks present) • Add vancomycin (possibly plus clindamycin) or linezolid alone to above (BIII)		

(Continu

TABLE 43.3. *(Continued)*

Opportunistic Infection	Preferred Therapy, Duration of Therapy, Chronic Maintenance	Alternative Therapy	Other Options/Issues
Bacterial enteric infections: Salmonellosis	Most specialists recommend treatment for all HIV-infected patients with salmonellosis due to the high risk of bacteremia in these patients (BIII)		The role of long-term secondary prophylaxis for patients with recurrent bacteremia is not well established; must weigh the benefit against the risks of long-term antibiotic exposure
	Preferred therapy for *Salmonella* gastroenteritis with or without symptomatic bacteremia • Ciprofloxacin 500–750 mg PO bid (or 400 mg IV bid) (AIII) Duration for mild gastroenteritis with or without bacteremia • If CD4+ count greater than or equal to 200/μL: 7–14 days (BIII) • If CD4+ count less than 200/μL: 2–6 weeks (CIII) • If recurrent symptomatic septicemia: may need 6 months or more (CIII)	Alternative therapy for *Salmonella* gastroenteritis with or without symptomatic bacteremia • Levofloxacin 750 mg or moxifloxacin (BIII) • TMP-SMX PO or IV (BIII), if susceptible • Third-generation cephalosporin such as ceftriaxone (IV) or cefotaxime (IV) (BIII), if susceptible	
Bacterial enteric infections: Shigellosis	Preferred therapy for *Shigella* infection • Fluoroquinolone IV or PO (AIII) Duration of therapy • For gastroenteritis: 3–7 days (AIII) • For bacteremia: 14 days (BIII)	Alternative therapy depending on antibiotic susceptibility *For gastroenteritis* • TMP-SMX DS 1 tab PO bid for 3–7 days (BIII); or • Azithromycin 500 mg PO on day 1, then 250 mg PO daily for 4 days (BIII)	Therapy is indicated both to shorten the duration of illness and to prevent spread of infection (AIII) *Shigella* infections acquired outside of the United States have high rates of TMP-SMX resistance
Bacterial enteric infections: Campylobacteriosis	For mild disease • Might withhold therapy unless symptoms persist for several days For mild to moderate disease • Ciprofloxacin 500 mg PO bid (BIII); or • Azithromycin 500 mg PO daily (BIII) • Consider addition of an aminoglycoside in bacteremic patients (CIII) Duration of therapy • Mild to moderate disease 7 days (BIII) • Bacteremia: at least 2 weeks (BIII)		There is an increasing rate of fluoroquinolone resistance; antimicrobial therapy should be modified based on susceptibility reports

TABLE 43.3. *(Continued)*

Opportunistic Infection	Preferred Therapy, Duration of Therapy, Chronic Maintenance	Alternative Therapy	Other Options/Issues
Bartonella infections	Preferred therapy for bacillary angiomatosis, peliosis hepatis, bacteremia, and osteomyelitis • Erythromycin 500 mg PO or IV qid (AII); or • Doxycycline 100 mg PO or IV q12h (AII) Duration of therapy: at least 3 months (AII) CNS infections and severe infections • Doxycycline 100 mg PO or IV q 12 h +/-rifampin 300 mg PO or IV q 12 h (AIII) Duration of therapy: 4 months (AII) Long-term suppression • With a macrolide or doxycycline for patients with relapse or reinfection as long as the CD4+ count remains less than 200 cells/μL (AIII)	Alternative therapy for bacillary angiomatosis infections, peliosis hepatis, bacteremia, and osteomyelitis • Azithromycin 500 mg PO daily (BIII) • Clarithromycin 500 mg PO bid (BIII)	Severe Jarisch-Herxheimer-like reaction can occur in the first 48 hours of treatment
Treponema pallidum infection (syphilis)	Preferred therapy early stage (primary, secondary, and early-latent syphilis) • Benzathine penicillin G 2.4 million units IM for 1 dose (AII)	Alternative therapy early stage (primary, secondary, and early-latent syphilis) (BIII) *For penicillin-allergic patients:* • Doxycycline 100 mg PO bid for 14 days (BIII); or • Ceftriaxone 1 g IM or IV daily for 8–10 days (BIII); or • Azithromycin 2 g PO for 1 dose (CII)	The efficacy of non-penicillin alternatives has not been evaluated in HIV-infected patients and should be undertaken only with close clinical and serologic monitoring (BIII) Combination of procaine penicillin and probenecid is not recommended for patients with history of sulfa allergy (DIII) The Jarisch-Herxheimer reaction is an acute febrile reaction accompanied by headache and myalgias that might occur within the first 24 hours after therapy for syphilis
	Preferred therapy late-latent disease (greater than 1 year or of unknown duration, CSF examination ruled out neurosyphilis) • Benzathine penicillin G 2.4 million units IM weekly for 3 doses (AIII)	Alternative therapy late-latent disease (without CNS involvement) *For penicillin-allergic patients:* • Doxycycline 100 mg PO bid for 28 days (BIII)	

(Continued)

TABLE 43.3. *(Continued)*

Opportunistic Infection	Preferred Therapy, Duration of Therapy, Chronic Maintenance	Alternative Therapy	Other Options/Issues
	Preferred therapy late-stage (tertiary-cardiovascular or gummatous disease) • Rule out neurosyphilis before therapy with 3 doses of benzathine penicillin and obtain infectious diseases consultation to guide management (AIII)		
	Preferred therapy neurosyphilis (including otic and ocular disease) • Aqueous crystalline penicillin G, 18–24 million units per day, administered as 3–4 million units IV q 4 h or by continuous IV infusion for 10–14 days (AII) +/- benzathine penicillin G 2.4 million units IM weekly for 3 doses after completion of IV therapy (CIII)	Alternative therapy neurosyphilis • Procaine penicillin 2.4 million units IM daily plus probenecid 500 mg PO qid for 10–14 days (BII) +/- benzathine penicillin G 2.4 million units IM weekly for 3 doses after completion of above (CIII); or *For penicillin-allergic patients:* • Desensitization to penicillin is the preferred approach (BIII); if not feasible, • Ceftriaxone 2 grams IM or IV daily for 10–14 days (CIII)	
Candidiasis (mucosal)	Preferred therapy oropharyngeal candidiasis: initial episodes (7–14 day treatment) • Fluconazole 100 mg PO daily (AI); or • Clotrimazole troches 10 mg PO 5 times daily (BII); or • Nystatin suspension 4–6 mL qid or 1–2 flavored pastilles 4–5 times daily (BII) • Miconazole mucoadhesive tablet PO daily (BII)	Alternative therapy oropharyngeal candidiasis: initial episodes (7–14 day treatment) • Itraconazole oral solution 200 mg PO daily (BI); or • Posaconazole oral solution 400 mg PO bid x 1, then 400 mg daily (BI)	Chronic or prolonged use of azoles might promote development of resistance Higher relapse rate of esophageal candidiasis with echinocandins than with fluconazole has been reported Patients with fluconazole refractory oropharyngeal or esophageal candidiasis who responded to echinocandin should be started on voriconazole or posaconazole for secondary prophylaxis until ART produces immune reconstitution (CI)

(Continued)

TABLE 43.3. *(Continued)*

Opportunistic Infection	Preferred Therapy, Duration of Therapy, Chronic Maintenance	Alternative Therapy	Other Options/Issues
	Preferred therapy esophageal candidiasis (14–21 days) • Fluconazole 100 mg (up to 400 mg) PO or IV daily (AI) • Itraconazole oral solution 200 mg PO daily (AI)	Alternative therapy esophageal candidiasis (14–21 days) • Voriconazole 200 mg PO or IV bid (BI) • Posaconazole 400 mg PO bid (BI) • Caspofungin 50 mg IV daily (BI) • Micafungin 150 mg IV daily (BI) • Anidulafungin 100 mg IV x 1, then 50 mg IV daily (BI) • Amphotericin B deoxycholate 0.6 mg/kg IV daily (BI)	Suppressive therapy is usually not recommended (DIII) unless patients have frequent or severe recurrences. If decision is to use suppressive therapy: Oropharyngeal candidiasis • Fluconazole 100 mg PO tiw (BI) • Itraconazole oral solution 200 mg PO daily (CI) Esophageal candidiasis • Fluconazole 100–200 mg PO daily (BI) • Posaconazole 400 mg PO bid (BII) Vulvovaginal candidiasis • Fluconazole 150 mg PO once weekly (CII) • Daily topical azole (CII)
	Preferred therapy uncomplicated vulvovaginal candidiasis • Oral fluconazole 150 mg for 1 dose (AII) • Topical azoles (clotrimazole, butoconazole, miconazole, tioconazole, or terconazole) for 3–7 days (AII)	Alternative therapy uncomplicated vulvovaginal candidiasis • Itraconazole oral solution 200 mg PO daily for 3–7 days (BII)	
	Preferred therapy fluconazole-refractory oropharyngeal candidiasis or esophageal candidiasis • Itraconazole oral solution greater than or equal to 200 mg PO daily (AII) • Posaconazole oral solution 400 mg PO bid (AII)	Alternative therapy fluconazole-refractory oropharyngeal candidiasis or esophageal candidiasis • Amphotericin B deoxycholate 0.3 mg/kg IV daily (BII) • Lipid formulation of amphotericin B 3–5 mg/kg IV daily (BII) • Anidulafungin 100 mg IV x 1, then 50 mg IV daily (BII) • Caspofungin 50 mg IV daily (CII) • Micafungin 150 mg IV daily (CII) • Voriconazole 200 mg PO or IV bid (CIII) Fluconazole-refractory oropharyngeal candidiasis (not esophageal) • Amphotericin B oral suspension 100 mg/ mL (not available in the US) – 1 mL PO qid (CIII)	

(Continued)

TABLE 43.3. *(Continued)*

Opportunistic Infection	Preferred Therapy, Duration of Therapy, Chronic Maintenance	Alternative Therapy	Other Options/Issues
	Preferred therapy complicated (severe or recurrent) vulvovaginal candidiasis • Fluconazole 150 mg q 72 h x 2–3 doses (AII) • Topical antifungal 7 or more days (AII)		
Cryptococcal meningitis	Preferred induction therapy • Amphotericin B deoxycholate 0.7 mg/kg IV daily plus flucytosine 100 mg/kg PO daily in 4 divided doses for at least 2 weeks (AI); or • Lipid formulation amphotericin B 4–6 mg/kg IV daily (consider for persons who have renal dysfunction on therapy or have high likelihood of renal failure) plus flucytosine 100 mg/kg PO daily in 4 divided doses for at least 2 weeks (AII)	Alternative induction therapy • Amphotericin B (deoxycholate or lipid for-mulation, dose as preferred therapy) plus fluconazole 400 mg PO or IV daily (BII) • Amphotericin B (deoxycholate or lipid formulation, dose as preferred therapy) alone (BII) • Fluconazole 400–800 mg/day (PO or IV) plus flucytosine 100 mg/kg PO daily in 4 divided doses for 4–6 weeks (CII): for persons unable to tolerate or unresponsive to amphotericin B	Addition of flucytosine to amphotericin B has been associated with more rapid sterilization of CSF and decreased risk for subsequent relapse Patients receiving flucytosine should have blood levels monitored; peak level 2 hours after dose should not exceed 75 μg/mL Dosage should be adjusted in patients with renal insufficiency Opening pressure should always be measured when a lumbar puncture (LP) is performed (AII). Repeated LPs or CSF shunting are essential to effectively manage increased intracranial pressure (BIII)
	Preferred consolidation therapy (after at least 2 weeks of successful induction: defined as significant clinical improvement and negative CSF culture) • Fluconazole 400 mg PO daily for 8 weeks (AI)	Alternative consolidation therapy • Itraconazole 200 mg PO bid for 8 weeks (BI), or until CD4+ count greater than or equal to 200 cells/μL for greater than 6 months as a result of ART (BII)	
	Preferred maintenance therapy • Fluconazole 200 mg PO daily (AI) lifelong or until CD4+ count greater than or equal to 200 cells/μL for greater than 6 months as a result of ART (BII)	Alternative maintenance therapy • Itraconazole 200 mg PO daily lifelong unless immune reconstitution as a result of potent ART: for patients intolerant of or who failed fluconazole (BI)	

(Continued)

TABLE 43.3. *(Continued)*

Opportunistic Infection	Preferred Therapy, Duration of Therapy, Chronic Maintenance	Alternative Therapy	Other Options/Issues
Histoplasma capsulatum infections	Preferred therapy for moderately severe–to–severe disseminated disease *Induction therapy* (for 2 weeks or until clinically improved) • Liposomal amphotericin B at 3 mg/kg IV daily (AI) *Maintenance therapy* • Itraconazole 200 mg PO tid for 3 days, then bid (AII)	Alternative therapy moderately severe–to–severe disseminated disease *Induction therapy* (for 2 weeks or until clinically improved) • Amphotericin B deoxycholate 0.7 mg/kg IV daily (BI) • Amphotericin B lipid complex 5 mg/kg IV daily (CIII) *Maintenance therapy* • same as "Preferred therapy"	
	Preferred therapy for less severe disseminated disease *Induction and maintenance therapy* • Itraconazole 200 mg PO tid for 3 days, then 200 mg PO bid (AII) Duration of therapy: at least 12 months Preferred therapy for meningitis *Induction therapy (4–6 weeks)* • Liposomal amphotericin B 5 mg/kg/day (AII) *Maintenance therapy* • Itraconazole 200 mg PO bid–tid for at least 1 year and until resolution of abnormal CSF findings (AII)		
	Preferred therapy for long term suppression therapy In patients with severe disseminated or CNS infection (AII) and in patients who relapse despite appropriate therapy (CIII) • Itraconazole 200 mg PO daily		

(Continued)

ABLE 43.3. *(Continued)*

Opportunistic Infection	Preferred Therapy, Duration of Therapy, Chronic Maintenance	Alternative Therapy	Other Options/Issues
Coccidioidomycosis	Preferred therapy for mild infections (focal pneumonia or positive coccidiodal serologic test alone) • Fluconazole 400 mg PO daily (BII); or • Itraconazole 200 mg PO tid x 3 days, then 200 mg bid (BII)		Certain patients with meningitis may develop hydrocephalus and require CSF shunting Therapy should be continued indefinitely for patients with diffuse pulmonary or disseminated diseases as relapse can occur in 25%–33% in HIV-negative patients (AIII) Therapy should be lifelong in patients with meningeal infections as relapse occurred in 80% of HIV-infected patients after discontinuation of triazole therapy (AII) Case reports of successful therapy with voriconazole and posaconazole are available
	Preferred therapy for severe, nonmeningeal infection (diffuse pulmonary or severely ill patients with extrathoracic disseminated disease): acute phase • Amphotericin B deoxycholate 0.7–1.0 mg/kg IV daily (AII) • Lipid formulation amphotericin B 4–6 mg/kg IV daily (AIII) Duration of therapy: until clinical improvement, then switch to azole	Alternative therapy for severe nonmeningeal infection (diffuse pulmonary or disseminated disease): acute phase • Certain specialists add triazole to amphotericin B therapy and continue triazole once amphotericin B is stopped (BIII)	
	Preferred therapy for meningeal infections • Fluconazole 400–800 mg PO or IV daily (AII)	Alternative therapy for meningeal infections • Itraconazole 200 mg PO tid x 3 days, then 200 mg PO bid (BII) • Intrathecal amphotericin B when triazole antifungals are not effective (AIII)	
	Maintenance therapy (for all cases) • Fluconazole 400 mg PO daily (AII); or • Itraconazole 200 mg PO bid (AII)		
Aspergillosis, invasive	Preferred therapy • Voriconazole 6 mg/kg q 12 h x 1 day, then 4 mg/kg q 12 h IV (BIII), followed by voriconazole PO 200 mg q 12 h after clinical improvement Duration of therapy: until CD4+ count greater than 200 cells/μL and with evidence of clinical response	Alternative therapy • Amphotericin B deoxycholate 1 mg/kg/day IV (AIII); or • Lipid formulation of amphotericin B 5 mg/kg/day IV (AIII) • Caspofungin 70 mg IV x 1, then 50 mg IV daily (BII) • Posaconazole 400 mg bid PO (BII)	Potential for significant pharmacokinetic interactions between PIs or NNRTIs with voriconazole; it should be used cautiously in these situations. Consider therapeutic drug monitoring and dosage adjustment if necessary.

(Continued)

TABLE 43.3. *(Continued)*

Opportunistic Infection	Preferred Therapy, Duration of Therapy, Chronic Maintenance	Alternative Therapy	Other Options/Issues
Cytomegalovirus (CMV) disease	Preferred therapy for CMV retinitis *For immediate sight-threatening lesions* • Ganciclovir intraocular implant + valganciclovir 900 mg PO (bid for 14–21 days, then once daily) (AI) • One dose of intravitreal ganciclovir may be administered immediately after diagnosis until ganciclovir implant can be placed (CIII) *For small peripheral lesions* • Valganciclovir 900 mg PO bid for 14–21 days, then 900 mg PO daily (BII)	Alternative therapy for CMV retinitis • Ganciclovir 5 mg/kg IV q 12 h for 14–21 days, then 5 mg/kg IV daily (AI); or • Ganciclovir 5 mg/kg IV q 12 h for 14–21 days, then valganciclovir 900 mg PO daily (AI); or • Foscarnet 60 mg/kg IV q 8 h or 90 mg/kg IV q 12 h for 14–21 days, then 90–120 mg/kg IV q 24 h (AI); or • Cidofovir 5 mg/kg/week IV for 2 weeks, then 5 mg/kg every other week with saline hydration before and after therapy and probenecid 2 g PO 3 hours before the dose followed by 1 g PO 2 hours after the dose, and 1 g PO 8 hours after the dose (total of 4 g) (AI). Note: This regimen should be avoided in patients with sulfa allergy because of cross hypersensitivity with probenecid.	The choice of initial therapy for CMV retinitis should be individualized, based on location and severity of the lesion(s), level of immunosuppression, and other factors such as concomitant medications and ability to adhere to treatment (AIII) Initial therapy in patients with CMV retinitis, esophagitis, colitis, and pneumonitis should include initiation or optimization of ART (BII) In patients with CMV neurological disease, localized morbidity might occur because of IRIS, a brief delay in initiation of ART until clinical improvement might be prudent (CIII) Maintenance therapy for CMV retinitis can be safely discontinued in patients with inactive disease and sustained CD4+ count (more than 100 cells/mm³ for at least 3–6 months); consultation with ophthalmologist is advised (BII)
	Preferred chronic maintenance therapy (secondary prophylaxis) for CMV retinitis • Valganciclovir 900 mg PO daily (AI); or • Ganciclovir implant (may be replaced every 6–8 months if CD4+ count remains less then 100 cells/μL) + valganciclovir 900 mg PO daily until immune recovery (BIII)	Alternative chronic maintenance (secondary prophylaxis) for CMV retinitis • Ganciclovir 5 mg/kg IV 5–7 times weekly (AI); or • Foscarnet 90–120 mg/kg body weight IV once daily (AI); or • Cidofovir 5 mg/kg body weight IV every other week with saline hydration and probenecid as above (AI)	Patients with CMV retinitis who discontinued maintenance therapy should undergo regular eye examination, optimally every 3 months, for early detection of relapse or immune recovery uveitis (IRU) (AIII) IRU might develop in the setting of immune reconstitution Treatment of IRU: periocular corticosteroid or short courses of systemic steroid

(Continue.

TABLE 43.3. *(Continued)*

Opportunistic Infection	Preferred Therapy, Duration of Therapy, Chronic Maintenance	Alternative Therapy	Other Options/Issues
	Preferred therapy for CMV esophagitis or colitis • Ganciclovir IV or foscarnet IV for 21–28 days or until resolution of signs and symptoms (BII) • Oral valganciclovir may be used if symptoms are not severe enough to interfere with oral absorption (BII) • Maintenance therapy is usually not necessary, but should be considered after relapses (BII)		
	Preferred therapy CMV pneumonitis • Treatment should be considered in patients with histologic evidence of CMV pneumonitis and who do not respond to treatment of other pathogens (AIII) • The role of maintenance therapy has not been established (CIII)		
	Preferred therapy CMV neurological disease *Treatment should be initiated promptly* • Combination of ganciclovir IV + foscarnet IV to stabilize disease and maximize response, continue until symptomatic improvement (BII) • Maintenance therapy (with valganciclovir PO + IV foscarnet) should be continued for life unless evidence of immune recovery is evident (BII)		
Herpes simplex virus (HSV) disease	Preferred therapy for orolabial lesions and initial or recurrent genital HSV • Valacyclovir 1 g PO bid, famciclovir 500 mg PO bid, or acyclovir 400 mg PO tid (AI) Duration of therapy • Orolabial HSV: 5–10 days (AII) • Genital HSV: 5–14 days (AI)		

TABLE 43.3. *(Continued)*

Opportunistic Infection	Preferred Therapy, Duration of Therapy, Chronic Maintenance	Alternative Therapy	Other Options/Issues
	Preferred therapy for severe mucocutaneous HSV infections • Initial therapy acyclovir 5 mg/kg IV q 8 h (AII); • After lesions began to regress, change to PO therapy as above (AI); continue therapy until lesions have completely healed		
	Preferred therapy for acyclovir-resistant mucocutaneous HSV infections • Foscarnet 80–120 mg/kg/day IV in 2–3 divided doses until clinical response (AI)	Alternative therapy for acyclovir-resistant mucocutaneous HSV infections (CIII) • Topical trifluridine • Topical cidofovir • Topical imiquimod Duration of therapy: 21–28 days or longer	Topical formulations of neither trifluridine nor cidofovir are commercially available in the US Extemporaneous compounding of topical products can be prepared using trifluridine ophthalmic solution and the intravenous formulation of cidofovir
	Preferred therapy for HSV encephalitis • Acyclovir 10 mg/kg IV q 8 h for 21 days (AII)		
	Suppressive therapy (for patients with frequent or severe recurrences of genital herpes) (AI) • Valacyclovir 500 mg PO bid (AI) • Famciclovir 500 mg PO bid (AI) • Acyclovir 400 mg PO bid (AI)		
HHV-6 infection	If HHV-6 has been identified as cause of disease in HIV-infected patients, use same drugs and doses as treatment for CMV disease (CIII) • Ganciclovir (or valganciclovir) • Foscarnet		

(Continued)

TABLE 43.3. *(Continued)*

Opportunistic Infection	Preferred Therapy, Duration of Therapy, Chronic Maintenance	Alternative Therapy	Other Options/Issues
Varicella zoster virus (VZV) disease	Varicella (chickenpox) *Uncomplicated cases* • Acyclovir (20 mg/kg body weight up to a maximum of 800 mg PO 5x daily), valacyclovir 1000 mg PO tid, or famciclovir 500 mg PO tid x 5–7 days (AIII) *Severe or complicated cases* • Acyclovir 10–15 mg/kg IV q 8 h x 7–10 days (AIII) • May switch to oral acyclovir, famciclovir, or valacyclovir after defervescence if no evidence of visceral involvement is evident (AIII) Herpes zoster (shingles) *Acute localized dermatomal* • Valacyclovir 1g tid or famciclovir 500 mg tid, or acyclovir 800 mg PO 5x daily x 7–10 days (AII), longer duration should be considered if lesions are slow to resolve *Extensive cutaneous lesion or visceral involvement* • Acyclovir 10–15 mg/kg IV q 8 h until clinical improvement is evident (AII) • Switch to oral therapy (valacyclovir 1000 mg tid or famciclovir 500 mg tid, or acyclovir 800 mg PO 5x daily) after clinical improvement is evident, to complete a 10–14 day course (AIII) Progressive outer retinal necrosis (PORN) • Ganciclovir 5 mg/kg IV q12h, plus foscarnet 90 mg/kg IV q 12 h, plus ganciclovir 2 mg/0.05mL intravitreal twice weekly, and/or foscarnet 1.2 mg/0.05 mL intravitreal twice weekly (AIII) • Optimization of ART (AIII) Acute retinal necrosis (ARN) • Acyclovir 10 mg/kg IV q 8 h x 10–14 days, followed by valacyclovir 1000 mg PO tid x 6 weeks (AIII)	Infection caused by acyclovir-resistant VZV • Foscarnet 90 mg/kg IV q 12 h (AII)	Involvement of an experienced ophthalmologist with management of VZV retinitis is strongly recommended (AIII) Corticosteroid therapy for herpes zoster is not recommended (DIII)

(Continued)

TABLE 43.3. *(Continued)*

Opportunistic Infection	Preferred Therapy, Duration of Therapy, Chronic Maintenance	Alternative Therapy	Other Options/Issues
HHV-8 diseases *(Kaposi's Sarcoma [KS], primary effusion lymphoma [PEL], multicentric Castleman's disease [MCD])*	Initiation or optimization of ART should be done for all patients with KS, PEL, or MCD (BII) Preferred therapy for visceral KS (BII), disseminated cutaneous KS (CIII), and PEL (BIII) • Chemotherapy + ART (BII) • Oral valganciclovir or IV ganciclovir might be useful as adjunctive therapy in PEL (BII)		
	Preferred therapy for MCD • Valganciclovir 900 mg PO bid (BII); or • Ganciclovir 5 mg/kg IV q 12 h (BII)	Alternative therapy for MCD Rituximab, 375 mg/m² given weekly x 4–8 weeks, may be an alternative to antiviral therapy (BII)	
Human papillomavirus disease	Treatment of condyloma acuminata (genital warts)		
	Patient-applied therapy • Podofilox 0.5% solution or 0.5% gel: apply to all lesions bid x 3 consecutive days, followed by 4 days of no therapy, repeat weekly for up to 4 cycles (BIII); or • Imiquimod 5% cream: apply to lesion at bedtime 2nd and remove in the morning on 3 nonconsecutive nights weekly for up to 16 weeks; each treatment should be washed with soap and water 6–10 hours after application (BII)	Provider-applied therapy • Cryotherapy (liquid nitrogen or cryoprobe): apply until each lesion is thoroughly frozen; repeat every 1–2 weeks; some providers allow the lesion to thaw, then freeze a second time in each session (BIII) • Trichloroacetic acid or bicloroacetic acid cauterization: 80–90% aqueous solution; apply to each lesion, repeat weekly for 3–6 weeks (BIII) • Surgical excision (BIII) or laser surgery (CIII) • Podophyllin resin 10–25% suspension in tincture of benzoin: apply to all lesions, then wash off a few hours later, repeat weekly for 3–6 weeks (CIII)	Intralesional interferon-α is usually not recommended because of high cost, difficult administration, and potential for systemic side effects (DIII) The rate of recurrence of genital warts is high, despite treatment

(Continue.

TABLE 43.3. *(Continued)*

Opportunistic Infection	Preferred Therapy, Duration of Therapy, Chronic Maintenance	Alternative Therapy	Other Options/Issues
Hepatitis B virus (HBV) disease	Therapy for patients who require ART • Patients should be treated with agents active against both HIV and HBV or with agents with independent activity against each virus (CIII) • Consider tenofovir + emtricitabine as part of HIV and HBV regimen (CIII) *Lamivudine or emtricitabine-naïve patients* • [Lamivudine 150 mg PO bid (or 300 mg PO daily) or emtricitabine 200 mg PO daily] + tenofovir (TDF) 300 mg PO daily (CIII) (+ additional agent[s] active against HIV) *Lamivudine or emtricitabine-experienced patients with detectable HBV DNA (assume lamivudine-resistance)* • *If not on TDF:* add TDF 300 mg PO daily as part of an ART regimen + lamivudine or emtricitabine (CIII); or • Adefovir 10 mg PO daily + lamivudine or emtricitabine + other combination ART (BII); or • Entecavir 1 mg PO daily can be considered in patients with complete HIV suppression (while on ART) who do not demonstrate YMDD (M204V/I) motif mutations in HBV DNA (CIII) Duration of therapy: because of the high rates of relapse, certain specialists recommend continuing therapy indefinitely (CIII)	Treatment for patients who do not require ART • Use agents with sole activity against HBV and with the least potential of selecting HIV resistance mutations (BIII) • Consider early initiation of ART, especially for patients with high HBV DNA *For patients with CD4+ count greater than 350 cells/µL, HBeAg (-), HBV DNA greater than 2000 IU/mL (greater than 20,000 copies/mL)* • Adefovir 10 mg PO daily (CIII) *For patients with CD4+ count greater than 350 cells/µL, HBeAg (+), HBV DNA greater than 2000 IU/mL (greater than 200,000 copies/mL), and elevated ALT* • Peginterferon α-2a 180 µg SQ weekly (CIII) x 48 weeks: with careful follow-up of HBeAg conversion	Emtricitabine, entecavir, lamivudine, or tenofovir should not be used for the treatment of HBV infection in patients who are not receiving combination ART (EII) Among patients coinfected with HIV, HBV, and HCV, consideration of starting ART should be the first priority; if ART is not required, an interferon-based regimen, which suppresses both HCV and HBV, should be considered (CIII) If IFN-based treatment for HCV has failed, treatment of chronic HBV with nucleoside or nucleotide analogs is recommended (CIII) Cross-resistance to emtricitabine or telbivudine should be assumed in patients with suspected or proven 3TC resistance When changing ART regimens, continue agents with anti-HBV activity because of the risk of IRIS If anti-HBV therapy is discontinued and a flare occurs, therapy should be reinstituted, as it can be potentially life saving (BIII)

(Continued)

TABLE 43.3. *(Continued)*

Opportunistic Infection	Preferred Therapy, Duration of Therapy, Chronic Maintenance	Alternative Therapy	Other Options/Issues
Hepatitis C virus (HCV) disease	Genotype 1, 4, 5, or 6 (AI) • Peginterferon α 2a 180 μg SQ weekly, or • Peginterferon α 2b 1.5 mg/kg SQ weekly + • Ribavirin PO (wt-based dosing) (AII) less than 75 kg: 600 mg qAM and 400 mg qPM; at least 75 kg: 600 mg qAM and 600 mg qPM Genotype 2 or 3 (AI) • Peginterferon α 2a 180 μg SQ weekly, or • Peginterferon α 2b 1.5 mg/kg SQ weekly + • Ribavirin (fixed dose) PO 400 mg qAM and 400 mg qPM Duration of therapy: • 48 weeks: genotypes 1 or 4, 5, or 6 (AI) and genotypes 2 and 3 (BII) • At least 24 weeks – treatment of acute HCV infection (less than 6 months from HCV exposure) (BIII)	In patients for whom ribavirin is contraindicated (e.g., unstable cardiopulmonary disease, preexisting anemia unresponsive to erythropoietin, renal failure, or hemoglobinopathy) • Peginterferon α 2a 180 μg SQ weekly (AII), or • Peginterferon α 2b 1.5 μg/kg SQ weekly (AII) In patients with decompensated liver disease • Liver transplantation if feasible (CIII)	For patients with CD4+ count less than 200 cells/μL, initiation of ART may be considered before HCV treatment (CIII) Didanosine + ribavirin may lead to increased mitochondrial toxicities; concomitant use is contraindicated (EI) HCV therapy is not recommended in patients with hepatic decompensation; liver transplantation, if feasible, should be the primary treatment option (CIII) Interferon is abortifacient in high doses and ribavirin is teratogenic; HCV treatment is not recommended in pregnant women or women who are not willing to use birth control (EIII)
Progressive multifocal leukoencephalopathy (JC virus infections)	Initiate antiretroviral therapy in ART-naïve patients (AII) Optimize ART in patients who develop PML in phase of HIV viremia on antiretroviral therapy (AIII)		Some patients might experience a remission after initiation of ART; although their neurological deficits frequently persist, disease progression remits Corticosteroids may be used in patients with progressive clinical deficits and neuroimaging features suggesting inflammatory disease (e.g., edema, swelling, and contrast enhancement) as a result of initiating ART (BIII)

(Continued)

TABLE 43.3. *(Continued)*

Opportunistic Infection	Preferred Therapy, Duration of Therapy, Chronic Maintenance	Alternative Therapy	Other Options/Issues
	Geographic opportunistic infections of specific consideration		
Malaria			
Uncomplicated malaria from *Plasmodium falciparum* or unknown malaria species	Preferred therapy for chloroquine-sensitive infection (north of the Panama Canal) • Chloroquine phosphate 1000 mg PO (=600 mg chloroquine base) once, then 500 mg PO (=300 mg chloroquine base) at 6, 24, and 48 hours • Total dose = chloroquine phosphate 2500 mg	Alternative therapy for chloroquine-sensitive infection (north of the Panama Canal) No alternative listed	
	Preferred therapy for chloroquine-resistant infections (all other malaria areas or unknown region) • Atovaquone-proguanil (250 mg/100 mg): 4 tablet PO daily x 3 days	Alternative therapy for chloroquine-resistant infections (all other malaria areas or unknown region) • Mefloquine 750 mg PO x 1, then 500 mg administered 12 hrs later, total dose = 1250 mg • Quinine sulfate 650 mg PO q 8 h x 3 days (infections acquired outside of southeast Asia) to 7 days (infections acquired in southeast Asia) + (doxycycline 100 mg PO q 12 h x 7 days or clindamycin 20 mg base/kg/day [in 3 divided doses] PO x 7 days)	Treatment recommendations for HIV-infected patients are the same as HIV uninfected patients For most updated treatment recommenda-tions for specific region, clinicians should refer to the following web link: www.cdc.gov/malaria or call the CDC Malaria Hotline: 770-488-7788 (M-F 8 AM-4:30 PM ET) 770-488-7100 (after hours)
Severe malaria from all regions	Preferred therapy • Quinidine gluconate 10 mg/kg IV over 1–2 hours, then 0.02 mg/kg/min infusion (quinidine 6.25 mg base/kg IV over 1–2 hours, then 0.0125 mg/kg/min) for at least 24 hours with cardiac monitoring + • Doxycycline 100 mg PO or IV q 12 h x 7 days; or • Clindamycin 20 mg base/kg/day (in 3 divided doses) PO or 10 mg base/kg loading dose IV followed by 5 mg base/kg IV q 8 h; switch to PO clindamycin (dose as above) as soon as patient can take PO medication, for a total course of 7 days	Alternative therapy • Artesunate 2.4 mg/kg IV bolus at 0, 12, and 24 hours, then daily Duration of therapy: 7 days for Southeast Asia and Oceania and 3 days for other areas When able to take PO, switch to: • Atovaquone-proquanil, mefloquine, or doxycycline (doses as listed above)	Intravenous artesunate is available from CDC quarantine stations (CDC Malaria Hotline 770-488-7788)

(Continued)

TABLE 43.3. *(Continued)*

Opportunistic Infection	Preferred Therapy, Duration of Therapy, Chronic Maintenance	Alternative Therapy	Other Options/Issues
Malaria from: *P. vivax* *P. ovale* *P. malariae*	All regions use the following regimens (except for Papua New Guinea, and Indonesia, in which case treat as for chloroquine-resistant *P. falciparum* malaria as above) • Chloroquine phosphate 1000 mg PO x 1, then 500 mg PO at 6, 24, and 48 hours, total dose = 2500 mg; then • Antirelapse therapy (after checking G6PD status): primaquine 30 mg base PO daily x 14 days		G6PD status should be checked before initiation of primaquine
Penicilliosis	Acute infection in severely ill patients • Amphotericin B deoxycholate 0.6 mg/kg/day IV for 2 weeks; followed by itraconazole 400 mg PO daily for 10 weeks (AII) Mild disease • Itraconazole 400 mg PO daily for 8 weeks (BII) Chronic maintenance therapy (secondary prophylaxis) • Itraconazole 200 mg PO daily (AI)		ART should be administered according to standard of care in the community; consideration should be given to simultaneously initiating ART and treatment for penicilliosis (CIII)
Leishmaniasis, visceral	Preferred therapy for initial infection • Liposomal amphotericin B or amphotericin B lipid complex (AII) 2–4 mg/kg IV daily x 10 days; or interrupted schedule (e.g., 4 mg/kg on days 1–5, 10, 17, 24, 31, 38) to achieve total dose of 20–60 mg/kg (BII)	Alternative therapy for initial infection • Amphotericin B deoxycholate 0.5–1.0 mg/kg IV daily for total dose of 1.5–2.0 grams (BII); or • Sodium stibogluconate (pentavalent antimony) (AII) 20 mg/kg body weight IV or IM daily for 3–4 weeks (Contact the CDC Drug Service at 404-639-3670 or drugservice@cdc.gov)	ART should be initiated or optimized (AII) Parenteral paromomycin has been proven effective in HIV-negative patients in India, may be available as an alternative in India in the future (BI)
	Preferred chronic maintenance therapy (secondary prophylaxis): especially in patients with CD4+ count less than 200 cells/µL • Liposomal amphotericin B 4 mg/kg every 2–4 weeks (AII)	Alternative chronic maintenance therapy (secondary prophylaxis) • Amphotericin B lipid complex (AII) 3–4 mg/kg every 2–4 weeks (AII) • Sodium stibogluconate 20 mg/kg IV or IM every 4 weeks (AII)	Alternative regimens for treatment failure Miltefosine 100 mg PO daily for 4 weeks (available in Europe via compassionate use) (CIII)

(Continued)

TABLE 43.3. *(Continued)*

Opportunistic Infection	Preferred Therapy, Duration of Therapy, Chronic Maintenance	Alternative Therapy	Other Options/Issues
Leishmaniasis, cutaneous	Preferred therapy for acute infection • Liposomal amphotericin B 2–4 mg/kg IV daily for 10 days or interrupted schedule (e.g., 4 mg/kg on days 1–5, 10, 17, 24, 31, 38) to achieve total dose of 20–60 mg/kg (BIII); or • Sodium stibogluconate 20 mg/kg IV or IM daily for 3–4 weeks (BIII)	Alternative therapy for acute infection choice dependent on species of *Leishmania* Other options include oral miltefosine, topical paromomycin, intralesional pentavalent antimony, and local heat therapy	
Chagas disease (American trypanosomiasis)	Preferred therapy for acute, early chronic, and reactivated disease • Benznidazole 5–8 mg/kg/day PO in 2 divided doses for 30–60 days (BIII) (not commercially available in the US; contact the CDC Drug Service at 404-639-3670 or drugservice@cdc.gov)	Alternative therapy • Nifurtimox 8–10 mg/kg/day PO for 90–120 days (CIII) (Contact the CDC Drug Service at 404-639-3670 or drugservice@cdc.gov)	Duration of therapy has not been studied in HIV-infected patients Initiation or optimization of ART in patients undergoing treatment for Chagas disease, once the patient is clinically stable (AIII)
Isospora belli infection	Preferred therapy for acute infection • TMP–SMX (AI) (160 mg/800 mg) PO (or IV) qid for 10 days (AII); or • TMP–SMX (160 mg/800 mg) PO (or IV) bid for 7–10 days (BI) • May increase daily dose and/or duration (up to 3–4 weeks) if symptoms worsen or persist (BIII)	Alternative therapy for acute infection • Pyrimethamine 50–75 mg PO daily plus leucovorin 10–25 mg PO daily (BIII); or • Ciprofloxacin 500 mg PO bid x 7 days (CI): as a second-line alternative	Fluid and electrolyte management in patients with dehydration (AIII) Nutritional supplementation for malnourished patients (AIII) Immune reconstitution with ART may result in fewer relapses (AIII)
	Preferred chronic maintenance therapy (secondary prophylaxis) In patients with CD4+ count less than 200/μL • TMP–SMX (160 mg/800 mg) PO tiw (AI)	Alternative chronic maintenance therapy (secondary prophylaxis) • TMP–SMX (160 mg/800 mg) PO daily or (320 mg/1600 mg) tiw (BIII) • Pyrimethamine 25 mg PO daily + leucovorin 5–10 mg PO daily (BIII) • Ciprofloxacin 500 mg tiw (CI): as a second-line alternative	

* Pyrimethamine and leucovorin doses: same as in "Preferred therapy" for toxoplasmosis

† All patients receiving INH should receive pyridoxine 25–50 mg PO daily (BIII)

ART = antiretroviral therapy, bid = twice a day, biw = twice weekly, g = gram, IM = intramuscular, IV = intravenous, μg = microgram, mg = milligram, PO = oral, qAM = every morning, qid = four times a day, q'n'h = every 'n' hour, qPM = every evening, SQ = subcutaneous, tid = three times daily, tiw = three times weekly

Source: Morbidity and Mortality Weekly Report, Centers for Disease Control and Prevention, 2009;58(RR-4):1–206.

REFERENCES

Lancet, 2004;363(9425):1965–76; *Retina,* 2005;25(5):633–49; *Curr Opin Pulm Med,* 2005;11(3):203–7; *Crit Care Med,* 2006;34 (9 Suppl):S245–50; *Clin Infect Dis,* 2005;40(3):480–2; *Br Med Bull,* 2005;72:99–118; *Curr Gastroenterol Rep,* 2000;2(4):283–93; *HIV Medicine,* 2011;12(Suppl s2):55–60; *MMWR Recomm Rep,* 2009;58(RR-4):1–207; *Am Fam Physician,* 2011;83(4):395–406; *N Engl J Med,* 1998;339(4):236–44.

CHAPTER 44

MENINGITIS

1. EPIDEMIOLOGY

- *Streptococcus pneumoniae, Neisseria meningitidis, H. influenzae* have traditionally accounted for 80% of bacterial meningitis cases; numbers decreasing with vaccinations
- Highest incidence of sporadic cases is in young children; 50–60% in children 3 months to 5 yo
- *Neisseria*: Gram-negative diplococci; human reservoir; communicated by respiratory droplet, mostly through exposure of asymptomatic carriers; incubation period is 1–10 days, usually less than 4 days; causes 10–40% of purulent meningitis
- *Haemophilus meningitis*: most common cause of bacterial meningitis outside of epidemic periods; annual incidence is 1–3 per 100,000; case fatality is 5–20%, 10–30% with sequelae, most common is hearing loss; incidence has virtually been eliminated with vaccination
- *Streptococcus pneumoniae*: annual incidence is 1–2 cases in 100,000 in developed countries; case fatality is several times higher than meningococcal and Hib meningitis; it often results in bilateral and profound hearing loss and accounts for 61% of all cases of bacterial meningitis
- *Listeria monocytogenes*: 2% incidence in the United States
- Viral meningitis: enteroviruses are most common cause of epidemics, generally occuring in late summer and early winter; affects infants and young children

2. PATHOPHYSIOLOGY

- *Neisseria meningitidis*: colonization of nasopharynx, unvaccinated status (though serogroup B, accounting for ⅓ of cases, not covered), complement deficiency
- Gram-negative Enterobacteriaceae: DM, cirrhosis, alcoholism, chronic UTI, neurosurgery
- *Listeria monocytogenes*: pregnancy, age older than 60, immunocompromised, contaminated foods
- *Staphylococcus aureus*: neurosurgery
- *S. pneumoniae* and *N. meningitidis* enter bloodstream from nasopharynx; capsule allows bacteria to evade immune detection and then invade CSF via choroid plexus; rapid proliferation in CSF due to relative lack of WBCs, complement, and immunoglobulins
  - Most neurologic injury is due to host immune response rather than direct bacterial injury; end result is increased ICP leading to herniation, then coma
  - Bacterial lysis causes meningeal inflammation, then cytokines increase permeability of blood-brain barrier leading to vasogenic edema
  - Protein-rich exudate in subarachnoid space
  - Obstructed CSF flow results in hydrocephalus
  - Vascular infiltration leads to thrombosis, then ischemia and obstruction
  - Neutrophils release cytotoxic substances, which cause cell injury, resulting in edema

3. CLINICAL PRESENTATION

- Fever, stiff neck, altered mental status *(less than ⅓ of patients have all 3, but more than 99% have at least one)*
- Other symptoms: photophobia, headache, nausea/vomiting, focal weakness, numbness
- Signs (all have poor diagnostic utility; LR+ 1, LR– 1)
  - Neck stiffness: difficulty in flexing neck forward
  - Kernig's sign: patient lies supine, flexes hip to 90°; knee is then extended (straightened); sign is positive if resistance or pain in the low back/posterior thigh is elicited
  - Brudzinski's sign: flexion of the neck; sign is positive if flexion of the hips and knees is induced
  - Jolt accentuation: head is rotated rapidly from side-to-side; sign is positive if headache is worsened

4. WORKUP OF PRESUMED MENINGITIS

- Perform blood cultures and lumbar puncture as quickly as possible
- See **Table 44.1** for typical CSF values for various causes of meningitis
- See **Table 44.2** for indications for head CT prior to lumbar puncture

TABLE 44.1.   Typical Cerebrospinal Fluid (CSF) Parameters

	Normal	Bacterial	Viral	Fungal	TB	Abscess
WBC/mL	0–5	Greater than 1000*	Less than 1000	100–500	100–500	10–1000
% PMN	0–15	Greater than 80*	Less than 50	Less than 50	Less than 50	Less than 50
% lymph	Greater than 50	Less than 50	Greater than 50	Greater than 80	Increased monos	Varies
Glucose (mg/dL)	45–60	Less than 40	45–65	30–45	30–45	45–60
CSF/Blood Glucose Ratio	Greater than or equal to 0.6	Less than or equal to 0.4	45–65	Less than 0.4	Less than 0.4	0.6
Protein (mg/dL)	15–45	150–1000	50–100	100–500	100–500	Greater than 50
Opening Pressure†	6–20	20–50	Variable	Greater than 20	Greater than 20	Variable

* Early meningitis may have lower numbers
† Opening pressure in cm H_2O, WBC = white blood cells
Source: Information from *Neurol Clinics,* 1999;17:675–89 and *JAMA,* 2006; 296(16): 2012–22.

TABLE 44.2.   Indications for CT Scan of Head Prior to Lumbar Puncture

Age older than 60 yo	Recent neurosurgical operation or procedure	Immunosuppressed state*
Seizure in last week		Dysphasia or aphasia
Gaze or facial palsy	Cognitive impairment†	Focal neurological deficits
Papilledema	Altered level of consciousness	Abnormal visual fields

* HIV infection, chronic steroids or posttransplantation
† Inability to answer 2 consecutive questions or follow 2 consecutive commands
Source: Adapted from *JAMA,* 2006; 296(16): 2012–22.

5. GENERAL GUIDELINES FOR MENINGITIS TREATMENT

- Start empiric antibiotics with or without adjunctive dexamethasone as soon as lumbar puncture and blood cultures obtained or prior to CT scan if this precedes a lumbar puncture
- Adjunctive dexamethasone administered prior to or concurrent with antibiotics
  - 10 mg IV q 6 h × 4 days for meningitis in adults if the CSF is purulent, CSF Gram stain is positive, or if CSF leukocytes are greater than 1000/mm³
  - Lower rates of severe hearing loss (RR 0.67) and severe neurological sequelae (RR 0.83)

- Little role for rapid bacterial antigen testing or *Limulus* lysate assays unless high likelihood of bacterial meningitis and patient has been receiving antibiotics
- Repeat CSF analysis if no clinical improvement after 48 hours of antibiotics
- Respiratory isolation × 24 h indicated for any suspected meningococcal meningitis
- Duration of IV antibiotics: 7 days for *N. meningitidis*, 7–14 days for *H. influenza*, 10–14 days for *S. pneumoniae*, 14–21 days for *Streptococcus agalactiae*, and 21 days for aerobic Gram-negative bacilli or *Listeria monocytogenes*, and unspecified 10–14 days

Cerebrospinal Fluid Tests to Identify Adult Bacterial Versus Aseptic Meningitis

- Individual predictors of bacterial meningitis: CSF glucose less than 34 mg/dL, CSF/blood glucose less than 0.23, CSF protein greater than 220 mg/dL, CSF with more than 1000 leukocytes/mm^3, CSF neutrophils greater than 1180/ mm^3, or CSF lactate greater than or equal to 31.5 mg/dL
- Serum C-reactive protein less than 1 mg/L excludes bacterial etiology with 99% accuracy
- CSF lactate greater than or equal to 27 mg/dL predicts bacterial meningitis in postoperative neurosurgical patients
- Acute meningoencephalitis: start IV acyclovir and send CSF for HSV RNA by PCR; check an MRI of the brain with gadolinium and an EEG to assess for temporal lobe encephalitis
- The workup of aseptic meningitis can be extensive and is beyond the scope of this text
- See **Table 44.3**

TABLE 44.3.   Empiric Antibiotic Therapy for Presumed Bacterial Meningitis

Clinical Condition/Age	Empiric Antibiotic Therapy
16–50 yo	Vancomycin 30–60 mg/kg/day* plus ceftriaxone 2 g IV q 12 h
Older than 50 yo, immunocompromised or presence of a Listeria risk factor†	Vancomycin 30–60 mg/kg/day* plus ceftriaxone 2 g IV q 12 h plus ampicillin 2 g IV q 4 h
Basilar skull fracture	Vancomycin 30–60 mg/kg/day* plus ceftriaxone 2 g IV q 12 h
Penetrating trauma, CSF shunt, postneurosurgical	Vancomycin 30–60 mg/kg/day* plus cefepime 2 g IV q 8 h **or** ceftazidime 2 g IV q 8 h
Hospital-acquired or neutropenic	Ceftazidime 2 g IV q 8 h or cefepime or meropenem **plus** vancomycin 30–60 mg/kg/day*

* Maintain serum trough levels 15–20 mcg/mL and give vancomycin as divided doses q 6–12 h
† Risk factors for listeria meningitis are alcoholism or immunocompromised state
Source: Adapted from *NEJM*, 2006: 354(1): 44–53.

6. COMPLICATIONS

- Altered mental status
- Increased intracranial pressure/cerebral edema result in herniation
- Seizures
- Neurological deficits such as paralysis/cranial nerve palsy
- Sensorineural hearing loss
- Fatality rate in bacterial meningitis is 25% in adults, higher in the elderly
- 1/3 of adults with bacterial meningitis will have cognitive impairments, especially in listeria meningitis
- In HIV-associated Cryptococcal meningitis, poor prognostic factors are altered mental status at presentation and high organism load, as determined by quantitative CSF culture or CSF antigen titer
- In Histoplasma meningitis, approximately 20% of patients fail initial therapy and as many as 40% may relapse
- In Coccidioidal meningitis, mortality ~30%, with high relapse if treatment is stopped

Management of Cerebral Edema Related to Meningitis
- 20% mannitol 1 g/kg IV q 4–6 h targeting Sosm 315–320 mOsm/L
- Head elevation greater than 30°

REFERENCES

Clin Infect Dis, 2004;39(9):1267–84; *New Engl J Med*, 2006;354(1):44–53; *JAMA*, 2006;296(16):2012–22; *Cochrane Database Syst Rev*, 2010;(9):CD004405; *Infect Dis Clin North Am*, 2009;23(4):925–43; *Clin Microbiol Rev*, 2010; 23(3): 467–92.

Attia J. Does this adult patient have acute meningitis? In: Simel D, Rennie D, eds. *The Rational Clinical Examination*. New York, NY: McGraw-Hill; 2009: 395–406.

CHAPTER 45

PNEUMONIA

COMMUNITY-ACQUIRED PNEUMONIA

1. **EPIDEMIOLOGY**
   - 2nd leading cause of hospitalization in the United States, after childbirth
   - 20% rehospitalization rate within 30 days after discharge per Medicare data
   - 6th leading cause of death; mortality is 14% in hospitalized patients and 1% in nonhospitalized patients
   - Mortality rate is 4.6 of 100 hospital discharges compared to heart disease (3.2 per 100 discharges) and all-cause mortality (4.2 per 100 discharges)
   - HAP is the 2nd most common nosocomial infection in the United States with mortality rate 30–70%
     - Mortality rate of HAP is 25–50%
     - Most common cause of septic shock

2. **PATHOPHYSIOLOGY**
   - Microaspiration (e.g., elderly, mechanically ventilated), frank aspiration (e.g., AMS), or inhalation of infected droplets introduce microbes into normally sterile alveoli
   - Failure of innate immunity (gag and cough reflexes, mucociliary clearance)
   - Alveolar macrophages become overwhelmed, causing inflammatory response
   - Cytokine release causes fever
   - Chemokines promote neutrophil recruitment, leukocytosis, and purulent sputum production
   - Leaky alveolar capillaries lead to exudate then crackles, poor lung compliance, infiltrate on CXR
   - Microbial inhibition of hypoxic vasoconstriction results in V/Q mismatch (alveoli perfused but not effectively ventilated), leading to hypoxia

3. **CLINICAL PRESENTATION**
   - Fever, productive cough, dyspnea, pleuritic chest pain, fatigue, anorexia, and myalgias
   - Inspect: asymmetric chest expansion [LR+ 44, but only 5% sensitive]
   - Palpate: fremitus (ball of hand is placed on the chest while the patient says 99, sign is positive when vibration increases over a section of the lung field)
   - Percuss: dullness to percussion [LR+ 3, LR− NS]
   - Auscultation
     - Bronchial breath sounds in the periphery [LR+ 3.3, L–R NS]
     - Crackles [LR+ 1.8, LR− 0.8]
     - Diminished breath sounds [LR+ 2.3, LR− 0.8]
     - Whispered pectoriloquy (whispered phrases become clearer)
     - Egophony (patient says "e," sounds like "a") [LR+ 4.1, LR− NS]

4. **DIAGNOSIS OF COMMUNITY-ACQUIRED PNEUMONIA (CAP)**
   - Acute symptoms (cough with or without sputum, dyspnea, fever, with or without pleuritic chest pain)
   - Exam: pulmonary rales or rhonchi with or without egophony or tactile fremitus
   - Chest X-ray or CT scan of the thorax with a pulmonary infiltrate
   - Exclude healthcare-associated pneumonia (HCAP); see page 202–203
   - Microbiology: *Streptococcus pneumoniae, Haemophilus influenzae, Moraxella catarrhalis, Mycoplasma pneumoniae, Chlamydia pneumonia*, and rarely *Legionella pneumophila*

5. **WORKUP FOR COMMUNITY-ACQUIRED PNEUMONIA**
   - Posteroanterior and lateral chest radiograph: examine for infiltrate/effusion
   - Pulse oximetry on room air or arterial blood gas (if any concern of adequate ventilation)

- Labs: CBCD, chemistry panel with or without C-reactive protein and HIV test (if 15–54 years old)
  - Consider urinary antigen tests for Legionella and *S. pneumoniae* if severe CAP
- Sputum culture and Gram stain and 2 sets of pretreatment blood cultures

6. INDICATIONS FOR HOSPITALIZATION

- PSI Class 4–5 (see below); CURB-65 score 2 or higher; oxygen saturation less than 90%; unstable comorbid conditions; poor psychosocial situation; failed outpatient therapy; inability to take oral medications; or active substance abuse

7. CRITERIA FOR SEVERE COMMUNITY-ACQUIRED PNEUMONIA

- Minor criteria: respiratory rate 30 or greater; PaO_2/FiO_2 250 or less; multilobar infiltrates; acute confusion/disorientation; BUN 20 mg/dL or higher; leukopenia (WBC less than 4000 cell/mm³); platelets less than 100K cells/mm³; temperature less than 36°C; hypotension resolved with fluid resuscitation; hypoglycemia (in absence of diabetes); acute alcohol intoxication or withdrawal; sodium 130 MEq/L or less; lactate greater than 2 mmol/L; underlying cirrhosis; or asplenia
- Major criteria: need for invasive mechanical ventilation and septic shock
- ICU admission for 1 or more major criteria; 3 or more minor criteria; CURB-65 score 3 or higher; or PSI class 5
  - Pneumonia Severity Index (PSI) available at www.mdcalc.com psi-port-score-pneumonia-severity-index-adult-cap/
  - See **Tables 45.1 and 45.2**

TABLE 45.1. CURB-65 Score

• Confusion (new-onset)
• Uremia (BUN greater than 20 mg/dL)
• Respiratory Rate 30 bpm or Higher
• Blood pressure (systolic less than 90 mmHg, diastolic 60 mmHg or less)
• 65 yo or older

1 point for the presence of each item; recommend ward care if score 2 and ICU care if score 3 or higher
Source: Adapted from *Thorax*, 2003; 58(5): 377–82.

TABLE 45.2. Empiric Antibiotic Therapy for Community-Acquired Pneumonia

Category	Empiric Therapy
Non-ICU inpatient	• β-lactam* **AND** macrolide† • Respiratory fluoroquinolone‡
ICU patient without pseudomonas risk factors§	• β-lactam* **AND** azithromycin **OR** doxycycline • β-lactam* **AND** respiratory fluoroquinolone‡ • Aztreonam **AND** respiratory fluoroquinolone‡ (penicillin allergic) • Add vancomycin‖ **OR** linezolid for MRSA risk factors¶
ICU patient with pseudomonas risk factors§	• Antipseudomonal β-lactam# **AND** either ciprofloxacin **OR** levofloxacin • Antipseudomonal β-lactam# **AND** aminoglycoside **AND** azithromycin • Add vancomycin‖ **OR** linezolid for MRSA risk factors¶

* Ceftriaxone, cefotaxime, ampicillin-sulbactam, or ertapenem
† Azithromycin or clarithromycin
‡ Levofloxacin, moxifloxacin, gatifloxacin, or gemifloxacin
§ Residence in a long-term care facility, underlying cardiopulmonary disease, multiple medical comorbidities, recent antibiotics more than 7 days or admission for at least 48 h in the last month, structural lung disease (severe COPD, cystic fibrosis, or bronchiectasis), malnutrition, immunosuppressive illness, or chronic prednisone use more than 10 mg/day
‖ Dose at 15 mg/kg/dose IV q 8–12 h with a goal trough of 15–20 mcg/mL (must be renally dosed)
¶ Residence in a long-term care facility, a history of intravenous drug use, postinfluenza, sickle cell disease, or a history of MRSA infection
# Piperacillin-tazobactam, ceftazidime, imipenem, meropenem, or cefepime (infuse each dose over 3 hours); use meropenem if patient is penicillin allergic
Note: Empiric antibiotics should be initiated within 4–8 h of triage into the emergency department
Source: Adapted from *CID*, 2007; 44(Suppl 2): S27–72.

8. **DURATION OF ANTIBIOTICS**

- Minimum of 5 days and afebrile 48 h or longer with no more than one sign of clinical instability: temperature higher than 37.8°C; HR faster than 100 beats/min; RR more than 24 breaths/min; SBP less than 90 mmHg; room air SaO$_2$ less than 90% or PaO$_2$ less than 60 mmHg; abnormal mentation; and inability to maintain oral intake
- Longer duration of IV antimicrobials is indicated for bacteremia with *S. aureus, Burkholderia*, fungal pneumonias, and for those with concomitant endocarditis or meningitis

Adjunctive Care for Community-Acquired Pneumonia

- Vaccinate patients for *Streptococcus pneumoniae* and influenza if indicated
- Smoking cessation counseling and pharmacotherapy to assist smoking cessation
- Follow-up chest X-ray in 4–6 weeks to assure resolution of infiltrate

9. **COMPLICATIONS**

- Pleural effusions: usually in form of parapneumonic effusions
- Empyema: risk increased in younger patients and drug abusers; higher incidence with *Streptococcus milleri*
- Lung abscess: risk increased in alcoholics, aspiration, patients with seizures, and poor oral hygiene; mortality increased in pediatric and geriatric population, multiple abscesses, large cavity size, prolonged symptoms prior to treatment, location in lower lobes, association with malignancy
  - Commonly associated with *Staphylococcus aureus, Pseudomonas aeruginosa, Klebsiella pneumoniae*
- ARDS
- Pneumothorax
- Cardiac arrhythmias
- CHF exacerbation
- Demand MI

HEALTHCARE-ASSOCIATED AND HOSPITAL-ACQUIRED PNEUMONIAS

1. **DEFINITIONS**

- Early-onset hospital-acquired pneumonia (HAP): starts 2–4 days after hospitalization
- Late-onset HAP: develops 5 or more days after hospitalization
- Healthcare-associated pneumonia (HCAP) if any of the following risk factors present
  - Hospitalization for 48 h or longer in last 90 days
  - Resident of a nursing home or long-term care facility
  - Received in the last 30 days: home infusion therapy or wound care, IV antibiotic therapy, chemotherapy, chronic dialysis, or has attended a hospital-based clinic
  - Family member or household contact with a multidrug-resistant pathogen
- See **Table 45.3** and **Figure 45.1**

TABLE 45.3.   MDR Infection Risk Factors in HCAP

Clinical Severity
- ICU admission
- Requires mechanical ventilation

Prior Antibiotic Therapy
- Antibiotics for more than 3 days in the past 6 months

Functional Status
- "Poor" functional capacity as defined by an ADL score greater than 12.5
- ADL score is based on 6 areas of activity: transfers, feeding, bathing, dressing, toileting, and continence; for each area, one point for independence, 2 points for partial dependence, and 3 points for total dependence

Source: Adapted from *CID*, 2008; 46 (Suppl 4): S296–S334.

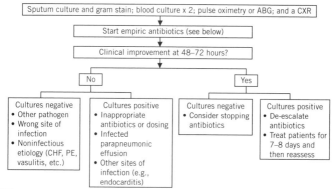

FIGURE 45.1. Management of Suspected HCAP or HAP

Source: Adapted from *Amer J Resp Crit Care Med*, 2005; 171(4): 388–416.

2. EMPIRIC ANTIBIOTIC THERAPY

- Early-onset HAP: treat as per CAP without pseudomonas risk factors as in Table 45.2
- Late-onset HAP or HCAP with MDR risk: see **Table 45.4**
- HCAP without MDR risk: see Table 45.4
- De-escalate therapy in 48–72 hours based on culture results and sensitivities
- Duration is usually 7–8 days; consider 15 days for nonfermenting GNRs (e.g., pseudomonas)

TABLE 45.4. Empiric Therapy for HCAP or Late-Onset HAP

HCAP with MDR Infection Risk or Late-Onset HAP	• Antipseudomonal cephalosporin (e.g., ceftazidime or cefepime) **OR** • Antipseudomonal carbapenem (e.g., imipenem or meropenem) **OR** • Piperacillin-tazobactam **AND** antipseudomonal fluoroquinolone (e.g., ciprofloxacin or levofloxacin) **OR** • Aminoglycoside (e.g., tobramycin or gentamicin) **AND** anti-MRSA therapy (e.g., vancomycin or linezolid)
HCAP Without MDR Infection Risk	• Respiratory fluoroquinolone (e.g., ciprofloxacin or levofloxacin) • Ceftriaxone **OR** • Ampicillin-sulbactam **OR** • Ertapenem **AND** azithromycin

3. PROGNOSIS

- All-cause mortality for HCAP is 30–70%

REFERENCES

Arch Intern Med, 2004(16);164(16):1807–11; *Am J Med*, 2004;117:51S–7S, *Clin Infect Dis*, 2007;44(Suppl 2): S27–S72, *Clin Infect Dis*, 2004;39(12):1783–90; *J Antimicrobial Chemother*, 2011;66(Suppl 3):3–9; *Am J Resp Crit Care Med*, 2005;171(4):388–416; *Clin Infect Dis*, 2008;46 (Suppl 4):S296–344; *Clin Infect Dis*, 2008;46:S378. *Ann Pharmacother*, 2007;41(2):235–44.

Simel D, ed. Does this adult patient have community-acquired pneumonia? In: Simel D, Rennie D, eds. *The Rational Clinical Examination*. New York NY: McGraw-Hill; 2009:527–34.

CHAPTER 46

MANAGEMENT OF INVASIVE FUNGAL INFECTIONS

1. ### <u>EPIDEMIOLOGY</u>
   Aspergillus
   - Neutropenia and chronic steroids are major risk factors
   - Overall mortality is 36% in 12 weeks and 75% in 1 year
   - Highest incidence among patients undergoing intensive chemotherapy for AML and allogenic hematopoietic stem cell transplant
   - Among solid organ transplants, lung transplantation has the highest incidence of invasive aspergillosis at 6–16%

   Candida
   - Leading cause of fungemia in hospitalized patients
   - Complicates solid organ transplantation, especially lung transplants, and tends to occur within 30 days

   Histoplasmosis
   - Mississippi valley, thermodimorphic fungi (mold in environment, yeast in host)
   - Incubation period and symptoms onset 5–17 days, average 10 days
   - Reservoir in soil with bird droppings and bat caves
   - Transmission by inhalation of spores (microconidia)
   - Dependent on T-cell mediated cellular immunity
   - Risk factors: spelunking, gardening, horticulture, construction

   Coccidioidomycosis
   - Arizona has about 60% of all cases in the United States: incidence in Arizona is 75 cases per 100,000
   - Spores (arthroconidia) reside a few inches below the soil surface; soil disruption contributes to increased incidence: construction sites (dust abatement), earthquakes, and landslides
   - Most posttransplant cocci infections are believed to be due to reactivation and 70% manifest within first 12 months
   - Overall incidence of this is about 4–8% with a dissemination rate of 75% and 50–63% mortality
     - Fluconazole prophylaxis decreases this incidence to 1–3% with 30% dissemination rate and 29% mortality

2. ### <u>PATHOPHYSIOLOGY</u>
   Aspergillus
   - Saprophytic mold, ubiquitous in environment; outbreaks usually due to contaminated hospital air
   - Most commonly *A. fumigatus* (occasionally *A. flavus, A. niger, A. terreus,* or *A. nidulans*)
   - Neutropenia, glucocorticoid use, and pulmonary disease are major risk factors for invasive aspergillosis

   Candida
   - Normal commensal yeasts that live on skin, GI tract, and female genital tract
   - Most commonly *C. albicans* but with advent of antifungals, increasing prevalence of non-*albicans* (e.g., *C. krusei, C. parapsilosis, C. tropicalis, C. lusitaniae, C. glabrata*) with different antifungal resistance patterns
   - Candidiasis results from hematogenous dissemination of *Candida* from mucocutaneous surfaces with transformation from blastospores to pseudohyphae form
   - Antibiotics decrease bacterial suppression of *Candida* leading to mucosal overgrowth
   - Abdominal or thoracic surgery, IV drug use, severe burns, indwelling catheters, and mechanical ventilators result in mucosal damage
   - Decreased CD_4 (HIV), DM increase mucocutaneous infection

- Decreased innate immunity (especially decreased neutrophils): IV corticosteroids, chemotherapy, immunosuppression

Coccidioidomycosis

- *Coccidioides immitis* is a dimorphic fungus endemic to the southwestern United States; mold form in soil produces airborne arthroconidia, which are small enough to bypass mucosal defenses upon inhalation
- Arthroconidia in bronchial tree leads to formation of spherules, which can grow, rupture, and produce new spherules
- Cell-mediated immune response determines extent of infection
  - Immunocompetent patients: granulomas contain spherules, so pulmonary infection is limited and often asymptomatic
  - Susceptible patients (African American or Filipino males, HIV with CD4 less than 250, gluco-corticoids, transplant recipients, TNF-α therapy, pregnancy: neutrophil response with minimal granulomatous inflammation)

Histoplasmosis

- *Histoplasma capsulatum* is a dimorphic fungus endemic to the Ohio and Mississippi river valleys, especially in soil contaminated with bird and bat feces
- Inhaled microconidia multiply within alveolar macrophages as budding yeasts, which then enter lymphatic system, then disseminate hematogenously
- Cell-mediated immune response 2 weeks after infection
  - Immunocompetent patients: calcified granulomas
  - Unlike TB, latent infection does not reactivate
  - Immunocompetent patients: infection disseminates to reticuloendothelial system (bone marrow, spleen, liver), adrenal glands, and skin
  - Underlying pulmonary disease: inflammation leads to necrosis then fibrosis, similar to pulmonary TB

3. CLINICAL PRESENTATION

Aspergillus

- Invasive pulmonary aspergillosis: fever with focal infiltrates, nodules, or wedge-shaped densities; cough, pleuritic pain, and hemoptysis; lesions may cavitate
- Acute *Aspergillus* sinusitis: fever, localized pressure, pain; eschars on nasal septum or turbinates
- Disseminated aspergillosis: most commonly involves CNS with abscesses and infarcts causing focal paresis, cranial nerve deficits, and seizures

Candida

- Disseminated candidiasis: microabscesses to multiple organs including eyes, kidneys, liver, spleen, brain; skin lesions can appear: papular/pustular, surrounded by a zone of erythema; retinal lesions are distinctive white exudates
- Risk factors for invasive candidiasis in ICU patients: host factors—neutropenia, candida colonization, necrotizing pancreatitis, GI perforation, acute renal failure, bacterial sepsis, hematologic malignancy, high APACHE II score, diabetes, advanced age; iatrogenic factors—immunosuppressive therapy, broad-spectrum antibiotic therapy, central venous catheters, mechanical ventilation, major surgical procedures (e.g., tumor resection), leaking intestinal anastomosis, antineoplastic chemotherapy, hemodialysis

Coccidioidomycosis

- Primary pulmonary infections: fever, weight loss, fatigue, dry cough, pleuritic chest pain, arthralgias ("desert rheumatism"), rash (nonpruritic, maculopapular)
- Extrapulmonary dissemination: destinations include skin (subcutaneous abscesses), joints (knees), bones, basilar meninges

Histoplasmosis

- Acute pulmonary histoplasmosis: fever, chills, fatigue, nonproductive cough, anterior chest pain, myalgias
- Chronic pulmonary histoplasmosis: fever, fatigue, anorexia, weight loss, purulent sputum, hemoptysis in elderly COPD patients

- Disseminated histoplasmosis: chills, fever, anorexia, weight loss, hypotension, dyspnea, hepatosplenomegaly, skin lesions

4. EVALUATION OF DIFFERENT FORMS OF ASPERGILLOSIS

- Risk factors: immunosuppression, neutropenia, chronic lung disease, and chronic steroid use
- Invasive aspergillosis may present as a necrotizing pneumonia, CNS infection, osteomyelitis, or extension to contiguous intrathoracic structures (e.g., pleura, pericardium, or arteries)
- Cutaneous aspergillosis should be treated as disseminated infection
- Chronic cavitary pulmonary aspergillosis: 1 or more pulmonary cavity with detectable Aspergillus antibodies; usually requires long-term, potentially lifelong, antifungal treatment
- Allergic bronchopulmonary aspergillosis (ABPA): episodic bronchial obstruction, eosinophilia, *Aspergillus* antibodies present, elevated IgE levels, episodic pulmonary infiltrates, and central bronchiectasis; can mimic adult-onset asthma
- Diagnosis: galactomannan assay of BAL fluid has more than 90% sensitivity and specificity for invasive aspergillosis
- See **Tables 46.1** through **46.3**

TABLE 46.1.   Recommended Initial Treatment of Aspergillosis

Condition	Primary Therapy	Alternative Therapy
Invasive aspergillosis of lungs, sinuses, tracheobronchial tree, CNS, skin, and peritoneum	• Voriconazole 6 mg/kg IV q 12 h × 2 doses, then 4 mg/kg IV q 12 h, then 200 mg PO bid	• LipAmB 3–5 mg/kg/day • Caspo 70 mg × 1, then 50 mg/day • Posaconazole 200 mg PO qid
Endocarditis or pericarditis	• Same medications as above	• Surgical resection required
Osteomyelitis or septic arthritis	• Same medications as above	• Surgical resection of devitalized bone/cartilage required
Endophthalmitis or keratitis	• Intraocular amphotericin B	• Partial vitrectomy often needed
Solitary aspergilloma	• No meds needed, but surgical extirpation needed at times	
Chronic cavitary pulmonary aspergillosis	• Itraconazole 200 mg PO bid • Voriconazole 200 mg PO bid	• LipAmB 3–5 mg/kg/day • Caspo 70 mg × 1, then 50 mg/day
Allergic bronchopulmonary aspergillosis	• Itraconazole 200 mg PO bid • Prednisone 0.5–1 mg/kg/day × 14 days, then taper × 3–6 months	• Voriconazole 200 mg PO bid • Posaconazole 400 mg PO bid
Allergic aspergillus sinusitis	• None if mild; itraconazole 200 mg PO bid if moderate–severe	

CNS = central nervous system, LipAmB = liposomal amphotericin B, Caspo = caspofungin

Source: Adapted from *CID*, 2008; 46(3): 327–60.

TABLE 46.2.   *Candida* Score to Identify ICU Candidates* for Empiric Antifungal Therapy

• Multifocal *Candida* colonization[†] • Surgery on ICU admission	• Severe sepsis • Use of total parenteral nutrition

* Applies only to nonneutropenic pts
† Surveillance cultures from urine, stomach, and trachea were obtained weekly
1 point for each risk factor, except for severe sepsis, which receives 2 points
Candida score of 3 or higher has an RR 6 for invasive candidiasis

Source: Adapted from *Crit Care Med* 2006; 34 (3):730–7 and *Crit Care Med*, 2009; 37(5): 1624–1633.

TABLE 46.3.   Recommended Empiric Treatment of Candidal Infections*

Condition	Primary Therapy	Alternative Therapy
Known or suspected candidemia, nonneutropenic, moderate–severe illness or shock	• Echinocandin†	• LipAmB 3–5 mg/kg/day • AmB 0.5–1 mg/kg/day • Voriconazole
Suspected candidemia, nonneutropenic, mild illness	• Fluconazole 800 mg IV load, then 400 mg/day	• Echinocandin†
Known or suspected candidemia, neutropenic	• Echinocandin† • LipAmB 3–5 mg/kg/day	• Fluconazole • Voriconazole
Candiduria, asymptomatic	• Remove urinary catheter	• Fluconazole 200–400 mg/day if neutropenic or undergoing a urologic procedure
Candiduria, symptomatic	• Fluconazole 200 mg/day for 2 weeks	• AmB 0.5 mg/kg bladder irrigation daily × 5–7 days
Pyelonephritis	• Fluconazole 200–400 mg/day for 2 weeks	• AmB 0.5–0.7 mg/kg IV daily with or without FC 25 mg/kg qid × 14 days
Chronic disseminated candidiasis	• Fluconazole 400 mg/day • LipAmB 3–5 mg/kg/day	• Echinocandin† • AmB 0.5–0.7 mg/kg/day
Osteomyelitis	• Fluconazole 400 mg/day × 6–12 months	• LipAmB 3–5 mg/kg/day or echinocandin† × 3 wks, then fluconazole
Septic arthritis	• Fluconazole 400 mg/day × 6 weeks	• LipAmB 3–5 mg/kg/day or echinocandin† × 3 wks, then fluconazole
CNS candidiasis	• LipAmB 3–5 mg/kg/day **plus** FC 25 mg/kg qid × 3 wks, then fluconazole	• Fluconazole 400–800 mg/day until CSF normal and clinical symptoms have resolved
Endocarditis	• LipAmB 3–5 mg/kg/day **or** AmB 0.6–1 mg/kg/day **plus** FC 25 mg/kg qid	• Fluconazole 400–800 mg/day as step-down therapy • Valve replacement usually needed
Pericarditis	• LipAmB 3–5 mg/kg/day • Fluconazole 400–800 mg/day	• Echinocandin†
Oropharyngeal candidiasis	• Clotrimazole troches • Nystatin swish and swallow	• Fluconazole 100–200 mg/day for moderate-severe disease × 7–14 days
Esophageal candidiasis	• Fluconazole 200–400 mg/day	• Echinocandin† × 14–21 days
Candida from airway aspirate	• None as a *Candida* pneumonia is exceedingly rare	

* Systemic antifungal may need to be changed based on the eventual *Candida* speciation and sensitivities.
† Caspofungin 70 mg IV load, then 50 mg/day; anidulafungin 200 mg IV load, then 100 mg/day; or micafungin 100 mg/day
Note: Patients with suspected candidemia should have vascular access devices removed if possible
LipAmB = liposomal amphotericin B, AmB = amphotericin B deoxycholate, FC = flucytosine, CSF = cerebrospinal fluid
Source: Adapted from *CID*, 2009; 48(5): 503–35.

5. <u>EVALUATION OF PATIENTS WITH COCCIDIOIDOMYCOSIS INFECTIONS</u>

- Risk factors for disseminated disease: HIV+; organ transplant pts; use of anti-TNF agents or steroids; lymphoma; DM and African, Filipino, Asian, Hispanic, or Native American ancestry
- Labs: serum cocci titer and CXR for all patients
  - Bone scan and LP for any risk factors or clinical suspicion of disseminated cocci

- Diagnosis: culture, histology, or serology
- See **Table 46.4**

TABLE 46.4.   Risk Factors for Invasive Candidiasis in ICU Patients

Risk Factors of the Host
Neutropenia
Candida colonization
Necrotizing pancreatitis
GI perforation
Acute renal failure
Bacterial sepsis
Hematologic malignancy
High APACHE II score
Diabetes
Advanced age

Iatrogenic Risk Factors
Immunosuppressive therapy
Broad-spectrum antibiotic therapy
Central venous catheters
Mechanical ventilation
Major surgical procedures (e.g., tumor resection)
Leaking intestinal anastomosis
Antineoplastic chemotherapy
Hemodialysis

Source: Adapted from Mycoses, 2010; 54: 420–433.

6. EVALUATION OF PATIENTS WITH SUSPECTED HISTOPLASMOSIS

- Labs: LDH, histoplasma antibody titers (HIV-negative) versus urine histo antigen (HIV-positive)
- Additional studies: CXR; head CT scan and LP if any meningismus or CNS symptoms
- Diagnosis: detection of *H. capsulatum* antigen, histopathology, CF titer of Histo antibody greater than or equal to 1:32, isolation in culture
- See **Table 46.5**

TABLE 46.5.   Initial Treatment of Coccidioidomycosis

Condition	Primary Therapy	Alternative Therapy
Acute pneumonia, mild	• None if uncomplicated in a nonpregnant, immunocompetent patient	
Pneumonia, moderate–severe	• Fluconazole 400 mg/day IV or PO • AmB 0.5–1.5 mg/kg/day IV if pregnant	• LipAmB 2–5 mg/kg/day IV • Itraconazole 400–600 mg/day PO
Chronic fibrocavitary pneumonia	• Fluconazole 400–800 mg/day	• AmB 0.5–1.5 mg/kg/day IV until stable, then fluconazole
Disseminated, nonmeningeal infection	• Fluconazole 800–1000 mg/day • AmB 0.5–1.5 mg/kg/day IV	• Itraconazole 400–800 mg/day PO
Coccidioidomycosis meningitis	• Fluconazole 800–1200 mg/day • AmB 0.5–1.5 mg/kg/day IV	• Itraconazole 400–600 mg/day PO • Shunt for hydrocephalus

AmB = amphotericin B deoxycholate, LipAmB = liposomal amphotericin B
Source: Adapted from *CID*, 2005;41(9):1217–23 and *Mayo Clin Proc*, 2008; 83(3):343–48.

TABLE 46.6. Recommended Treatment of Histoplasmosis

Condition	Treatment
Acute (less than 4 weeks) pulmonary histoplasmosis, mild; or pulmonary nodule	• None required
Acute (less than 4 weeks) pulmonary histoplasmosis, moderate–severe	• LipAmB 3–5 mg/kg/day **or** AmB 0.7–1 mg/kg/day **or** ABLC 5 mg/kg/day, then itraconazole 200 mg PO bid × 12 weeks • With or without methylprednisolone 0.5–1 mg/kg/day × 1–2 wks
Chronic (more than 4 weeks) pulmonary histoplasmosis, mild–moderate	• Itraconazole 200 mg PO tid × 3 day, then 200 mg bid × 6–12 weeks
Chronic cavitary pulmonary histoplasmosis	• Itraconazole 200 mg PO bid × 12–18 months
Pericarditis, mild	• NSAIDs alone
Pericarditis, moderate–severe	• Itraconazole 200 mg PO tid × 3 days, then bid × 6–12 wks • Prednisone 0.5–1 mg/kg/day tapered over 1–2 wks
Mediastinal lymphadenitis/granuloma, mild	• NSAIDs or no treatment
Mediastinal lymphadenitis/granuloma with obstructive or compressive complications	• Prednisone 0.5–1 mg/kg/day tapered over 1–2 wks • Itraconazole 200 mg PO tid × 3 days, then × 6–12 wks
Fibrosing mediastinitis	• Stenting of any obstructed vessels, no antifungals
Disseminated histoplasmosis, mild–moderate	• Itraconazole 200 mg PO bid for at least 12 months
Disseminated histoplasmosis, moderate–severe	• LipAmB 3 mg/kg/day **or** AmB 0.7–1 mg/kg/day **or** ABLC 5 mg/kg/day × 1–2 weeks, then itraconazole 200 mg PO bid for at least 12 months
CNS histoplasmosis	• LipAmB **or** ABLC 5 mg/kg/day × 4–6 wks, then itraconazole 200 mg PO bid–tid for at least 12 months

LipAmB = liposomal amphotericin B (Ambisome); AmB = amphotericin B deoxycholate, ACLC = Abelcet, NSAIDs = nonsteroidal anti-inflammatory drugs, CNS = central nervous system

Source: Adapted from *CID*, 2007;45(7):807–25 and *Proc Am Thorac Soc*, 2010(3);7:169–72.

7. COMPLICATIONS

Aspergillus

- CNS aspergillosis causes seizures, focal neurological deficits, cerebral infarction, local extension into cerebral vasculature that results in cavernous sinus thrombosis; poor prognosis
- Aspergillus endophthalmitis results in vision loss
- Aspergillus endocarditis has a higher incidence in IV drug use and indwelling central line; carries a high mortality rate

Candida

- Invasive candidiasis/candidemia: increased risk in immunocompromised/ICU patients
- Chronic disseminated candidiasis, also called hepatosplenic candidiasis; almost exclusively associated with neutropenia in patients with hematologic malignancies
- Endophthalmitis: mechanism includes hematogenous seeding of retina and choroid
- Osteoarticular candidiasis: from hematogenous seeding, direct trauma/injection; most commonly at vertebrae for adults and long bones for children; symptoms of pain and decreased ROM may manifest months up to a year after inoculation
- Meningitis: more commonly seen in premature newborns or patients with ventricular draining devices; diagnosis via large volume lumbar puncture due to scarcity of organisms within CSF
- Endocarditis/pericarditis

Coccidioidomycosis

- Pulmonary cavity formation that can be further complicated by rupture of cavity, followed by broncho-pleural fistula/pneumothorax
- Chronic fibrocavitary pneumonia: complication of primary coccidioidal pneumonia especially in diabetics
- Disseminated coccidioidomycosis: less than 1% incidence, more commonly in immunocompromised patient (e.g., HIV, long-term steroid treatment, pregnancy)
- Coccidioidal meningitis further complicated by hydrocephalus (associated with mortality rate of 40%) and infectious arteritis (which may cause occlusion of vessels from inflammatory exudates leading to stroke)
- Septic shock due to disseminated coccidioidomycosis

Histoplasmosis

- Fibrosing mediastinitis: rare pulmonary complication; usually unilateral; further complicated by development of obstruction of pulmonary arteries and veins/bronchiectasis and bacterial superinfection
- Broncholithiasis (erosion of calcified lymph nodes into bronchi) manifested in expectoration of blood and calcified particles
- Pericarditis

8. <u>PROGNOSIS</u>

- Mortality for systemic candidiasis ranges from 25–60%; comorbidities time to treatment, as well as appropriate antifungal treatment, contribute to mortality
- Chronic coccidioidomycosis develops in 5–8% of patients following primary pulmonary disease
  - Fewer than 1% of patients progress to disseminated disease, and this is usually in immunocompromised patients
  - Mortality is only 0.07% among all cocci infections, but can be as high as 70% in immunocompromised patients
- Acute pulmonary histoplasmosis is generally associated with a good outcome, but relapse occurs in 50% of patients and is associated with acute progressive disseminated histoplasmosis

REFERENCES

Curr Opin Pulm Med, 2011;17(3):160–6; *Crit Care Med*, 2010;38(8 suppl):S380–7; *Mycoses,* 2011; 54(5): 420–33.

CHAPTER 47

SKIN, SOFT TISSUE, BONE, AND JOINT INFECTIONS

1. ## EPIDEMIOLOGY
   - Increased SSTI incidence is due to increased prevalence of CA-MRSA, which accounts for 38–75% of all community-acquired Staph infections
   - HA-MRSA accounts for 28% of all hospital isolates of Staph aureus
   - Necrotizing SSTI carries a mortality of of 9–73% (mean 24%)
   - Most common organism in SSTI is *S. aureus* (44%)

2. ## PATHOPHYSIOLOGY
   - Infecting microbes may be commensal (*Staphylococcus*) or exogenous (*Pseudomonas*)
   - Even minimal inoculum may cause cellulitis, due to effect of bacterial toxins
   - Staphylococcal infection usually starts as localized infection (e.g., abscess) and spreads gradually
   - Streptococcal infection spreads rapidly via lymphatics leading to erysipelas
   - Microbes may gain access to deeper tissue via compromised epidermis (burns, trauma, surgery, ulcers, skin disease, catheters), hair follicles, lymphatics
   - Infection by *Streptococcus pyogenes*, MRSA, and *Clostridium perfringens* may cause dermal vessel thrombosis and infection of deep fascia resulting in rapid spread via fascia through lymphatics leading to necrotizing fasciitis

3. ## CLINICAL PRESENTATION
   - Cellulitis: erythema (well demarcated border), warmth, pain, edema
   - Furuncles: purulence surrounding a hair follicle
   - Abscess: erythema with fluctance on palpation, may have pustule
   - Impetigo: crusted exudates with pustules or vesicles
   - Erysipelas: intense erythema, well demarcated, painful plaques
   - Necrotizing: clinical clues include tense edema, grayish wound drainage, bullae, necrosis, crepitus, pain that extends past visible margin of infection, induration that extends beyond erythema, pain out of proportion to physical findings, anesthesia at site of infection, signs of systemic illness

4. ## DIAGNOSIS
   - Diagnosis is clinical

5. ## WORKUP
   - Labs: CBCD, basic metabolic panel, CK, blood cultures, and wound cultures (if pus)
   - Radiology: plain X-rays for soft tissue gas or foreign body; CT scan for equivocal cases to detect deep abscesses and provide early diagnosis of necrotizing infections
   - **See Table 47.1 and Figure 47.1**

TABLE 47.1.   Management of Skin and Soft Tissue Infections

Infection	Clinical Presentation	Microbiology	Preferred Treatment	Alternative Treatment
Cellulitis (no MRSA risk factors)	Erythema, warmth, tenderness; swelling with or without fever, leukocytosis, and indistinct infection borders	*Streptococcus* species, *Staphylococcus aureus*	• Nafcillin infections refractory to β-lactam antibiotics • Vancomycin	• Cefazolin infections refractory to β-lactam antibiotics • Linezolid
Cellulitis (MRSA risk factors)	Above; purulent drainage	*Staphylococcus aureus*	• Vancomycin	• Linezolid • Daptomycin
Soft tissue infection in neutropenic patients	Red, maculopapular lesions; focal cellulitis; or ecthyma gangrenosum	*E. coli, Klebsiella, P. aeruginosa, Staphylococcus, Streptococcus, Enterococcus,* and rarely *Clostridium*	• Piperacillin-tazobactam • Carbapenem	• Nafcillin and aminoglycoside • Cefepime
Erysipelas	Bright red, tender, edematous, and raised border with a sharp demarcation; 80% involves legs; marked lymphatic involvement	Group A *Streptococcus pyogenes*; MRSA possible for facial erysipelas	• Penicillin G • Nafcillin Facial erysipelas • Vancomycin	• Cefazolin • Erythromycin (penicillin allergy) Facial erysipelas • Linezolid
Uncomplicated cellulitis or infected foot ulcer in diabetic patient	As per cellulitis description above	*Streptococcus* species, *Staphylococcus aureus*	• Nafcillin	• Cefazolin
Limb-threatening or life-threatening diabetic foot infection	Ulcer with purulent exudate, surrounding cellulitis, tissue necrosis, and gangrene	Streptococcus, *Staphylococcus aureus,* Enterobacteriaceae, and nonfermenting Gram-negative rods (GNRs)	• Vancomycin and piperacillin-tazobactam	• Linezolid and carbapenem • Vancomycin, ciprofloxacin, and clindamycin
Necrotizing, malodorous DM foot infection	Tissue necrosis, gangrene, crepitus, and foul odor	Polymicrobial with nonfermenting GNRs and anaerobes	• Vancomycin and piperacillin-tazobactam	• Linezolid and carbapenem
Infection after a human or animal bite	Puncture marks; surrounding edema and cellulitis	Oral anaerobes, *Pasteurella* (animals), *Eikenella* (humans)	• Ampicillin-sulbactam	• Clindamycin and moxifloxacin
Infection after ocean or river exposure		*Vibrio* sp., *Aeromonas hydrophila,* pseudomonas	• Ceftazidime and doxycycline	• Ciprofloxacin

MRSA risk factors: IVDU, purulent drainage, recent hospitalization or antibiotics, hemodialysis, DM, incarceration, contact sports, homosexual men, soldiers, history of "spider bite," Native Americans, Pacific Islanders, or prior MRSA

Source: Information from *CID,* 2004; 39(7): 885–910, *CID,* 2005; 41(10): 1373–406, *NEJM,* 2007; 357(4): 380–90, *Ann Int Med,* 2009:151(3); ITC-2.

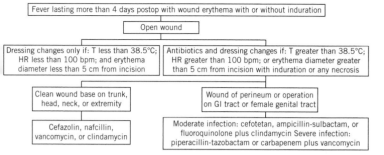

FIGURE 47.1. Management of Surgical Site Infections

Source: Adapted from *CID*, 2005; 41(10): 1373–406.

6. COMPLICATIONS

- Abscess
- Facial infections can be complicated by septic cavernous thrombosis (due to lack of valves in these veins)
- Gangrene formation
- Necrotizing fasciitis
- Bacteremia/sepsis

NECROTIZING SOFT TISSUE INFECTIONS (NSTI)

1. RISK FACTORS

- Injection drug use, diabetes, immunosuppression, and obesity

2. CLINICAL PRESENTATION

- Tense edema or pain outside the area of erythematous skin, pain disproportionate to appearance, violaceous skin discoloration, blisters/bullae, tissue necrosis, crepitus, cutaneous anesthesia, subcutaneous gas, fever, tachycardia, hypotension, delirium, AKI, and shock
- Progression is usually rapid (especially for group A *Streptococcus* or *Clostridium* species)
- See **Table 47.2**

TABLE 47.2. Laboratory Risk Indicator for Necrotizing Fasciitis (LRINEC) Score

Score	C-Reactive Protein (mg/dL)	WBC (cells/mm³)	Hemoglobin (g/dL)	Sodium (mmol/L)	Creatinine (mg/dL)	Glucose (mg/dL)
0	Less than 15	Less than 15	Greater than 13.5	Greater than or equal to 135	Less than or equal to 1.6	Less than or equal to 180
1	–	15–25	11–13.5	–	–	Greater than 180
2	–	Greater than 25	Less than 11	Less than 135	Greater than 1.6	–
4	Greater than 15	–	–	–	–	–

LRINEC score 5 or lower is low risk for NF (less than 50%); score 6–7 = intermediate risk (50–75%); score 8 or higher = high risk (greater than 75%)

Source: Adapted from *CID*, 2007; 44(5): 705–10.

3. **TREATMENT**

- Early surgical debridement, source control, and scheduled debridement every 6–24 hours recommended until no further necrosis or infected tissue is seen
- Empiric antibiotics
  - Mixed NSTI
    - Ampicillin plus clindamycin plus ciprofloxacin or gentamicin **OR**
    - High-dose penicillin G or clindamycin plus ciprofloxacin or gentamicin **OR**
    - Monotherapy: carbapenems or piperacillin-tazobactam
    - Add vancomycin, linezolid, or daptomycin to above regimen until MRSA excluded
  - Streptococcal NSTI or clostridial myonecrosis: high-dose penicillin G plus clindamycin
    - Consider hyperbaric oxygen therapy for clostridial myonecrosis
- Consider adjunctive use of drotrecogin-α and IVIG for severe NSTIs associated with severe sepsis or septic shock (especially in streptococcal toxic shock syndrome)

4. **PROGNOSIS**

- Mortality is approximately 100% without source control; mortality is 34% with best care

OSTEOMYELITIS

1. **CLASSIFICATION OF OSTEOMYELITIS**

- Acute: evolves in 3 weeks or less
- Chronic: evolves over months to year(s)

2. **DIAGNOSIS OF OSTEOMYELITIS**

- Chronic osteomyelitis and vertebral osteomyelitis require bone cultures to guide therapy
- Labs: WBC is a poor predictor of bone infection
  - ESR and CRP are typically greatly increased and more reliable markers of active bone infection
- Imaging procedures
  - X-rays: bone destruction, periosteal elevation, joint space widening after 10–21 days
  - MRI scan: detects early osteomyelitis and soft tissue disease better than CT; appears superior to CT for vertebral osteomyelitis, epidural abscesses, and for DM foot infections
  - Tc-99m bone scan: uptake with bone infection
    - More than 90% NPV and 80% PPV for bone infection under decubiti
    - Sensitivity 69–100%/specificity 88% if done with gallium scan for acute osteomyelitis

3. **TREATMENT OF OSTEOMYELITIS**

- Acute osteomyelitis: requires 4–6 weeks IV antibiotics
- Chronic osteomyelitis: requires bone debridement, removal of hardware, and 4-6 wks therapy
- DM foot ulcers with exposed bone: requires bone debridement and possible revascularization
- PEDIS assessment: *p*erfusion (arterial inflow), *e*xtent, *d*epth, *i*nfection, and *s*ensation
- See **Table 47.3**

TABLE 47.3.   Duration of Antibiotics for Diabetic Foot Osteomyelitis

Bone involvement After Debridement	Soft Tissue Involvement After Debridement	Duration of Antibiotic Therapy
Entire infected bone removed	No infected tissue remains	2–3 days
Entire infected bone removed	Residual soft tissue infection	7–14 days
Viable remnant of infected bone remains	With or without residual soft tissue infection	4–6 weeks
Dead infected bone remains	With or without residual soft tissue infection	3 or months (suppressive therapy)

Source: Adapted from *CID*, 2004; 39: 885–910.

4. PROSTHESIS-ASSOCIATED OSTEOMYELITIS

- Generally requires a 2-stage exchange arthroplasty, removal of infected prosthesis, placement of an antibiotic spacer, 4–6 weeks IV antibiotics; repeat arthroplasty with antimicrobial-impregnated cement

5. VERTEBRAL OSTEOMYELITIS

- 6–12 weeks optimal duration of antibiotics for vertebral osteomyelitis
- See **Table 47.4**

TABLE 47.4.   Antibiotic Treatment for Osteomyelitis

Organism	First-Line Therapy	Alternative Choices
MSSA	• Nafcillin 2 g IV q 4–6 h	• Cefazolin 1 g IV q 6 h • Vancomycin 30–45 mg/kg/day*
MRSA	• Vancomycin IV 30–45 mg/kg/day*	• Linezolid 600 mg IV/PO q 12 h
Streptococcus	• Penicillin G 4 MU IV q 4 h	• Clindamycin 600 mg IV q 6 h • Ceftriaxone 2 g IV daily
Enteric GNRs	• Ciprofloxacin 400 mg IV q 12 h	• Ceftazidime 2 g IV q 8 h
Anaerobes	• Clindamycin 600 mg IV q 6 h	• Ampicillin-sulbactam 3 g IV q 6 h
Polymicrobial	• Piperacillin-tazobactam 4.5 g IV q 6 h **PLUS** vancomycin 30–45 mg/kg/day* **or** linezolid 600 mg IV/PO q 12 h	• Imipenem 500 mg IV q 6 h **PLUS** vancomycin 30–45 mg/kg/day* **or** linezolid 600 mg IV/PO q 12 h

MSSA = methicillin-susceptible S. *aureus*, MRSA = methicillin-resistant *S. aureus*, GNR = Gram-negative rod
* Dose vancomycin q 6–12 h to achieve a serum vancomycin trough level of 15–20 mcg/mL

Source: Information from *NEJM*, 1997; 336(14): 999–1007 and *Lancet*, 2004; 364(9431): 364: 369–71.

SEPTIC ARTHRITIS

1. CLINICAL PRESENTATION

- Warm, swollen, exquisitely tender joint; fever; usually monoarticular of hips or knees
- Gonococcal arthritis may be migratory and associated with tenosynovitis or skin rash

2. RISK FACTORS

- Age older than 80 yo, diabetes, rheumatoid arthritis, recent joint surgery, hip or knee prosthesis, overlying skin infection, HIV-1 infection, fever, and IV drug use

3. EVALUATION

- Labs: WBC greater than 10,000/mm^3, ESR greater than 30 mm/h, CRP greater than 10 mg/dL, and send blood cultures × 2
- Arthrocentesis: joint fluid WBC greater than 25,000/mm^3 (usually greater than 50,000/mm^3 with 90% or more neutrophils), Gram stain with organisms, with or without fluid for crystal analysis

4. TREATMENT

- Arthroscopic joint irrigation and drainage
- Aggressive physical therapy to prevent joint contracture or muscle atrophy
- Antibiotic duration is based on the isolated organism, presence of bone involvement, and the presence or absence of retained hardware
- See **Table 47.5**

TABLE 47.5.   Empiric Antibiotics for Septic Arthritis Based on Synovial Fluid Gram Stain

Synovial Fluid Gram Stain	Empiric Antibiotic
Gram-positive cocci (no MRSA risk factors)	• Cefazolin 2 g IV q 8 h
Gram-positive cocci (MRSA risk factors)	• Vancomycin 30 mg/kg/day IV in divided doses
Gram-negative cocci (presumed Neisseria)	• Ceftriaxone 2 g IV q 24 h
Gram-negative bacilli	• Cefepime 2 g IV q 8 h or piperacillin-tazobactam 4.5 g IV q 6 h
No organisms (no MRSA risk factors)	• Cefazolin 2 g IV q 8 h
No organisms (MRSA risk factors)	• Vancomycin plus piperacillin-tazobactam or cefepime

Source: Adapted from *Infect Dis Clin N Amer*, 2005; 19(4): 799–817.

REFERENCES

Clin Infect Dis, 2007;44(5):705–10; *Clin Infect Dis*, 2005;41(10):1373–406; *N Engl J Med*, 2007;357(4):380–90; *Clin Infect Dis*, 2004;39(7):885–910; *Curr Opin Crit Care*, 2007;13(4):433–9; *Am Fam Physician*, 2010;81(7):893–9; *Infect Dis Clin North Am*, 2009;23(3):571–91; *J Antimicrob Chemotherap*, 2010;65(Suppl 3):iii35–44; *Am Fam Physician*, 2003;68(2):323–8; *Infect Dis Clin North Am*, 2005;19(4):799–817; *Am J Emerg Med*, 2007;25(7):749–52; *Ann Emerg Med*, 2008;52(5):567–9; *JAMA*, 2007;297(13):1478–88;

CHAPTER 48

MANAGEMENT OF CATHETER-RELATED BLOODSTREAM INFECTIONS (CRBSI)

1. DEFINITION OF CRBSI

- Bacteremia, fungemia, or clinical sepsis with no other source of infection
- Most common microorganisms recovered in at least 2 blood cultures (1 from peripheral draw and 1 from catheter): *Staphylococcus, Enterococcus*, Gram-negative bacilli, or *Candida* species
  - Growth of more than 15 colony-forming units of same organism from 5-cm segment of catheter tip
- Signs and symptoms of localized infection at the vascular insertion site
- The vascular catheter has been used in the 48 hours preceding a CRBSI

2. INTERVENTIONS THAT MINIMIZE THE RISK OF A CRBSI

- Good hand hygiene prior to insertion of catheter or accessing catheter ports
- Maximal barrier precautions (sterile gown and gloves, cap, and face mask)
- Chlorhexidine skin antisepsis of insertion area preferred over povidone-iodine
- Optimal site selection (subclavian and internal jugular preferred over femoral vein)
- Daily review of line necessity
- Consider antimicrobial-impregnated catheters if rate of infection is greater than 3/1000 line days
- *Avoid* antibiotic ointments to catheter entry sites
- Cover all catheters with a wide, transparent sterile dressing
- See **Figures 48.1** through **48.3**

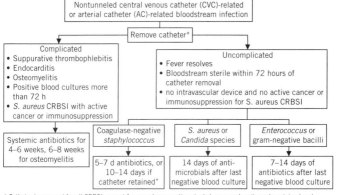

* Catheter is removed for all CRBSI, except for coagulase-negative *staphylococcus* when it can be retained and treated with systemic antibiotics **plus** antibiotic lock therapy

FIGURE 48.1. Management of Nontunneled Catheter-Related Bloodstream Infections (CRBSI)

Source: Adapted from *CID*, 2009; 49(1): 1–45.

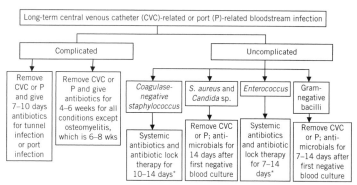

FIGURE 48.2.   Management of Long-Term Central Venous Catheter-Related or Port-Related Bloodstream Infections

Source: Adapted from *CID*, 2009; 49(1): 1–45.

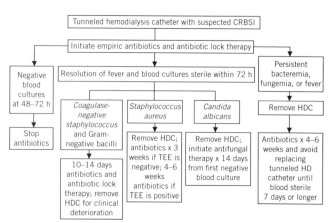

HDC = hemodialysis catheter, TEE = transesophageal echocardiogram

FIGURE 48.3.   Management of Tunneled Hemodialysis Catheter-Related Bloodstream Infections

Source: Adapted from *CID*, 2009; 49(1): 1–45.

CHAPTER 49

TUBERCULOSIS

1. **EPIDEMIOLOGY**
   - Global annual incidence for active disease is about 10.4 million, with 1.8 million deaths in 2007
   - Prevalence for latent disease is about 2 billion, or 30% of the world's population
   - In the United States, prevalence of active infection declined from 6.2 cases per 100,000 in 1998 to 4.2 cases per 100,000 in 2008
   - TB is the most common opportunistic infection among HIV patients
   - 25% of TB-related deaths are associated with HIV infection
   - Chemoprophylaxis with 6–9 months of INH or 4 months of rifapentine and INH can reduce progression from latent TB infection to active disease by 60%
   - Risks for progression (arranged from higher to lower): 10% annual risk for untreated HIV > close contacts of smear-positive contacts > patients with reticulonodular infiltrate > recent PPD converters in last 2 years > treatment of more than 15 mg/day prednisone > CKD > treatment with a TNF-α inhibitor > DM

2. **PATHOPHYSIOLOGY**
   - *Mycobacterium tuberculosis* (occasionally *M. bovis* from unpasteurized milk) is an aerobic acid-fast bacillus with heavily cross-linked mycolic acid–rich cell wall (impermeable to most antibiotics)
   - Initial asymptomatic infection
   - Bacilli from infectious droplets inhaled into alveoli are phagocytosed by macrophages; bacilli prevent normal maturation of phagosomes and reproduce within them until macrophage ruptures and releases bacilli, which infect new macrophages
   - During repeated cycles of macrophage lysis and infection, dendritic cells present mycobacterial antigens to T cells in lymph nodes, initiating host immune response
   - CD_4+ T cells critical to immune defense against tuberculosis (which is why patients with AIDS have a higher mortality rate compared with normal hosts)
   - Macrophage-activating response (majority): cell-mediated response contains bacilli within relatively anaerobic tubercles (granulomas) with central caseous necrosis and dormant bacilli, representing latent Tb infection (which may later reactivate in lungs, bone, CNS, and kidneys)
   - Tissue-damaging response (minority): delayed-type hypersensitivity results in progressive tissue damage and liquefaction of tubercles, leading to relatively aerobic cavities with rapid proliferation of bacilli
   - Erosion of bronchi results in infectious sputum causing active, infectious (smear-positive) TB
   - Erosion of blood vessel walls leads to hematogenous dissemination, which results in extrapulmonary TB

3. **CLINICAL PRESENTATION**
   - Pulmonary: fever, night sweats, cough (productive; hemoptysis in advanced disease), weight loss, anorexia, malaise
   - Extrapulmonary
     - Meningitis: headache, fever, malaise, eventually altered mental status, and focal neuro deficits (especially cranial nerves)
     - Pleural effusion: mild-to-moderate in size, unilateral except in military disease
     - Pericardial effusion
     - Genitourinary tract: often occult, dysuria would be a late finding
     - Osteomyelitis (Pott's disease): spinal tenderness, most often lower thoracic or lumbar, can progress to cord compression; rarely systemically ill

- Latent
  - Simon's focus (apical fibrosis or calcification)
  - Ghon's complex (calcified granuloma near a fissure)
  - Ranke complex (Ghon focus plus calcified hilar lymph node)

4. DIAGNOSIS

Latent Tuberculosis
- Positive PPD
- Positive IGRA: has no cross-reactivity with the BCG vaccine
- Both PPD and IGRA assays rely on T-cell immunity and therefore false-negatives more likely with immunodeficiency syndromes and at extremes of age

Active Pulmonary Tuberculosis
- Induced morning sputum positive for acid-fast bacilli
- Sputum culture growth of *Mycobacterium tuberculosis*
- Tissue biopsy

Extrapulmonary Tuberculosis
- Positive AFB RNA by PCR or AFB culture of CSF, pleural fluid, or ascitic fluid
- Tissue biopsy positive for acid-fast bacilli

5. WORKUP OF SUSPECTED TUBERCULOSIS

- See **Figure 49.1**

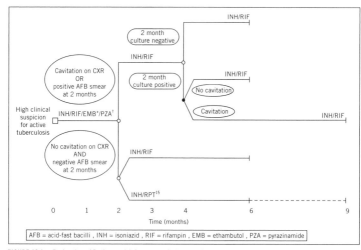

FIGURE 49.1.   Evaluation of Patients with Suspected Pulmonary Tuberculosis

Source: CDC/ATS/IDSA Guidelines for Treatment of Tuberculosis in *MMWR*, 2003; 52(RR-11): 1–77.

6. TREATMENT OF LATENT TUBERCULOSIS

- Isoniazid 300 mg PO daily × 9 months
- Rifampin 600 mg PO daily × 6 months
- INH plus rifapentine × 4 months

Initial Treatment of Pulmonary or Miliary Tuberculosis

- Isoniazid 300 mg PO daily
- Rifampin 600 mg PO daily
- Pyrazinamide 20–25 mg/kg PO daily (max 2000 mg PO daily)
- Ethambutol 15–25 mg/kg PO daily (max 2500 mg PO daily)

COMPLICATIONS

- Pulmonary fibrosis, emphysema, bronchiectasis, empyema, pneumothorax, ARDS
- Right middle lobe syndrome is the collapse of RML from compression by enlarged lymph nodes, which increases risk of pneumonia
- Hepatosplenomegaly
- Pancreatitis
- Cholecystitis
- Meningitis/tuberculoma
- Tuberculosis cutis miliaris disseminata
- Pericarditis
- Adrenal insufficiency
- Osteomyelitis/arthritis
- Emergence of multidrug resistance
- IRIS (immune reconstitution inflammatory syndrome) in AIDS patients

PROGNOSIS

- Without treatment the mortality rate of pulmonary TB exceeds 50%
- Poor prognostic factors include increased age, delay in diagnosis of TB, extent of radiographic involvement, mechanical ventilation, chronic renal failure, diabetes, and immunocompromised state

CHAPTER 50

URINARY TRACT INFECTIONS: CYSTITIS AND PYELONEPHRITIS

1. ## EPIDEMIOLOGY
   - Asymptomatic bacteriuria: always higher risk in women; risks: female sex, sexual activity, diabetes, advanced age, institutionalization, catheter
   - 71% of women under age 50 yo with symptoms consistent with UTI also have bacteriuria
   - Risk of UTI increases by 60 times within 48 hours after sexual intercourse
   - 97% of nosocomial UTIs are associated with instrumentation of urinary tract; it accounts for up to 40% of all nosocomial infections annually in the United States

2. ## PATHOPHYSIOLOGY
   - Ascending bacteria (usually Gram-negative Enterobacteriaceae) from urethra spreads to bladder (cystitis), then to ureter, then to kidneys (pyelonephritis)
   - Factors promoting colonization and infection: intercourse, catheter, stone, urinary retention, urinary stasis, vesicoureteral reflux, altered ecology of vaginal flora (nonoxynol-9, postmenopausal state), bacterial virulence factors (e.g., P fimbriae on *E. coli*), pregnancy, urethral length (female versus male)
   - Hematogenous spread to kidneys is relatively rare, except for *Candida* and *Staphylococcus aureus.*

3. ## CLINICAL PRESENTATION
   - Cystitis with dysuria, urinary urgency and frequency, and suprapubic pain; fever, nausea, vomiting, and flank pain suggest pyelonephritis
   - Microbiology: Enterobacteriaceae, *Enterococcus*, and rarely *Staphylococcus saprophyticus*

4. ## DIAGNOSIS
   - Urinalysis with negative nitrite **and** leukocyte esterase (LE) has a 90% NPV excluding UTI
   - Symptomatic patient with positive nitrite **or** LE: 75% sensitivity; 82% specificity for UTI
   - Cystitis if urine culture is greater than or equal to 10^5 colonies/mm^3 or greater than or equal to 10^4 colonies/mm^3 in catheterized specimen
   - Pyelonephritis typically has either full field WBCs in urine or WBC casts

5. ## WORKUP
   - Urinalysis, urine culture and Gram stain, blood culture × 2, CBCD, and basic metabolic panel
   - Renal ultrasound or CT urogram (for stones, renal abscess, or emphysematous pyelonephritis) indicated for pain out of proportion to exam or lack of clinical response within 72 hours
   ### Risk Factors for Cystitis and Pyelonephritis in Women
   - Frequent intercourse, obesity, sickle cell disease, urinary calculi, DM or other immunocompromised state, incontinence, pregnancy, neurogenic bladder, and recent instrumentation
   ### Risk Factors for UTI in Men
   - Immunocompromised, uncircumcised, age older than 65 yo, institutionalized, prostatism, neurogenic bladder, recent urinary tract surgery or instrumentation, and engages in anal intercourse

6. ## TREATMENT OF COMPLICATED CYSTITIS OR PYELONEPHRITIS
   - Urology consultation for emphysematous pyelonephritis, renal or perinephric abscess, or pyelonephritis with an obstructing stone: may need a ureteral stent or nephrostomy tube
   - Aggressive IV hydration; analgesia with oral acetaminophen and opioids or IV opioids
   - Empiric antibiotics for community-acquired *complicated* cystitis or pyelonephritis
     - Ceftriaxone, ampicillin and gentamicin, or fluoroquinolone; antibiotic duration 7–10 days with a fluoroquinolone; 10–14 days with TMP-SMX or β-lactam or if patient has DM, is immunocompromised, or is pregnant
     - Switch to narrowest spectrum oral antibiotics based on culture and sensitivity results when clinically improved, afebrile 24 h or longer, and good oral intake

- Empiric antibiotics for nosocomial complicated UTI (risk of pseudomonas or enterococcus)
  - Ampicillin and gentamicin, piperacillin-tazobactam, levofloxacin, and imipenem
- Prostatitis: age younger than 35 yo ceftriaxone 250 mg IM × 1 and doxycycline 100 mg PO bid × 10 days
  - Age 35 yo or older: fluoroquinolone or Bactrim DS for 2–4 wks (acute) or 4–8 wks (chronic)

7. **COMPLICATIONS**

- Renal abscess carries a 20–50% mortality
- Infected renal calculus serving as nidus of infection
- Xanthogranulomatous pyelonephritis
- Emphysematous pyelonephritis
- Renal parenchymal scarring leading to CKD
- Acute renal failure
- Sepsis/septic shock
- ARDS
- Multiorgan failure

8. **PROGNOSIS**

- Emphysematous pyelonephritis (20–80% mortality rate)
- Perinephric abscess (20–50% mortality rate)
- The mortality for urosepsis is 16.1%

REFERENCES

Clin Infect Dis, 1999;29(4):745–58; *J Fam Pract,* 2007;56(8):657–8; *Am J Med Sci,* 2007;333(2):111–6; *Am J Med,* 1999;106(3):327–34; *Obstet Gynecol,* 2005;106(5 Pt 1):1085–92, *Clin Infect Dis,* 2011;52(5):561–4; *Am Fam Physician,* 2005;71(5):933–42.

SECTION 6

NEUROLOGY

CHAPTER 51

ACUTE ISCHEMIC STROKE

1. EPIDEMIOLOGY

- 20% of patients with a TIA or minor stroke have a recurrent vascular event within 1 year
- Risk of recurrent ischemic stroke is highest within first week after a minor stroke or TIA
- Ischemic strokes account for 85% of all strokes (thrombotic 20%, lacunar 25%, cardioembolic 20%, cryptogenic 30%, other 5%)
  - Less than 5% get tPA within 3 hours
  - Cryptogenic is most likely embolic and often paradoxical through a PFO
  - Other causes: hypercoagulable states, dissection, vasculitis, endocarditis, complicated migraine, stimulant drugs, neurosyphilis, paradoxical embolus through a PFO, sickle cell crisis, or cerebral vein or cerebral sinus thrombosis

2. PATHOPHYSIOLOGY

- Occlusion of blood vessel decreases cerebral blood flow, resulting in necrosis and apoptosis, then focal infarction
- Extent of infarction depends on extent of collateral vessels
- Around infarcted area is a reversibly ischemic penumbra that is the target of potential revascularization
- Hyperglycemia and hyperthermia worsen cell death
- Sources of occlusion
  - Arterial embolism
  - Atherosclerosis (most commonly from carotid bifurcation), carotid, or vertebral artery dissection
  - Cardioembolism: MCA, PCA, or branches
  - Atrial fibrillation, MI, prosthetic valves, mitral stenosis, paradoxical embolism from venous circulation via patent foramen ovale, infective endocarditis

3. CLINICAL PRESENTATION

- See **Table 52.1**
- Embolic: patients generally experience a sudden onset of maximal deficit
- Thrombotic: patients generally have a stuttering or stepwise progression
- Paradoxical embolus presents as a sudden neurologic deficit after a Valsalva maneuver
- Hemorrhagic strokes are managed as an acute intracranial hemorrhage (see **Table 51.1**)
- Acute unprovoked onset of focal weakness and/or speech disturbance
- Symptoms: facial paresis, arm/leg weakness (pronator drift), arm/leg paresthesias, dizziness, visual field defects, cranial nerve abnormalities
- Cincinnati Prehospital Stroke Scale: facial paresis, arm drift, abnormal speech
  - 3 present = LR+ 14
  - 2 present = LR+ 4.2
  - 1 present = LR+ 5.2
  - 0 present = LR+ 0.4
- Oxfordshire Ischemic Stroke Subtypes
  - Total anterior circulation infarct (TACI): combination of new higher cerebral dysfunction (e.g., dysphasia, dyscalculia, visuospatial disorder); homonymous visual field defect and ipsilateral motor and/or sensory defect of at least 2 areas of the face, arm, or leg
  - Partial anterior circulation infarct (PACI): patients with only 2 of 3 TACI components, with higher cerebral dysfunction alone, or with a motor/sensory deficit more restricted than those classified as LACI (e.g., confined to 1 limb or to face and hand, but not the whole arm)

- Lacunar infarct (LACI): pure motor or pure sensory symptoms, sensorimotor stroke, or ataxic hemiparesis; face-arm and arm-leg syndromes included
- Posterior circulation infarct (POCI): any one of the following: ipsilateral cranial nerve palsy with contralateral motor and/or sensory deficit, bilateral motor and/or sensory deficit, disorder of conjugate gaze, cerebellar dysfunction without ataxic hemiparesis, isolated homonymous visual field defect
- See **Tables 51.2** and **51.3** and **Figure 51.1**

TABLE 51.1.   Clinical Presentation of Acute Ischemic Strokes

Clinical Presentation of Strokes in Carotid Distribution	Vascular Area
Face and arms affected more than legs, aphasia, hemiparesis, hemianesthesia, contralateral homonymous hemianopsia, and ipsilateral gaze deviation	MCA (dominant)
Face and arms affected more than legs, neglect, hemiparesis, hemianesthesia, contralateral homonymous hemianopsia, and ipsilateral gaze deviation	MCA (nondominant)
Legs are affected more than face and arms, hemiparesis, hemianesthesia, incontinence, personality change, and altered grasp and suck reflexes	ACA
Clinical Presentation of Strokes in Posterior Circulation	
Homonymous hemianopsia with or without difficulty with colors	PCA
Ipsilateral cranial nerve palsies and contralateral hemiparesis	Brainstem
Headache, vertigo, vomiting, ataxia, dysarthria, and nystagmus	Cerebellum
Cranial nerve deficits, quadriparesis, somnolence, ophthalmoplegia, dysphonia, dysphagia, and dysarthria	Basilar artery
Vertigo, facial pain, dysphagia, postural instability, hoarseness, ipsilateral Horner syndrome, impaired pain/temperature of face, and limb ataxia and contralateral impaired pain/temperature of limbs	Lateral medullary infarct
Clinical Presentation of Penetrating Artery Strokes	
Hemiparesis where legs, arms, and face are equally affected is a pure motor lacunar stroke	IC
Hemianesthesia where legs, arms, and face are equally affected is a pure sensory lacunar stroke	Thalamus
Ipsilateral weakness and limb ataxia represent an ataxia hemiparesis lacunar stroke	Pons and posterior IC
Clumsy hand-dysarthria lacunar stroke	Pons
Hemiparesis and hemianesthesia where legs, arms, and face are equally affected represent a sensorimotor lacunar stroke	Posterior IC and thalamus

MCA = middle cerebral artery, ACA = anterior cerebral artery, PCA = posterior cerebral artery, IC = internal capsule

TABLE 51.2.   ABCD* Risk Score for 7-Day Stroke Risk After Transient Ischemic Attack

ABCD Risk Score	7-Day Stroke Risk (%)	95% Confidence Interval
3 or lower	0	0
4	2.2	0–6.4%
5	16.3	6–26.7%
6	35.5	18.6–52.3%

* ABCD Risk Score is the total combined points: age 60 yo or older = 1 point; blood pressure elevation at presentation (SBP 140 mmHg or higher and/ or DBP 90 mmHg or higher) = 1 point; clinical features (unilateral weakness = 2 points, speech disturbance without weakness = 1 point, other = 0 points); and duration of symptoms (60 minutes or longer = 2 points, 10–59 minutes = 1 point, less than 10 minutes = 0 points)

Source: Adapted from *Lancet,* 2005(9479); 366: 29–36.

TABLE 51.3.   Secondary Prevention of Ischemic Strokes

Modifiable Risk Factor	Therapeutic Goals/Recommendations
Hypertension	BP less than 140/90 (less than 130/80 for DM or CKD)
DM	Hemoglobin A1c 7% or less
Sympathomimetic abuse	Abstinence
Smoking	Smoking cessation
Daily alcohol use	Men less than 2 drinks, nonpregnant women 1 drink or less
Obesity	Weight loss until waist circumference is less than 35 inches for women and less than 40 inches for men
Physical inactivity	30 minutes or more moderate exercise most days
Symptomatic severe CAS	CEA recommended for stenosis 70–99%
Symptomatic moderate CAS	Consider CEA for stenosis 50–69%
Left ventricular thrombus	Warfarin anticoagulation to INR 2.5 (2–3) for 3–12 months
Atrial fibrillation/flutter	Warfarin anticoagulation to INR 2.5 (range 2–3)
Rheumatic MV disease	Warfarin anticoagulation to INR 2.5 (range 2–3)
Dilated cardiomyopathy	Warfarin anticoagulation or antiplatelet therapy
HMG-CoA peductase inhibitors (statins)	Statins beneficial even with normal cholesterol levels and no CAD • Desire LDL less than 100 mg/dL or less than 70 mg/dL for very high risk patients* with multiple risk factors
Antiplatelet therapy (aspirin clopidogrel or ASA–extended-release dipyridamole)	All patients after a noncardioembolic stroke
Prosthetic heart valves	Chronic anticoagulation to INR 2.5 (range 2–3)
Mitral valve prolapse/aortic stenosis	Antiplatelet therapy
Sickle cell disease	Exchange transfusion until Hgb S less than 30%
Cerebral vein thrombosis	Anticoagulation to INR 2.5 (range 2–3) for 6 months
Antiphospholipid syndrome	Antiplatelet therapy or chronic anticoagulation to INR 2.5 (range 2–3) if multiple organs involved

DM = diabetes mellitus, CKD = chronic kidney disease, HMG CoA = 3-hydroxy-3-methylglutaryl-CoA, CAD = coronary artery disease, CAS = carotid artery stenosis, CEA = carotid endarterectomy, INR = international normalized ratio, MV = mitral valve, HMG CoA = 3-hydroxy-3-methylglutaryl-CoA, CAD = coronary artery disease, ASA = aspirin
* CAD plus diabetes, metabolic syndrome, uncontrolled risk factors, or progressive cardiac ischemia

Source: Adapted from *Stroke*, 2006; 37(2); 577–617.

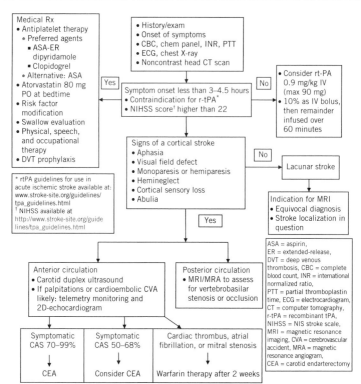

FIGURE 51.1.   Management of Patients with an Ischemic Stroke

Source: Information from *Mayo Clin Proc*, 2004;79(8):1071–86; *NEJM*, 2006;355(6): 549–59 and *Stroke*, 2009;40:2945–48

4. EVALUATION OF STROKE IN YOUNG ADULTS (YOUNGER THAN 50 YO) WITH FEW VASCULAR RISK FACTORS

- Studies: drug screen, blood cultures, echocardiogram with bubble study, serum for VDRL, lupus anticoagulant, anticardiolipin antibody, lipoprotein (a) level, homocysteine level, ANA, ESR, ECG, duplex ultrasound of neck (arterial dissection), sickle cell prep (if patient is African American or of Mediterranean or Southeast Asian descent)

5. DIFFERENTIAL DIAGNOSIS

- Complex migraine
- Todd's paralysis
- Focal seizures
- Conversion disorder
- Malingering
- Severe hypoglycemia
- Brain mets
- Brain abscess

COMPLICATIONS

- Intraparenchymal hemorrhage
- Myocardial infarction, arrhythmias
- Seizure
- Cerebral edema/herniation
- Dysphagia
- Aspiration pneumonia/pneumonitis
- DVT/PE from stasis/immobility
- Pressure sores/ulcers from immobility and decreased sensation
- Development of contractures to paralyzed extremity
- Delirium: increased risk with preexisting cognitive impairment, infection, or increased stroke severity
- Recurrence or extension of stroke
- Urinary tract infection due to indwelling Foley catheter
- Constipation
- Depression
- Falls secondary to unstable gait

PROGNOSIS

- Mortality following ischemic stroke is 8–12%
- Clinical stroke severity is the strongest predictor of outcome; advanced age, female sex, and medical comorbidities, especially diabetes and hyperglycemia, are poor prognostic factors

REFERENCES

Am Fam Physician, 2009;80(1):33–40; *Lancet,* 2005;366(9479):29–36; *Stroke,* 2006;37(2):577–617; *Mayo Clin Proc,* 2004;79(8):1071–86; *N Engl J Med,* 2006;355(6):549–59; *Stroke,* 2007;38(5):1655–711

Simel D. Is this patient having a stroke? In: Simel D, Rennie D, eds. *The Rational Clinical Examination.* New York, NY: McGraw-Hill; 2009:627–41.

CHAPTER 52

ACUTE HEMORRHAGIC STROKE

1. **EPIDEMIOLOGY**
   - Accounts for 10–20% of all strokes; 30-day mortality of 35–52%
   - Only 21% of patients with ICH are expected to be independent in 6 months
   - In-hospital mortality reduction of only 6% between 1990 and 2000
   - Chronic HTN is responsible for 60% of cases
2. **PATHOPHYSIOLOGY**
   - Hypertensive intraparenchymal hemorrhage: small penetrating artery bursts spontaneously or due to anticoagulant therapy, most commonly in basal ganglia, thalami, cerebellum, and pons
   - Mass effect may compress brain tissue leading to herniation
   - Blood may enter ventricles leading to hydrocephalus
3. **CLINICAL PRESENTATION**
   - Acute onset followed by gradual progression of neurologic deficits
   - Frequently, patient has a decreased level of consciousness
   - Headache
4. **DIAGNOSIS**
   - Noncontrast CT scan of the head

- History/exam
- Onset of symptoms
- GCS score
- CBC, chem panel, PT, PTT
- Noncontrast head CT scan

For GCS 8 or lower or increased ICP
- Intubate, then PaCO$_2$ 35 plus or minus 2 mmHg
- Head of bed elevated to 30–45°
- Isotonic fluids until euvolemic
- Consider mannitol 0.5–1 g/kg IV q 4 h (if sOsm is less than 320 mOsm/L)
- Recommend intracranial pressure monitoring
- Sedation and neuromuscular blockade for refractory ICP greater than 20 mmHg

- Maintain normothermia and euvolemia
- Keep glucose less than 180 mg/dL
- Sequential compression devices
- H$_2$-blocker or proton pump inhibitor
- Consider antiepileptic therapy x 7 days for lobar hemorrhages
- Correct coagulopathy with FFP, PCC, or cyroprecipitate
- Platelet transfusion if PLT less than 50 K (or recent antiplatelet use)

SAH

ICH

Medical management
- Keep MAP below 130 mmHg and SBP below 160 mmHg
  - Labetalol, esmolol, or nicardipine
- Nimodipine 60 mg PO q 4 h x 21 days

Medical management
- Acute BP management
  - Keep MAP below 130 mmHg or SBP below 180 mmHg if preexisting HTN or if suspected/known increased ICP
    - Labetalol, hydralazine, or nicardipine
  - Keep MAP at 110 mmHg or lower or SBP below 160 mmHg if no history of HTN, if postcraniotomy, or normal ICP
- Recombinant FVIIa does not improve survival and is not recommended

- Cerebral angiogram to locate aneurysm
  - 4-vessel cerebral angiogram
  - Digital subtraction CT angiogram
- Surgical clipping or endovascular coiling within 72 hours

Indications for surgical evacuation
- Infratentorial ICH larger than 3 cm or smaller with neurological deterioration
- Superficial supratentorial ICH with neurological deficits
- Young patient with lobar ICH and GCS 13 or lower

FIGURE 52.1. Management of Patients with a Nontraumatic Intracranial Hemorrhage

Sources: *Stroke* 2007; 38(6): 2001–23, *Lancet* 2005; 365(9457): 387–97, *Ann Emer Med*, 2008; 51(Suppl 3): S24–7, *Mayo Clin Proc* 2005; 80(3): 420–33, *Cochrane Database*, 2007, July 18;Issue 3:CD000277 and *NEJM*, 2008; 358(20): 2127–37.

TABLE 52.1. Glasgow Coma Scale

Score	Eye Opening	Verbal Response	Motor Response
6	–	–	Follows commands
5	–	Normal conversation	Localizes pain
4	Spontaneous	Disoriented/inappropriate	Withdraws to pain
3	To voice	Incoherent	Decorticate posturing
2	To pain	Moans	Decerebrate posturing
1	None	None	No movement

5. **INDICATIONS FOR INTUBATION IN ACUTE HEMORRHAGIC STROKE**
   - GCS of 8 or lower or a rapidly declining GCS, hemodynamic instability, respiratory instability, a combative patient precluding the safe completion of studies, or the need for surgery

6. **INDICATIONS FOR INTRACRANIAL PRESSURE (ICP) MONITORING**
   - GCS of 8 or lower and either an abnormal CT scan **OR** 2 of following: age older than 40 yo, motor posturing or focal lateralizing signs, SBP less than 90 mmHg, GCS 9–12 and need for a prolonged extracranial operation

7. **MANAGEMENT OF INCREASED ICP**
   - Keep ICP less than or equal to 20 mmHg and cerebral perfusion pressure greater than or equal to 60 mmHg (CPP = MAP − ICP)
   - Assure proper patient positioning (head of bed elevated at least 30 degrees), adequate sedation, no fever, avoid a tight cervical collar, and assure a good ICP waveform
   - Hyperosmolar therapy: mannitol 1 g/kg load, then 0.25–0.5 g/kg IV 2 h prn increased ICP if Sosm is less than 320 mosm; or 3% saline at 50 mL/hr to maintain Na at around 150 MEq/L
   - Ventriculostomy with CSF drainage
   - Refractory elevated ICP management: consider short-term paralysis, pentobarbital 1 mg/kg/h or propofol therapy (if blood pressure allows), or decompressive craniectomy
     - Consider a norepinephrine drip to maintain a CPP 60 mmHg or greater if necessary for increased ICP

8. **COMPLICATIONS**
   - Hydrocephalus
   - Seizure
   - Cerebral edema/herniation
   - Dysphagia
   - Aspiration pneumonia/pneumonitis
   - DVT/PE from stasis/immobility
   - Pressure sores/ulcers from immobility and decreased sensation
   - Development of contractures to paralyzed extremity
   - Delirium: increased risk with preexisting cognitive impairment, infection, or increased stroke severity
   - Recurrence or extension of stroke
   - Urinary tract infection due to indwelling Foley catheter
   - Constipation
   - Depression
   - Falls secondary to unstable gait

. PROGNOSIS

- FUNC score (see **Figure 52.2**) identifies patients who will attain functional independence by 90 days after a primary ICH

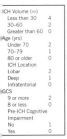

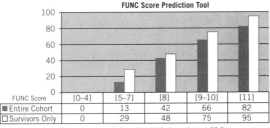

IGURE 52.2.   FUNC Score Prediction Tool That Predicts 90-Day Functional Independence After an Intracranial Hemorrhage

*ource: Stroke, 2008; 39(8): 2304–2309. Printed with permission from Wolters Kluwer Health.

EFERENCES

*troke, 2007;38(6):2001–23; *Lancet*, 2005;365(9457):387–97; *Ann Emerg Med*, 2008;51(Suppl 3):S24–7; *Mayo :lin Proc*, 2005;80(3):420–33; *Cochrane Database Syst Rev*, 2005;(1):; *N Engl J Med*, 2008;358(20):2127–37; *troke*, 2008;39(8):2304–9.

CHAPTER 53

DEMENTIA

1. **EPIDEMIOLOGY**
   - Community dwellers with dementia have a 30% prevalence of having concomitant behavioral or psychological symptoms; prevalence is 80% in an SNF

2. **PATHOPHYSIOLOGY**
   - Large-scale neuronal dysfunction with neurotransmitter imbalances
   - Behavior and mood: noradrenergic, serotonergic, dopaminergic
   - Attention and memory: cholinergic pathways
   - Alzheimer's dementia
     - Amyloid oligomers lead to progressively accumulate as neuritic plaques (Aβ) and neurofibrillary tangles (tau), which spread to the medial temporal lobe, then the hippocampus, then the temporal and parietal neocortex
     - Genetic factors: APP gene (chromosome 21) increases amyloid production, apo ε4 decreases amyloid clearance
     - Primary neurotransmitter defect is decreased acetylcholine
   - Vascular dementia
     - Multi-infarct dementia: successive strokes, especially involving left hemisphere, lead to stepwise neurologic deterioration
     - Diffuse white matter disease (Binswanger disease): hypertension leads to microangiopathy, then chronic ischemia
   - Frontotemporal dementia: tau inclusions result in atrophy of frontal, insular, and temporal cortex; serotonergic defect with relative preservation of cholinergic signaling
   - Parkinson's disease: Lewy bodies (α-synuclein) in substantia nigra result in loss of dopaminergic innervation

3. **CLINICAL PRESENTATION**
   - Cognitive or behavioral impairments: recall of new information, reasoning, visuospatial ability, language, personality
   - Visual hallucinations may indicate Lewy body dementia
   - Disinhibition may indicate frontotemporal dementia
   - Tremor, cogwheeling may indicate Parkinson-related dementia
   - Alcohol abuse history may indicate alcoholic dementia

4. **DEFINITION OF DEMENTIA**
   - Acquired, persistent cognitive impairment that interferes with daily functioning and affects 3 or more cognitive domains: memory, language, visuospatial skills, emotional or personality changes, and poor executive functioning
   - Folstein Mini-Mental Status Exam (MMSE) less than or equal to 23/30 indicative of dementia
     - Less accurate for age younger than 50, low level of education or non-Caucasians
     - Other tests: memory impairment score, clock drawing, or word-list acquisition

   Alzheimer's Dementia (50–80% of dementias)
   - Gradually progressive deterioration following Functional Assessment Staging (FAST) Scale available at www.ec-online.net/Knowledge/articles/alzstages.html
   - Additional features: personality changes (extreme passivity to severe hostility), psychotic symptoms (50% with delusions and 25% with hallucinations), mood disorders (40% depressed or anxious), and 30% with Parkinsonian features

Vascular Dementia (10–20% of dementias)

- Progression of cognitive decline that usually follows a stroke
- Urinary incontinence, gait disturbance, and language impairment are common

Parkinson's Disease Dementia (PDD) and Lewy Body Dementia (5–10% of dementias)

- Parkinsonism and graphic, recurrent hallucinations and delusions are common

Frontotemporal Dementia (12–25% of dementias)

- Initiation, goal setting, and planning more than memory loss
- Apathy, disinhibited behavior, conduct problems, poor hygiene, and poor grooming
- Language impairments (logorrhea, echolalia, and palilalia)

5. DIFFERENTIAL DIAGNOSIS

- Depression
- Delirium
- Encephalitis
- Encephalopathy

6. COMPLICATIONS

- Malnutrition due to loss of interest in food/drink
- Aspiration pneumonitis/pneumonia due to loss of control/coordination in muscles/swallow
- Decreased ability to perform ADLs (i.e., bathing, dressing, eating, ambulating, toileting)
- Medication administration error
- Behavioral changes: depression, aggression, confusion, frustration, anxiety, inhibition
- Delirium: especially in demented patients admitted to hospital or with surrounding changes/activities/routines
- Insomnia and other disruptive sleep patterns such as restless leg syndrome and sleep apnea
- Falls/motor vehicle crash
- Autonomic dysfunction such as orthostatic hypotension, urinary incontinence or retention, impotence
- Constipation
- See Table 53.1

TABLE 53.1.   Reversible Causes of Dementia

B_{12} Deficiency	Hypothyroidism	HIV Dementia	Neurosyphilis
Normal pressure hydrocephalus (triad of dementia, ataxia, and urinary incontinence)			

REFERENCES

N Engl J Med, 2004;351(1):56–67; Ann Intern Med, 1956;44(5):925–37; Neurology, 2001; 56(9): 1133–42; JAMA, 2007;297(21):2391–404; J Psychopharmacol, 2006;20(6):732–55; Ann Intern Med, 2008;148(5):370–8; Am Fam Physician, 2011;84(8):895–902.

CHAPTER 54

DELIRIUM

1. ## EPIDEMIOLOGY

   - 31% of all ICU patients, and 82% of intubated patients; causes 3-fold reintubation rate; increased risk of inpatient mortality; 39% increase in ICU cost per patient and 31% increase in hospital cost alone
   - Each additional day of delirium increases hospital mortality by 10% and hospital length of stay by 20%
   - 46% of cases are misdiagnosed by nonpsychiatric hospital staff
   - 10–24% of patients with persistent delirium may have long-term cognitive deficits and develop PTSD as a result of the experience and hallucination

2. ## PATHOPHYSIOLOGY

   - Generalized cortical and subcortical dysfunction
   - Nonspecific symmetric slowing on EEG
   - Acute imbalances in neurotransmitter imbalances (decreased acetylcholine, increased dopamine) with underlying predisposition
   - May be precipitated by anticholinergic medications, especially in patients with underlying acetylcholine deficiency (Alzheimer's disease, Lewy Body dementia)
   - Antipsychotic medications used to treat delirium decrease dopamine activity

3. ## CLINICAL PRESENTATION

   - Acute, fluctuating change in cognition and attention precipitated by acute medical illness
   - Possible presenting symptoms
     - Altered mental status (acute and fluctuating)
     - Inattention
     - Disorganized thinking (hallucinations or visual misperceptions)
     - Altered level of consciousness (lethargic or hyperalert)
     - Alterations in sleep–wake cycle or mood lability

4. ## DIAGNOSIS OF DELIRIUM REQUIRES THESE 3 CONDITIONS

   - Disturbance of consciousness: decreased awareness of environment, poor attention span leading to poor information recall
   - Cognitive change: confusion, disorientation, language impairment, with or without psychosis
   - Sudden onset, fluctuating severity, disturbed sleep–wake cycle, and transient in nature

5. ## DIFFERENTIAL DIAGNOSIS

   - Drug intoxication
   - Psychosis
   - Mania
   - Dementia
   - Encephalitis

6. ## RISK FACTORS FOR DELIRIUM

   - Advanced age, dementia, medical comorbidities, psychiatric disorder, polypharmacy, depression, social isolation, history of substance abuse, and severity of acute illness
   - See **Table 54.1**

TABLE 54.1. Etiologies of Delirium

Categories	Specific Etiologies (mnemonic = AEIOUMITS)
Alcohol (or illicit drugs)	Alcohol or illicit drug intoxication or withdrawal
Endocrine/electrolytes/ environmental	Hyper-/hyponatremia, hypercalcemia, hyper/ hypothyroidism, Addison's disease, Cushing syndrome, and hyper-/hypothermia
Infection/infarct	Myocardial infarction, hypertensive encephalopathy, hyperviscosity, or any infection
Oxygen (gases)	Hypoxia, hypercarbia, or carbon monoxide poisoning
Uremia	Usually blood urea nitrogen greater than 100 mg/dL
Metabolic/mental (psychiatric) or meds (see below)	B_{12} deficiency, Wilson's disease, Wernicke's and/or Korsakoff's syndrome, hepatic encephalopathy, or psychiatric disease (diagnosis of exclusion)
Insulin	Severe hypoglycemia or hyperglycemia
Trauma/toxins/TTP	Head trauma, toxins (organophosphates, etc.), or thrombotic thrombocytopenic purpura
Seizures, space-occupying lesion, stroke	Stroke, intracranial bleed, brain tumor, hydrocephalus, or seizure

Commonly Implicated Medications

Anticholinergics, amiodarone, α blockers, amantadine, amphotericin B, anticonvulsants, antihistamines, antiparkinsonian meds, aspirin, baclofen, barbiturates, benzodiazepines, β blockers, bromocriptine, cephalosporins, chlorpromazine, clonidine, colchicine, digoxin, disopyramide, fluoroquinolones, GI antispasmodics, glucocorticoids, histamine receptor$_2$ blockers, levodopa, lithium, methyldopa, metoclopramide, neuroleptics, nifedipine, NSAIDs, opioids, oseltamivir, penicillins, pentamidine, pergolide, pramipexole, procainamide, prochlorperazine, promethazine, quinidine, ropinirole, sedatives, sympathomimetics, theophylline, tricyclic antidepressants, tuberculosis meds, zalcitabine, zidovudine, and zolpidem

Source: Information from *Emer. Med. Clin. N. Amer.*, 2000; 18(2): 243–52 and *AFP.* 1997; 55(5): 1773–80.

TREATMENT OF DELIRIUM

- Detailed history, exam, and lab evaluation for above conditions
- Pharmacologic interventions
  - Discontinue all nonessential medications and treat underlying condition(s)
  - Low-dose haloperidol (0.5–2.5 mg IM/IV q 0.5–1 h prn agitation or psychotic symptoms)
  - Control pain with scheduled analgesics
  - Minimize use of benzodiazepines
- Nonpharmacologic interventions
  - Quiet room with familiar objects, family/friends to calm and reorient patient
  - Maintain adequate hydration and avoid hypoxia
  - Early mobilization with physical and occupational therapy
  - Use sensory aids to correct visual or auditory impairments
  - Maintain consistent caregivers and constantly reorient/reassure patient
  - Avoid overstimulation and change lighting to cue day and night

COMPLICATIONS

- Deterioration of memory and skills especially if underlying dementia or chronic/serious illness exists
- In the setting of serious medical illness, delirium may lead to poor or delayed recovery, increased mortality, and need for institutional care
- Mistaking delirium for dementia or psychiatric illness

REFERENCES

Emerg Med Clin North Am, 2000;18(2):243–52; *Am Fam Physician*, 1997;55(5):1773–80; *Chest*, 2007;132(2):624–36; *Am Fam Physician*, 2008;78(11):1265–70.

CHAPTER 55

SEIZURES

1. **EPIDEMIOLOGY**
   - 20% of epileptic pts have only nocturnal seizures
   - 60% of seizures have good prognosis for long-term remission with AED; number of seizures within 6 months of diagnosis have good predictive value for long-term remission
   - 40% with persistent seizures require further evaluation
   - 20–30% have intractable seizures requiring further intervention
   - 6.3% acute seizure risk within first 24 hours after stroke

2. **PATHOPHYSIOLOGY**
   - Initiation
     - Ca influx into neuron opens Na channels, resulting in depolarization, then repetitive action potential bursts, which cause hyperpolarization via GABA receptors and K channels
     - Synchronized bursts from cluster of neurons cause spike on EEG
     - Recruitment of surrounding neurons results in propagation
   - Increased Ca in presynaptic terminals increases neurotransmitter release
   - NMDA activation increases Ca influx
   - Changes in osmolality lead to extracellular electric fields
   - Common pathway for decreased seizure threshold is increased neuronal excitability, which is influenced by neurotransmitters, extracellular ions, ion channel conductance, structural alterations of neuronal pathways, etc.
   - Focal seizures involve one cerebral hemisphere; generalized seizures involve both cerebral hemispheres

3. **CLINICAL PRESENTATION**
   - Generalized: loss of consciousness
     - Whole-body tonic and/or clonic movements
       - Tonic: rigid muscle contraction
       - Clonic: jerking, frequency of about 4 per second
     - Loss of bowel/bladder function
     - Followed by a postictal phase of sedation or confusion
   - Partial, simple
     - Focal: clonic movements or paresthesias of a single limb, aphasia, and/or visual changes
     - Consciousness is unimpaired
     - May evolve into a generalized seizure
   - Partial, complex
     - Partial seizure symptoms, but with alteration of consciousness
   - Status epilepticus
     - Defined as either recurrent seizures without recovery between or a prolonged seizure lasting 30 minutes or longer
   - See **Table 55.1**

TABLE 55.1. Classification of Seizures

Seizure Type	Consciousness Impaired	Tongue Biting or Incontinence	Aura*	Hyperventilation Triggers	Automatisms†	Postictal Duration
Simple partial seizure	No	No	Yes	No	No	Seconds
Complex partial seizure	Yes	No	Yes, 1st	No	Yes (after aura)	Minutes
Secondary generalized partial seizure	Yes	Yes	Yes, 1st	No	Possibly	Minutes–hours
Grand mal seizure	Yes	Yes	No	No	No	Minutes–hours

Jerking movements, epigastric discomfort, fear, bad smell, focal sensory, or psychic symptoms
Facial grimacing, gesturing, chewing, lip smacking, snapping fingers, walking, or undressing

WORKUP

- Chemistry panel, drug screen, electroencephalogram, thyroid-stimulating hormone, lumbar puncture if immunocompromised or for possible meningoencephalitis, and a pregnancy test
- Imaging: noncontrast head CT scan for head trauma, new severe headache, and anticoagulated patients; MRI preferred for focal neuro deficits, new partial seizures, persistent headaches or altered mental status, history of cancer, HIV-positive pts, or unprovoked seizures in patients older than 40 yo or younger than 2 yo
- Risk factors for recurrent seizures: history of closed head injury, structural brain lesion, focal neuro exam, cognitive impairment, partial seizures, abnormal electroencephalogram (EEG), or positive family history

TREATMENT

- Indications for chronic antiepileptic drug (AED) use (see **Table 55.2**)
  - Start after 1st seizure and either abnormal EEG or 2 risk factors as above
  - Start after 2nd seizure
- Miscellaneous: check state requirements for mandatory Department of Motor Vehicles reporting and driving limitations (see www.epilepsyfoundation.org)
- Discontinuation of therapy: wean AED 25% every 2–4 weeks; can attempt once seizure-free for **at least** 2–3 years; increased risk of recurrent seizures if risk factors present (see above), abnormal EEG, or abnormal neuroimaging
- See **Figure 55.1**

TABLE 55.2.   Antiepileptic Medications for Adults with Seizures

Medication	PS	GS	Starting Dose (mg)*	Therapeutic Dose (mg)*	Side Effects/Monitoring
Carbamazepine†	1st	1st	200 bid	400 tid‡	Hyponatremia, osteopenia, hepatitis, rash, dizziness, leukopenia/follow levels, liver panel, CBC
Clonazepam			0.5 tid	1–5 tid	Sedation, confusion, ataxia, anemia, leukopenia
Gabapentin	•		300 at bedtime	300–1200 tid	Somnolence, ataxia, headache, weight gain, fatigue
Lacosamide	•		50 bid	100–300 bid	AV block, dizziness, nausea, diplopie, headache
Lamotrigine†	1st	•	25 daily	200 bid	Rash, headache, tremor, vomiting, insomnia, diplopia
Levetiracetam†	•	•	500 bid	500–1500 bid	Somnolence, asthenia, headache, dizziness, anxiety
Oxcarbazepine†	1st	1st	300 bid	600 bid	Dizziness, headache, nausea, ataxia, hyponatremia
Phenytoin†	1st	1st	1 g load	300 daily‡	Fatigue, rash, gingival hyperplasia, ataxia, hepatitis, osteopenia/follow drug levels, liver panel
Pregabalin	•		75 bid	150–300 bid	Weight gain, pedal edema, dizziness, fatigue
Tiagabine	•	•	4 mg daily	4–8 bid–qid	Dizziness, tremor, confusion, asthenia, fatigue
Topiramate†	•	•	25 daily	200 bid	Ataxia, confusion, dizziness, fatigue, paresthesias, acidosis, nephrolithiasis, weight loss, nervousness
Valproic acid/ divalproex†	1st	1st	250 bid	500–750 tid‡	Weight gain, tremors, hair loss, sedation, ataxia, nausea, thrombocytopenia, confusion/ follow levels
Zonisamide	•	•	50–100 daily	400 daily	Fatigue, mental slowing, nephrolithiasis, anorexia, nausea, ataxia, headache, tremor, hyperhidrosis

PS = partial seizures including partial complex seizures with secondary generalization, GS = generalized seizures including tonic-clonic, tonic, clonic, myoclonic or atonic seizures, 1st = first-line therapy, CBC = complete blood count, • Alternative or adjunctive medication

* Oral doses

† Appropriate for monotherapy

‡ Adjust based on serum drug levels

Source: Adapted from *Arch. Neurology,* 2004; 61(9): 1361–5. *JAMA,* 2004; 291(5): 605–20. *Ann Emer Med,* 2004; 43(5): 605–25 and *NEJM,* 2008; 359(2): 166–76.

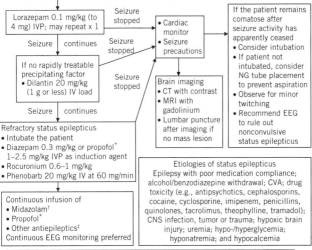

General measures
- Ensure adequate airway; provide respiratory support if necessary
  - Most patients have adequate ventilation if airway is clear
  - Consider placing a nasal trumpet when the seizure has abated
- Position patient so they do not harm themselves
- Check blood sugar: give glucagon 1 mg IM if less than 60 and no IV access
  - With IV access, give thiamine 100 mg followed by 1 ampule D$_{50}$ IV
- Assure stable IV access
- Keep core temperature below 40°C
- Rule out reversible causes (see etiologies below)

Lorazepam 0.1 mg/kg (to 4 mg) IVP; may repeat x 1 → **Seizure stopped** → Cardiac monitor / Seizure precautions

Seizure continues

If no rapidly treatable precipitating factor
- Dilantin 20 mg/kg (1 g or less) IV load → **Seizure stopped**

Seizure continues

Refractory status epilepticus
- Intubate the patient
- Diazepam 0.3 mg/kg or propofol* 1–2.5 mg/kg IVP as induction agent
- Rocuronium 0.6–1 mg/kg
- Phenobarb 20 mg/kg IV at 60 mg/min

Continuous infusion of
- Midazolam†
- Propofol*
- Other antiepileptics‡
Continuous EEG monitoring preferred

Brain imaging
- CT with contrast
- MRI with gadolinium
- Lumbar puncture after imaging if no mass lesion

If the patient remains comatose after seizure activity has apparently ceased
- Consider intubation
- If patient not intubated, consider NG tube placement to prevent aspiration
- Observe for minor twitching
- Recommend EEG to rule out nonconvulsive status epilepticus

Etiologies of status epilepticus
Epilepsy with poor medication compliance; alcohol/benzodiazepine withdrawal; CVA; drug toxicity (e.g., antipsychotics, cephalosporins, cocaine, cyclosporine, imipenem, penicillins, quinolones, tacrolimus, theophylline, tramadol); CNS infection, tumor or trauma; hypoxic brain injury; uremia; hypo-/hyperglycemia; hyponatremia; and hypocalcemia

* Propofol 1–2.5 mg/kg load, then 1–4 mg/kg/hr titrated to seizure suppression by EEG; titrate down by 50% over next 12 h, then off over subsequent 12 h
† Midazolam 0.2 mg/kg load, then 0.1–0.2 mg/kg/h to produce seizure suppression by EEG
‡ Other options include levetiracetam, high-dose thiopentone or pentobarbital, IV valproate, topiramate, ketamine, isoflurane, lidocaine, and tiagabine

GURE 55.1.   Management of Status Epilepticus

urce: Information from Chest 2004; 126(2): 582–91 and J Neurol Neurosurg Psychiatry 2008; 79(5): 588–9. Adapted with permission from Mark Lepore, M.D.

COMPLICATIONS

- Cognitive impairment (consequence of recurrent seizures/hypoxia)
- Anxiety/depression
- Seizure-related injuries such as falls and fractures
- Seizure-related death such as motor-vehicle crash and drowning
- Sudden unexplained death in epilepsy (SUDEP): more common in people with uncontrolled seizures

PROGNOSIS

- Status epilepticus mortality rate is 20%

EFERENCES

pilepsia, 2001;42(10):1255–60, 1387; N Engl J Med, 2001;344(15):1145–51; Am Fam Physician, 007;75(9):1342–7.

CHAPTER 56

WEAKNESS

1. <u>PATHOPHYSIOLOGY</u>
   - Upper motor neuron: spasticity, hyperactive reflexes, Babinski sign
     - Corticospinal tract: distal greater than proximal weakness, peripheral greater than axial weakness
     - Corticobulbar tract: lower greater than upper face weakness
     - Hemiparesis: UMN lesion above cervical spinal cord
     - Lower motor neuron: hypotonic, hypoactive reflexes, no Babinski, muscle fasciculations and atrophy
   - Myopathy: normal tone, normal reflexes, no Babinski, some atrophy, proximal greater than distal weakness
   - Peripheral neuropathies
     - Symmetric
       - Sensory loss without weakness: DM, medications, toxins, inherited neuropathies, vitamin deficiencies (B_{12}, E, copper)
       - Sensory loss and weakness: GBS, CIDP, DM, medications, toxins, inherited neuropathies
       - Weakness without sensory loss: SMA, inherited neuropathy
     - Asymmetric
       - Sensory loss without weakness: paraneoplastic, Sjögren's syndrome, cisplatin, pyridoxine toxicity, H
       - Sensory loss with weakness: vasculitis, cryoglobulinemia, amyloidosis, sarcoidosis, infections, neoplasm, mononeuropathy, plexopathy, radiculopathy
       - Weakness without sensory loss: motor neuron disease
     - Autonomic: hereditary, amyloidosis, DM, porphyria, HIV, vincristine
   - Channelopathy: periodic paralysis
   - Toxic metabolic causes
   - Myopathies
     - Structural or functional disorders of muscle, generally with symmetric proximal weakness, normal sensation, and normal reflexes
     - Inherited myopathy: muscular dystrophies (Duchenne, Becker, limb-girdle, myotonic), glycogen storage disease, lipid metabolism defects, mitochondrial myopathies
     - Endocrine myopathy: hypothyroidism, hyperparathyroidism, hyperparathyroidism, steroids, Vitamin D deficiency
     - Systemic illness myopathy: critical illness, CKD
     - Drug-induced myopathy: statins, steroids, neuromuscular blockers, alcohol
     - Inflammatory myopathies: dermatomyositis, polymyositis, inclusion body myositis
   - Radiculopathies/plexopathies
     - Injury to nerve root is called radiculopathy
     - Cervical nerve roots exit above correspondingly named vertebral body
     - Thoracic and lumbar nerve roots exit below correspondingly named vertebral body
     - Since spinal cord ends at L1–L2; lumbar nerve roots have a long course and are thus more susceptible to injury
     - Radicular pain radiates within dermatome of nerve root
     - Most common cause of radicular pain is herniation of intervertebral disk with subsequent impingement on nerve root
     - Plexopathies: multiple motor and sensory deficits in multiple nerve distributions in one extremity
     - Brachial: immune-mediated, compression from neoplasms, iatrogenic (perioperative)
     - Lumbosacral: psoas abscess, neoplasms, retroperitoneal masses/bleeding, radiation, sarcoidosis, DM, iatrogenic (positioning during surgery, obstetric)

CLINICAL PRESENTATION

Peripheral Neuropathies

- Asymmetric distal symptoms
  - Loss of sensation (numbness or tingling)
  - Pain (often "burning" in a stocking/glove distribution)
  - Weakness
  - Diminished reflexes

Myopathies

- Dermatomyositis
  - Gottron's papules: scaly, erythematous, flat papules with central atrophy on the dorsum of MCP and IP joints
  - Heliotrope rash: violaceous erythema on eyelids
  - Respiratory symptoms of interstitial lung disease

Toxic Metabolic Causes

- Variable presentation of global muscle weakness, easy fatigability

Radiculopathies/Plexopathies

- Pain, paresthesias, weakness, loss of reflex in a nerve-root distribution
- Special tests
  - Spurling's test (for cervical radiculopathy): patient flexes head toward the painful side, and the examiner applies an axial load on the top of the head; a positive test is reproduction of the patient's symptoms
  - Straight leg raise (for lumbar radiculopathy): leg is raised straight, a positive test provokes pain in the leg (*not the back*)

Plexopathies

- Brachial: pain, weakness, numbness, distribution depending on level of plexus injury
- Femoral: iliopsoas or quadriceps weakness, sensory deficits over anteromedial leg
- Obturator: hip abductor weakness
- Sciatic: leg pain radiating to low back and buttock, advancing down posterolateral leg; numbness and weakness follow; often include foot drop, sensory changes on top of foot

Patterns of Weakness

- Upper motor neuron (UMN): increased tone, hyperreflexia, positive Babinski sign, and spastic
- Lower motor neuron (LMN): hypotonia, hyporeflexia, negative Babinski sign, severe atrophy, fasciculations, fibrillations, and flaccid paralysis
- Myopathic: mild atrophy, proximal weakness, normal DTRs, and negative Babinski sign

3. **WORKUP OF WEAKNESS**

- Is the weakness generalized or does it fit one of the weakness syndromes in **Table 56.1**?

TABLE 56.1.   Weakness Syndromes

Defect Location	Clinical Features	Diagnosis
Cortex	Contralateral hemiparesis and hemianesthesia and upper motor neuron pattern present	CT/MRI
Internal capsule	"Pure motor" lacunar syndrome and UMN pattern present	CT/MRI
Brainstem	Ipsilateral cranial nerve palsies, contralateral hemiparesis, and UMN pattern present	MRI
Spinal cord lesion	Sensory level, bilateral weakness, and UMN pattern present	Spinal MRI
Brown-Sequard syndrome	Hemiparesis, ipsilateral decreased proprioception, and contralateral decreased pain/temperature	Spinal MRI
Radiculopathy	Back and dermatomal pain/weakness, hyporeflexia	Spinal MRI
Anterior horn cells (polio)	Asymmetric monoparesis, lower motor neuron pattern present, and normal sensation	Clinical
Amyotrophic lateral sclerosis	Any combination of LMN and UMN weakness in bulbar, cervical, thoracic, or lumbosacral innervated muscles	Clinical
Peripheral nerves	Nerve distribution, lower motor neuron pattern present	EMG/NCS
Myopathies	Proximal muscle weakness	EMG and muscle biopsy
PMR	Pain and stiff hip/shoulder girdles, and ESR greater than 50	Clinical
Rhabdomyolysis	Increased CK and sore muscles	Elevated CK

CT = computed tomography, MRI = magnetic resonance imaging, UMN = upper motor neuron, LMN = lower motor neuron, EMG = electromyogram, NCS = nerve conduction studies, PMR = polymyalgia rheumatica, ESR = erythrocyte sedimentation rate, CK = creatinine phosphokinase

Evaluation of Generalized Weakness
- Assess for depression or chronic cardiopulmonary disease
- Labs: CHEM 7 panel, magnesium, phosphate, calcium, thyroid-stimulating hormone (TSH) level, and complete blood count
- Cosyntropin stimulation test for any suspicion of adrenal insufficiency
- Consider a chest X-ray for adult smokers or those with a chronic cough

Evaluation of Weakness Syndromes
- Start with the diagnostic test of choice as outlined in Table 56.1
- For myopathies or myositis, check an erythrocyte sedimentation rate, creatine kinase, antinuclear antibody test, and EMG, and consider an open muscle biopsy of the affected muscle for routine pathology and electron microscopy

Evaluation of Peripheral Neuropathies
- See **Table 56.2**
- Examine for any medication culprits
- Routine labs: CHEM 7 panel, TSH, B_{12} and folate levels, serum protein electrophoresis, and a venereal disease research laboratory (VDRL) test
- Additional labs if the history and exam are suggestive: antinuclear antibody, anti-SSA and anti-SSB (Sjögren's syndrome A and B) antibodies, serum cryoglobulins, angiotensin-converting enzyme (ACE) level, and HIV test

TABLE 56.2.   Causes of Peripheral Neuropathies (mnemonic = MOVESTUPID)

Metabolic	B$_{12}$, thiamine, pyridoxine, or folate deficiencies
Other	Rare familial disorders, amyloidosis
Vasculitis	Systemic lupus erythematosus, Sjögren's, cryoglobulinemia, or polyarteritis nodosa
Endocrine	Diabetes or hypothyroidism
Syphilis or sarcoidosis	Neurosyphilis or neurosarcoidosis
Tumor-related	Paraneoplastic
Uremia	Blood urea nitrogen usually greater than 100 mg/dL
Paraproteinemia	Porphyria or polycythemia vera
Infectious/idiopathic	Lyme disease, leprosy, mononucleosis, AIDS, or chronic inflammatory demyelinating polyneuropathy

Drugs/toxins: alcohol, amiodarone, arsenic, β-lactams, carboplatin, chloroquine, cisplatin, colchicine, dapsone, didanosine, disulfiram, fluoroquinolones, herbicides, hydralazine, isoniazid, lead, mercury, metronidazole, niacin, nitrofurantoin, pentazocine, pesticides, phenytoin, statins, stavudine, suramin, tacrolimus, taxanes, thalidomide, vincristine, zalcitabine, and zidovudine

CAUSES OF MYOPATHIES

- Alcohol, dermatomyositis, hyperparathyroidism, inclusion body myositis, medications, myotonic or limb-girdle muscular dystrophies, polymyositis, postviral, or thyrotoxicosis, (amiodarone, chloroquine, cimetidine, colchicine, fenofibrate, gemfibrozil, hydroxychloroquine, interferon, lamivudine, leuprolide acetate, methimazole, penicillamine, penicillins, propylthiouracil, statins, steroids, sulfonamides, and zidovudine)

TOXIC-METABOLIC CAUSES OF GENERALIZED WEAKNESS

- Electrolytes: low levels of potassium, phosphate, magnesium, or sodium; or elevated levels of sodium or calcium
- Periodic paralysis (look for hypokalemia or hyperthyroidism)
- Depression
- Medical problems: anemia, chronic ischemic or congestive cardiomyopathy, COPD, adrenal insufficiency, thyroid disorders, anorexia nervosa, cachexia of malignancy, AIDS
- See **Table 56.3** and **Figure 56.1**

TABLE 56.3.   Spinal Root and Peripheral Nerve Lesions

Root	Disc	Muscles	Weakness	Reflex Loss
C4	C3–4	Trapezius, scalene	Shoulder shrugging	None
C5	C4–5	Deltoid, biceps, brachioradialis	Shoulder abduction, external rotation of arm, elbow flexion	Biceps, brachioradialis
C6	C5–6	Brachioradialis, biceps, pronator teres, extensor carpi radialis	Elbow flexion, arm pronation, finger and wrist extension	Biceps, brachioradialis
		Radial nerve injuries produce similar findings except brachioradialis function is normal		
C7	C6–7	Triceps, pronator teres, extensor digitorum	Elbow extension, finger and wrist extension	Triceps
C8	C7–T1	Flexor digitorum, flexor/abductor pollicis, interossei	Long flexors of fingers, intrinsics of hand (finger abduction, palmar abduction of thumb)	Finger flexor
		Ulnar nerve injuries similar but also weaken thumb adductor		
T10	T9–10		Beevor's sign (situp results in umbilicus pulled upward)	
L2	L1–2	Iliopsoas	Hip flexion	Cremaster
L3	L2–3	Iliopsoas, adductors	Hip flexion, thigh adduction	Knee jerk
L4	L3–4	Quadriceps, sartorius, tibialis anterior	Knee extension, ankle dorsiflexion, and inversion	Knee jerk
		Femoral nerve injury limited to knee extension, associated hip flexion and adduction weakness localized to plexus		
L5	L4–5	Glutei, hamstrings, tibialis, extensor hallux/digiti, peronei	Thigh adduction and internal rotation, knee flexion, plantar and dorsiflexion of ankle and toes	None
		Deep peroneal nerve weakness limited to ankle/toe extensors, posterior tibial nerve lesions weaken foot inversion		
S1	L5–S1	Gluteus maximus, hamstrings, soleus, gastrocnemius, extensor digitorum, flexor digitorum	Hip extension, knee flexion, plantar flexion of ankle and toes	Ankle jerk
S2	S1–2	Interossei	Cupping and fanning of toes	

Source: Reproduced from the *Tarascon Internal Medicine & Critical Care Pocketbook*, 4th Edition, Tarascon Publishing.

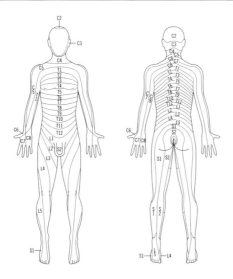

Motor Level	Motor Function	Motor Level	Motor Function
C1–2	Neck flexion	T7–L1	Abdominal muscles
C3	Side neck flexion	T12	Cremasteric reflex
C4	Spontaneous breathing	L1/L2	Hip flexion, psoas
C5	Shoulder abduction/deltoid	L2/L3/L4	Hip adduction, quads
C6	Biceps (elbow flexion), wrist extension	L4	Foot dorsiflexion, foot inversion
C7	Triceps, wrist flexion	L5	Great toe dorsiflexion
C8	Thumb ext, ulnar deviation	S1	Foot plantar flexion foot eversion
C8/T1	Finger flexion		
T1–T12	Intercostal and abdominal muscles	S2–S4	Rectal tone

FIGURE 56.1.   Dermatomal Map

Source: Reproduced from the *Tarascon Adult Emergency Pocketbook*, 4th Edition, Tarascon Publishing.

GUILLAIN-BARRE SYNDROME (GBS)

1. PATHOPHYSIOLOGY

- Autoimmune destruction of gangliosides on host nerves due to molecular mimicry; antibodies originally directed against exogenous antigens (*Campylobacter jejuni*, CMV, EBV, vaccinations)
- Deposition of complement on Schwann cell with macrophage recruitment leads to demyelination, then decreased nerve conduction (but axonal connections preserved, unless severe)

2. CLINICAL PRESENTATION

- Subacute onset of ascending paralysis, areflexia or severe hyporeflexia with or without paresthesias/ numbness, dysautonomia, and muscle aches
- Miller Fisher variant is characterized by the triad of ophthalmoplegia, ataxia, and areflexia

- Progressive symmetric motor paralysis; sometimes with sensory and autonomic disturbances
- Weakness: begins in proximal muscles, legs more than arms, progresses to distal
  - Deep tendon reflexes disappear within first few days
  - Cranial nerve involvement: airway maintenance, facial muscles, eye muscles, swallowing
  - Respiratory muscle involvement: 30% end up needing a ventilator
- Stocking-glove paresthesias/dysesthesias
- Pain: severe, most in shoulder girdle, back, posterior thighs; deep, aching muscle pain
- Autonomic involvement: brady- or tachyarrhythmias, hypo- or hypertension

3. DIAGNOSIS

- Clinical, CSF with increased protein and normal WBCs; electromyography and nerve conduction studies confirm the diagnosis, antecedent URI or *C. jejuni* infection in ⅔ of cases

4. MONITORING

- Serial forced vital capacity, consider elective intubation if FVC is less than 15 mL/kg

5. TREATMENT

- Plasma exchange × 5 sessions or IVIG 0.4 g/kg/day × 5 days are equally efficacious

MYASTHENIA GRAVIS CRISIS (MGC)

1. PATHOPHYSIOLOGY

- Autoantibodies (T-cell dependent IgG) directed against acetylcholine receptors at neuromuscular junctions
- Cross-linking and endocytosis of receptors
- Complement-mediated destruction of postsynaptic membrane
- Prevention of receptor binding to acetylcholine
- Associated with hyperplastic thymus (65%), thymoma (10%) due to molecular mimicry by acetylcholine receptor-bearing myoid cells in thymus
- Normal release of acetylcholine but decreased in available receptors decreases neuromuscular transmission, which then decreases muscle action potentials, which then decreases activation with subsequent nerve stimulation, leading to fatigability
- Myasthenic crisis can lead to respiratory muscle failure

2. CLINICAL PRESENTATION

- Ocular, bulbar, or generalized fatigable weakness with diplopia, ptosis, dysphagia, dysarthria, dyspnea, difficulty chewing, with or without proximal limb weakness
- Painless muscle weakness
- Fatigable: weakness worsens with muscle use, improves after rest
  - Diplopia and ptosis fluctuate
  - Peek sign: gentle closure of eyelids; a positive sign is muscle fatigue leading to separation of the eyelids and the sclera showing within 30 seconds [LR+ 30, LR− 1]
  - Speech becomes less intelligible after prolonged speaking
- Usually starts with eye muscles (double vision, ptosis), facial muscles
- Limb muscles involved later, proximal more than distal
- Respiratory involvement is uncommon but can be life threatening
- Reflexes are brisk

3. DIAGNOSIS

- Improvement with edrophonium, positive α-acetylcholine receptor antibodies

PRECIPITANTS

- Infection, aspiration, surgery, trauma, stress, meds (aminoglycosides, β blockers, botulinum toxin, calcium channel blockers, cisplatin, clindamycin, colchicines, corticosteroids, diphenhydramine, erythromycin, lithium, penicillamine, phenothiazines, phenytoin, procainamide, quinidine, quinine, tricyclic antidepressants, and trihexyphenidyl)

MANAGEMENT OF MYASTHENIC CRISIS

- Rapid-sequence intubation with etomidate; add **low-dose** rocuronium (if necessary)
- Plasma exchange × 5 sessions or IVIG 0.4 g/kg/day × 5 days
- Evaluate for and treat any underlying infection
- No role for anticholinesterase-inhibitor therapy or steroids **during an acute crisis**
- Consider a thymectomy once the patient is stable

ULTIPLE SCLEROSIS EXACERBATIONS

PATHOPHYSIOLOGY

- Infiltration of white matter by inflammatory cells results in breakdown in blood-brain barrier, followed by myelin destruction then gliosis
- Destruction of axons causes neuronal death, leading to progressive neurologic disability
- Demyelination results in conduction block
- Relapsing-remitting course: redistribution of sodium channels from nodes of Ranvier to axon allows conduction in demyelinated segments

CLINICAL PRESENTATION

- The presentation can vary from focal weakness, numbness, paresthesias, impaired vision, diplopia, imbalance, or impaired coordination
- Episodic presentations with numbness, weakness, visual impairment, loss of balance, dizziness, urinary urgency, fatigue, sexual dysfunction, or depression
- Lhermitte's sign: electrical sensation down the spine on neck flexion
- Classic presentation: young, white woman with acute/subacute onset of impaired vision or sensation; first episode is often mild enough that patient does not seek care
- Initial symptoms usually resolve spontaneously; relapses may occur in months or years
- See **Table 56.4**

TABLE 56.4.   2010 Revised McDonald Criteria for MS Diagnosis

Clinical Presentation	Additional Data Needed
• 2 or more attacks (relapses) • 2 or more objective clinical lesions	• None • Clinical evidence will suffice
• 2 or more attacks • 1 objective clinical lesion	Dissemination in space (DIS), demonstrated by • Positive CSF and 2 or more MRI lesions consistent with MS • Further clinical attack involving different site • The presence of 1 or more T2 lesions on MRI in at least 2 of 4 of the following areas of the CNS: periventricular, juxtacortical, infratentorial, or spinal cord
• 1 attack • 2 or more objective clinical lesions	Dissemination in time (DIT), demonstrated by • A second clinical attack • Dissemination in time, demonstrated by: simultaneous presence of asymptomatic gadolinium-enhancing and nonenhancing lesions at any time; or a new T2 and/or gadolinium-enhancing lesion(s) on follow-up MRI, irrespective of its timing with reference to a baseline scan

• 1 attack
• 1 objective clinical lesion
(clinically isolated syndrome)
	Dissemination in space and time, demonstrated by
	• For DIS
	    ◦ 1 or more T2 lesion in at least 2 of 4 MS-typical regions of the CNS (periventricular, juxtacortical, infratentorial, or spinal cord)
	    ◦ A second clinical attack implicating a different CNS site
	• For DIT
	    ◦ Simultaneous presence of asymptomatic gadolinium-enhancing and nonenhancing lesions at any time
	    ◦ A new T2 and/or gadolinium-enhancing lesion(s) on follow-up MRI, irrespective of its timing with reference to a baseline scan
	    ◦ A second clinical attack

• Insidious neurological progression suggestive of MS (primary progressive MS)	One year of disease progression (retrospectively or prospectively determined) and 2 or more of the following • Evidence for DIS in the brain based on 1 or more T2 lesions in the MS-characteristic (periventricular, juxtacortical, or infratentorial) regions • Evidence for DIS in the spinal cord based on 2 or more T2 lesions in the cord • Positive CSF (isoelectric focusing evidence of oligoclonal bands and/or elevated IgG index)

Source: Adapted from Polman C et al. *Ann Neurology.* 2011; 69(2): 292–302.

3. **MANAGEMENT**
- Evaluate and treat any precipitating infection
- Methylprednisolone 1 g IV daily × 3–5 days, then prednisone 1 mg/kg/day × 11 days, then taper

4. **COMPLICATIONS**
Peripheral Neuropathies
- Numbness/decreased sensation increases susceptibility to trauma, burns, infection
- Infected extremity complicated by neuropathy may lead to necrosis/amputation
- Reduced quality of life secondary to pain, gait instability, weakness

Myopathies
- Exacerbation of weakness such as falls/fractures
- Muscular atrophy
- Renal tubular necrosis due to precipitation of myoglobin in renal tubules
- Cardiomyopathy: commonly seen in Duchenne dystrophy
- Infection, especially respiratory due to impaired lung function from progressive weakness

- Dyspnea due to impaired lung function
- Aspiration due to dysphagia
- Increased association with gastric dilation, cardiac arrhythmias/heart block, hypertension, endocrinopathies (i.e., Addison's/Conn syndrome, thyroid disease), and cataracts

Toxic-Metabolic Causes

- Certain drugs (i.e., amphetamines) can cause rhabdomyolysis

Radiculopathies/Plexopathies

- Incomplete neurologic recovery of affected limb
- Loss of full range of motion of affected extremity
- For cervical radiculopathy, persistent loss of cervical lordosis leading to pain issues

Guillain-Barre

- 2–12% die from complications; mortality increases with age
  - Poor prognostic indicators include more severe weakness, rapid onset, older age, muscle wasting, and preceding diarrheal illness
- Respiratory failure and ARDS/pneumonia in ventilator-dependent patients
- Venous thromboembolism
- Autonomic instability/cardiac arrest
- Persistent weakness, areflexia, imbalance, sensory loss in 7–15% of patients (i.e., footdrop, intrinsic muscle wasting, dysesthesia)
- Incomplete recovery of paralysis, tetraplegia in some cases
- Constipation/urinary retention from neurogenic bowel/bladder
- Persistent fatigue
- Depression/anxiety

Myasthenia Gravis

- Aspiration leading to pneumonia/weight loss due to dysphagia
- Nasal regurgitation (especially liquids) due to weakness of palatal muscles
- Respiratory insufficiency/failure due to bulbar muscle weakness, diplopia/visual occlusion from extraocular muscle/eyelid weakness
- Myasthenic crisis: life-threatening condition in which severe muscle weakness necessitates intubation
- Mortality rate is 3–4%, from aspiration, respiratory compromise, and falls from lack of muscle strength

Multiple Sclerosis

- Primary progressive MS has the worst prognosis
- Cognitive dysfunction can manifest as memory impairment, difficulty with problem solving, speech, comprehension
- Depression
- Fatigue can be worsened by MS exacerbation or elevated temperature
- Gait impairment due to weakness, imbalance, and spasticity
- Pain due to demyelination and muscle spasticity
- Spasticity, which may affect functionality/mobility
- Sexual dysfunction either secondary to lesions on motor/sensory pathways or to psychological effects of the disease
- Sphincter dysfunction results in urinary incontinence/incomplete bladder emptying and higher risk for UTI; also causes constipation (more than fecal incontinence), partly due to decreased mobility
- Seizures: usually benign/transient and therapy responsive
- Tremor

REFERENCES

JAMA, 1998;279(11):859–63; Semin Neurol, 2004;24(2):155–63; Emerg Med Clin North Am, 1999;17(1):265–78; Am Fam Physician, 2005;71(7):1327–36; South Med J, 2008;101(1):63–9; Am Fam Physician, 2004;70(10):1935–44; Clin Neuropharmacol, 2006;29(1):45–51; Curr Opin Neurol, 2008;21(5):547–54.

SECTION 7

ONCOLOGY

CHAPTER 57

ADVERSE EFFECTS OF CHEMOTHERAPEUTIC AGENTS

ADVERSE EFFECTS OF CHEMOTHERAPY MEDICATIONS BY PROBLEM

- **Allergic/hypersensitivity reactions**: asparaginase, bleomycin, carboplatin, cetuximab, cisplatin, dacarbazine, daunorubicin, docetaxel, doxorubicin, etoposide, oxaliplatin, paclitaxel, procarbazine, rituximab, teniposide, and trastuzumab
- **Alopecia**: bleomycin, bolus fluorouracil, busulfan, cisplatin, cyclophosphamide, dactinomycin, daunorubicin, docetaxel, doxorubicin, etoposide, gemcitabine, idarubicin, ifosfamide, irinotecan, melphalan, methotrexate, mitomycin C, mitoxantrone, paclitaxel, topotecan, vinblastine, vincristine, and vinorelbine
- **Cardiomyopathy**: daunorubicin, doxorubicin, epirubicin, idarubicin, mitoxantrone, sunitinib, and trastuzumab
- **CNS neurotoxicity**: altretamine, asparaginase, bevacizumab, carmustine, cisplatin, cytarabine, eribulin, etoposide, ifosfamide, interferon α, methotrexate, and procarbazine
- **Constipation**: nilutamide, thalidomide, vinblastine, vincristine, and vinorelbine
- **Diarrhea**: bicalutamide, cabazitaxel, capecitabine, cetuximab, dacarbazine, erlotinib, fluorouracil, flutamide, imatinib, irinotecan, and methotrexate
- **Gynecomastia**: bicalutamide, estramustine, flutamide, goserelin, ketoconazole, leuprolide, nilutamide, and triptorelin
- **Hemorrhagic cystitis**: cyclophosphamide (more than 1500 mg) and ifosfamide
- **Hepatotoxicity**: asparaginase, bicalutamide, carmustine, cytarabine, dacarbazine, docetaxel, estramustine, etoposide, flutamide, gemcitabine, ifosfamide, irinotecan, ketoconazole, lomustine, mercaptopurine, methotrexate, mitomycin, nilutamide, paclitaxel, plicamycin, streptozocin, tamoxifen, and thioguanine
- **Hypogonadism**: bleomycin, cisplatin, cyclophosphamide, epirubicin, estramustine, goserelin, ifosfamide, ketoconazole, leuprolide, temozolomide, triptorelin, vinblastine, vincristine, vindesine, and vinorelbine
- **Moderate extravasation reactions (ulceration rare)**: cisplatin, etoposide, oxaliplatin, paclitaxel, teniposide, vinblastine, vincristine, vindesine, and vinorelbine
- **Myelosuppression**: bolus fluorouracil, busulfan, carboplatin, carmustine, cisplatin, cyclophosphamide, cytarabine, dacarbazine, daunorubicin, doxorubicin, etoposide, idarubicin, ifosfamide, interferon α, melphalan, 6-mercaptopurine, methotrexate, mitoxantrone, oxaliplatin, paclitaxel, streptozocin, taxanes, and vinblastine
- **Nephrotoxicity**: azacitidine, carboplatin, carmustine, cisplatin, denileukin diftitox, gefitinib, gemcitabine, ifosfamide, imatinib, interferon, interleukin-2, lomustine, methotrexate, mitomycin C, pentostatin, plicamycin, and streptozocin
- **Ototoxicity**: carboplatin, cisplatin, vinblastine, vincristine and vinorelbine
- **Palmar-plantar dysesthesia**: capecitabine, cytarabine, infusional fluorouracil, irinotecan, liposomal doxorubicin, sunitinib, and sorafenib
- **Peripheral/autonomic neuropathy**: altretamine, bortezomib, carboplatin, cisplatin, docetaxel, fluorouracil, ifosfamide, ixabepilone, oxaliplatin, paclitaxel, procarbazine, thalidomide, vinblastine, vincristine, and vinorelbine
- **Pulmonary toxicity**: aldesleukin, bleomycin, busulfan, carmustine, chlorambucil, cyclophosphamide, cytarabine, fludarabine, gemcitabine, melphalan, methotrexate, paclitaxel, procarbazine, and temsirolimus
- **Severe extravasation reactions (ulceration common)**: daunorubicin, doxorubicin, epirubicin, idarubicin, mechlorethamine, and mitomycin C
- **Severe vomiting**: carboplatin, carmustine, cisplatin, cyclophosphamide, cytarabine, dacarbazine, dactinomycin, doxorubicin, epirubicin, etoposide, ifosfamide, lomustine, mechlorethamine, high-dose methotrexate, procarbazine, and streptozocin
- **Skin rashes/discoloration**: bleomycin, busulfan, capecitabine, cetuximab, docetaxel, doxorubicin, epirubicin, erlotinib, fluorouracil, gemcitabine, ketoconazole, and trastuzumab

- **Stomatitis/mucositis**: bleomycin, bolus fluorouracil, capecitabine, cytarabine, dactinomycin, daunorubicin, doxorubicin, everolimus, idarubicin, irinotecan, methotrexate, mitoxantrone, and oxaliplatin
- **Syndrome of inappropriate antidiuretic hormone secretion**: cisplatin, cyclophosphamide, ifosfamide, vinblastine, vincristine, and vinorelbine
- See **Table 57.1**

TABLE 57.1. Adverse Effects of Chemotherapeutic Agents by Medication

Alkylating agents	Interact structurally with DNA molecules to interfere with replication and function, causing death of rapidly dividing cells; generally dose-limiting bone marrow toxicity and lesser extent GI toxicity; reproductive toxicity in male and female. Leukemogenic and myelodysplasia are long-term effects. Nausea and vomiting can be severe and preventable with 5HT3 antagonists.
Cisplatin	Neuro: ototoxicity, peripheral neuropathy Nephrotoxic: prevented by chloride diuresis Electrolyte disturbances (especially hypomagnesemia) Renal metabolism, 90% protein bound
Carboplatin	Generally better tolerated than cisplatin Electrolyte abnormal Ototoxic, hypersensitivity, elevated alkaline phosphatase Renal metabolism, less protein bound
Oxaliplatin (colorectal and gastric cancers)	Peripheral neuropathy (dose limiting, can decrease with Mag and Ca) Delayed pulmonary fibrosis, hypersensitivity Renal metabolism
Cyclophosphamide	GI ulceration Alopecia ADH secretion Hemorrhagic myocardial necrosis (rare with very high doses) Nephrotoxic Hemorrhagic cystitis (if greater than 1500 mg): Mesna and hydration can prevent Hepatic metabolism
Ifosfamide	Alopecia CNS toxicity Renal impairment Hemorrhagic cystitis (**Mesna and hydration must be given in all doses**) Liver
Topoisomerase inhibitors	All have mucositis, alopecia, and nausea and vomiting All cause myelosuppression Can cause irreversible delayed cardiac damage by injuring myofibrils
Irinotecan	Diarrhea can be dose-limiting and delayed; start loperamide with first loose BM following infusion to prevent severe diarrhea (if more than 6 BM/day needs evaluation and hydration) Pain/anorexia Cholinergic syndrome, bradycardia, asthenia, dizziness, acute diarrhea (atropine will reverse) Transaminitis Dyspnea, pain, fever and febrile neutropenia, cough
Doxorubicin	Nausea and vomiting/anorexia/constipation Cardiotoxicity Fever, headache, pain, fever
Daunorubicin	As above

(Continued)

Table 57.1. *(Continued)*

Etoposide	Stomatitis Hepatic toxicity
Antimitotics	Interfere with microtubules, then mitosis, phagocytosis, neuronal transport and structure Bone marrow suppression is dose-limiting Neurotoxicity and neuropathies can be dose-limiting
Vincristine	Constipation (treated prophylactically) Alopecia Neurotoxicity can be severe Modest leukopenia Hepatic (dose reduction if elevated bilirubin)
Vinblastine	Anorexia, nausea and vomiting, diarrhea Infrequent alopecia, dermatitis, stomatitis Mild neurotoxicity Rare SIADH Hepatic (dose reduction if elevated bilirubin)
Paclitaxel (Taxol)	Cardiac arrhythmias Anaphylaxis—**needs dexamethasone before therapy**
Nab-paclitaxel (Abraxane)	Albumin-bound paclitaxel (reduces anaphylaxis) Peripheral neuropathy (reversible)
Docetaxel (Taxotere)	Fluid retention, myelosuppression Anaphylaxis—**needs dexamethasone before therapy**
Antimetabolites	
Cytarabine	GI upset Dermatitis, stomatitis, conjunctivitis Seizure, coma, arachnoiditis, myelopathy Potent myelosuppression Pulmonary edema
Gemcitabine	Posterior leukoencephalopathy syndrome, asthenia Myelosuppression HUS, flulike syndrome, interstitial pneumonitis
Mercaptopurine	Bile stasis, hepatic necrosis (monitor LFTs), anorexia, nausea and vomiting Rare stomatitis Myelosuppression, sometimes delayed Opportunistic infections
Fluorouracil, Capecitabine	Anorexia, nausea, diarrhea, mucosal ulcers Stomatitis, alopecia, dermatitis, hand-foot syndrome, skin atrophy Coronary artery vasospasm Myelosuppression (only with bolus 5-FU)
Methotrexate	Intestinal Alopecia, dermatitis Nephrotoxicity Myelosuppression Cirrhosis, transaminitis Teratogen, gametogenesis
Hormonal agents	
Tamoxifen	Estrogen receptor blockade with multiple side effects Increases risk of uterine cancer 2.5-fold due to estrogen-like effect on endometrium (usually low-grade malignancy) VTE

(Continued)

Table 57.1. *(Continued)*

Monoclonal antibodies and enzyme inhibitors	
Letrozole	Decreased bone density and increased fractures Arthralgias 2.5-fold increased risk of carpal tunnel syndrome
Miscellaneous	
Bleomycin	Nausea and vomiting Dermatitis, ulceration Cardiorespiratory collapse in 1% Pulmonary fibrosis, hyperthermia

REFERENCES

Semin Nephrol, 2010;30(6):570–81.

CHAPTER 58

BREAST CANCER

1. ## EPIDEMIOLOGY
   - Most common cancer in women
   - DCIS: malignant cells of ductal epithelium without invasion; 50–60% develop cancer in ipsilateral breast if not resected; 5–10% develop cancer in contralateral breast
   - LCIS: 40% progress to cancer in either breast; 70% of CAs are ductal cancer
   - Breast cancer risk: 1 in 8 women; screening decreases mortality by 25%; 10% of breast cancers have negative mammogram and ultrasound; mammography has up to a 90% sensitivity/specificity (depending on age group, less in younger women)
   - Ductal cancer is 85% of all breast cancer; lobular cancer is 10% of all breast cancer
   - Male breast cancer: less than 1% of all breast cancer, usually ductal cancer, BRCA-2 gene
     - BRCA-2–positive has 7% lifetime risk of breast CA and 5% risk of pancreatic CA

2. ## PATHOPHYSIOLOGY
   - Accumulation of somatic and/or germline mutations in epithelial cell results in acquired clonality
   - Tumor suppressor genes: p53, BRCA-1, BRCA-2, PTEN
   - Loss of heterozygosity of BRCA-1 or BRCA-2 leads to loss of tumor suppressor activity
   - Oncogenes (gain-of-function mutations): HER2/*neu*
   - Hormone-driven disease
   - Cumulative hormonal exposure dependent on age of menarche, age of 1st full-term pregnancy, and menopause (which explains 80% of variation in disease frequency worldwide)

3. ## CLINICAL PRESENTATION
   - Most often identified during routine screening
   - May present as a palpable mass, asymmetry, nipple discharge, or skin or nipple changes
   - Clinical breast exam is 54% sensitive for detecting cancer
   - Breast self-examination has not been shown to reduce mortality, but women should be aware of abnormal findings and taught proper technique if interested
   - Inflammatory breast cancer: erythema, warmth, edema; do not mistake it for mastitis!
   - Paget's disease: adenocarcinoma that presents as nipple excoriation

4. ## DIAGNOSIS
   - Screening studies
     - Mammogram
     - Breast ultrasound can differentiate cystic from solid masses
     - Breast MRI can be considered for women who are BRCA-positive, have very strong family histories, have had prior chest radiation therapy, or have very dense breasts
       - More than 75% dense breasts have 5.5-fold risk of breast CA and higher false-negative rate on mammography
   - Definitive diagnosis is with tissue analysis after a core needle biopsy or an excisional biopsy or fluid analysis after fine needle aspiration of a cystic mass

5. ## WORKUP
   - Assessment of axillary lymph node status at the time of lumpectomy or mastectomy
     - Patients with clinically palpable axillary lymphadenopathy should undergo a full axillary lymph node dissection
     - Patients with **no** axillary lymphadenopathy can undergo a sentinel lymph node biopsy

- Assess estrogen receptor (ER), progesterone receptor (PR), and human epidermal growth factor (HER2) status of all invasive breast cancers
- Workup for metastatic disease is indicated for any weight loss, headache, bone pain, inflammatory breast CA, or locally advanced disease
  - MRI of brain with gadolinium
  - CT scan of chest, abdomen, and pelvis
  - Radionuclide bone scan or PET scan
  - CEA, CA27–29

6. STAGING

TABLE 58.1. Staging of Breast Cancer

Stage	Tumor Size	Nodal Status		Mets
Stage 0	TIS (in situ)	N0		
Stage I	T1 (2 cm or smaller)	N0		
Stage IIA	T0	N1	(1–3 ax nodes +/– microscopic int mammary nodes)	
	T1	N1		
	T2 (2–5 cm)	N0		
Stage IIB	T2	N1		
	T3	N0		
Stage IIIA	T0	N2		
	T1	N2		
	T2	N2		
	T3 (larger than 5 cm)	N1, N2		
Stage IIIB	T4 (locally invasive to chest wall, inflammation, or ulceration)	Any N		
	Any T			
Stage IIIC	Any T	N3 (10 or more ax nodes; 3 or more ax plus microscopic int mammary; 1 or more ax plus clinically apparent int mammary; subcarinal)		
Stage IV	Any T	Any N		M1 (any distant metastasis, including supraclavicular nodes)

7. TREATMENT

DCIS

- Lumpectomy followed by radiation therapy × 5–6 weeks
- Simple mastectomy: no sentinel node biopsy or radiation required and 10-year survival rate higher than 97%

Localized Breast Cancer (Stage I/II or nonbulky axillary lymph nodes and easily resectable primary tumor)

- Lumpectomy
- Calculate the recurrence risk using prognosis calculator at www.adjuvantonline.com

- Combination chemotherapy for triple negative or tumor larger than 1 cm or lymph nodes positive
  - Anthracycline- or taxane-based chemo regimens
- Trastuzumab for HER2/*neu*–positive patients with chemotherapy
- Hormone therapy in ER-/PR-positive patients
  - Tamoxifen × 5 years for premenopausal patients
  - Aromatase inhibitors (letrozole, anastrozole, or exemestane) for menopausal patients
  - Fulvestrant
  - In adjuvant setting, node negative, HR+ patients should have tumor genetics-based Oncotype DX testing to determine benefit of adding chemotherapy
- Adjuvant whole breast radiation therapy is indicated for T3 tumors, 4 or more positive lymph nodes, or 1–3 positive nodes with extracapsular extension following combination chemotherapy

Invasive Breast Cancer (T3 or T4 tumors or bulky axillary lymphadenopathy)

- Neoadjuvant combination chemotherapy, then surgery and radiation therapy
- Aromatase inhibitors for menopausal patients who are ER-/PR-positive
- Neoadjuvant trastuzumab in HER2/*neu*–positive patients
  - Lapatinib for trastuzumab-refractory disease
  - Consider adding lapatinib to trastuzumab for disease progression

Inflammatory Breast Cancer

- Combination chemotherapy, then mastectomy, and adjuvant radiation therapy mandatory

Metastatic Breast Cancer

- ER-/PR-positive tumors: hormonal therapy with or without systemic chemotherapy
- ER-/PR-negative and HER2/*neu*–positive: trastuzumab plus chemotherapy
- Options for prevention of skeletal-related events
  - Zoledronic acid 4 mg IV monthly for bony metastases
  - Denosumab may be preferred if renal insufficiency present
  - Calcium and Vitamin D
- Single-agent palliative chemotherapy
  - Eribulin for heavily pretreated metastatic disease
  - Consider the addition of bevacizumab to first- or second-line chemotherapy in advanced breast cancer (not FDA-approved, does not change overall survival)

8. **COMPLICATIONS**

- Recurrence (locally: i.e., ipsilateral breast/chest wall, or regionally, i.e., axillary/supraclavicular lymph nodes, or distant metastasis)
- Metastasis (especially to bones, liver, lungs, pleura, or brain)

9. **PROGNOSIS**

- Prognosis depends on ER/PR receptor status, HER2/*neu* status, size of tumor, Ki67 status, etc.
- In patients with lymph nodes that are positive for cancer, the recurrence rates at 5 years are as follows
  - 1–3 positive nodes: 30–40%
  - 4–9 positive nodes: 44–70%
  - More than 10 positive nodes: 72–82%

REFERENCES

Barton M. Does this patient have breast cancer? In: Simel D, Rennie D, eds. *The Rational Clinical Examination.* New York, NY: McGraw-Hill; 2009:87–98.

N Engl J Med, 2000;343(15):1086–94; *Breast Cancer,* 2011;18(3):165–73; *Endocrinol Metab Clin North Am,* 2011;40(3):519–32; *J Clin Invest,* 2011;121(10):3797–803; *Hematol Oncol Clin North Am,* 2007;21(2):207–22; *NICE Clinical Guideline,* 2009;80:1–37.

CHAPTER 59

COLORECTAL CANCER

1. ## EPIDEMIOLOGY
   - Second leading cause of cancer mortality; nodal spread first
   - Sites of metastasis: liver is primary site through the portal vein; lung is secondary site through the iliac vein
   - If liver is the only site of metastasis and able to leave 25% disease-free segment postresection, the cure rate is 25–45%
   - Gardner's syndrome is a variant of familial adenomatous polyposis (FAP) with colon cancer and desmoid tumors/osteomas
   - Turcot syndrome is a variant of FAP with colon cancer and brain tumors

2. ## PATHOPHYSIOLOGY
   - Precursor lesion is an adenomatous polyp (but less than 1% become malignant)
   - Risk increase in sessile versus pedunculated polyps, villous versus tubular adenomas, large versus small polyps
   - Accumulation of genetic changes
   - Point mutations in oncogenes: K-ras
   - Loss of tumor suppressor allele: APC, DCC, p53
   - Epigenetic changes: abnormal DNA methylation leads to gene activation
   - Risk factors: diet (increased animal fat consumption), family history, IBD, *Streptococcus bovis* bacteremia, ureterosigmoidostomy
   - Familial adenomatous polyposis: autosomal dominant; deletion in APC gene; 100% patients with FAP develop cancer by 40 yo
   - Hereditary nonpolyposis colon cancer (Lynch syndrome): autosomal dominant, errors in DNA mismatch repair result in microsatellite instability in 90–95%

3. ## CLINICAL PRESENTATION
   - Common presentations include: rectal bleeding, anemia, abdominal pain, change in bowel function (decrease in stool caliber)
   - Signs of metastatic disease
     - Virchow's nodes (supraclavicular lymph nodes)
     - Sister Mary Joseph's node (periumbilical mass)
     - Ascites
     - Enlarged liver (most common site of metastasis)

4. ## DIAGNOSIS
   - Screening studies
     - Colonoscopy
     - Flexible sigmoidoscopy and air-contrast barium enema
     - Fecal occult blood testing
     - Fecal immunochemical testing
     - CT colonography
   - Definitive diagnosis with a tissue biopsy

5. ## EVALUATION
   - Chest X-ray
   - CT scan of chest/abdomen/pelvis

- PET/CT scan is occasionally used for preoperative staging to exclude systemic metastases other than liver metastases
- Endoscopic ultrasound most accurate modality to assess T and N stage for rectal CA
- MRI pelvis is also useful in staging for rectal CA
- Baseline CEA and assessment of tissue for the Kras mutation
- Surgical staging requires dissection of at least 12 lymph nodes; sentinel node mapping is being studied and does increase the stage of many cancers, but long-term benefit has not yet been established

6. **STAGING**

- See **Table 59.1**

TABLE 59.1.   Staging of Colon Cancer

TNM Stage	Primary Tumor	Lymph Metastasis	Distant Metastasis
0	Tis (in situ)	N0	M0
I	T1 (submucosa)	N0	M0
	T2 (muscularis propria)	N0	M0
IIA	T3 (subserosa or pericolic tissues)	N0	M0
IIB/C	T4 (through visceral peritoneum or invades other organs)	N0	M0
IIIA	T1, 2	N1 (1–3 regional LN)	M0
IIIB	T3, 4	N1	M0
IIIC	Any T	N2 (4 or more regional nodes)	M0
IV	Any T	Any N	M1 (any metastasis)

7. **TREATMENT**

- Subtotal colectomy with resection of more than 12 nodes
- Consider adjuvant chemotherapy for high-risk Stage II colon CA: obstruction, perforation, inadequate node sampling, lymphovascular invasion, poorly differentiated, or local cancer adherence
- FOLFOX chemotherapy for Stage III colon CA
- Metastatic colorectal CA treated with palliative chemotherapy
  - FOLFOX or FOLFIRI plus bevacizumab
  - Consider adjunctive EGFR antibody therapy (cetuximab) for Kras-wild type CA (40% of colon CA will be Kras-mutated)
  - Isolated liver metastases can be resected in patients if patient has a good performance score

Treatment of Rectal CA

- T1 rectal CA can undergo endoscopic mucosal resection
- Stage II/III rectal CA should have neoadjuvant chemoradiation therapy followed by total mesorectal excision

8. **COMPLICATIONS**

- Bleeding/iron-deficiency anemia
- Intestinal obstruction/perforation (more common with sigmoid/left-sided tumor)
- Bleeding/diarrhea (more common with right-sided tumor)

9. PROGNOSIS

- About half of patients presenting with symptoms have advanced local (Stage III) or metastatic disease (Stage IV) at diagnosis
- Overall, 5-year survival rates for colorectal cancer are
  - 93–97% for Stage I disease
  - 72–85% for Stage II disease
  - 44–83% (depending on nodal involvement) for Stage III disease
  - Less than 8% for Stage IV disease

REFERENCES

Drugs, 2011;71(7):869–84 and *Gastroenterol Clin North Am*, 2010;39(3):601–13.

CHAPTER 60

CHRONIC LEUKEMIAS

1. EPIDEMIOLOGY

Chronic Myelogenous Leukemia
- Incidence of 1–2 cases per 100,000 per year with median age at diagnosis around 60 yo
- More than 90% of patients are diagnosed in the chronic phase
- Splenomegaly present in more than 50% of patients in initial chronic phase and 50% are asymptomatic
- Philadelphia chromosome with balanced translocation of t(9;22)

Chronic Lymphocytic Leukemia
- Most common leukemia with incidence of 4.2 per 100,000 per year
- For age older than 80 yo, incidence increases to more than 30 per 100,000 per year with median age at diagnosis of 72 yo
- 10% of patients are younger than 55 yo

2. PATHOPHYSIOLOGY

Chronic Myelogenous Leukemia
- t(9;22) translocation (Philadelphia chromosome) forms bcr/abl fusion protein, which promotes clonal hematopoietic stem cell
- Transformation to blast crisis requires additional genetic abnormalities

Chronic Lymphocytic Leukemia
- Clonal proliferation of mature CD5+ B cells (equivalent to small B-cell lymphocytic lymphoma)
- Increased expression of antiapoptotic protooncogene bcl-2
- Defective B-cell function associated with autoimmune hemolytic anemia (AIHA), ITP, hypogammaglobulinemia with frequent infections

3. CLINICAL PRESENTATION

Chronic Myelogenous Leukemia
- Often asymptomatic, discovered on routine blood test or exam
- Symptoms (anemia, splenomegaly): fatigue, weight loss, malaise, early satiety, LUQ fullness, pain
- Signs: splenomegaly, stigmata of anemia; hepatomegaly and lymphadenopathy are uncommon

Chronic Lymphocytic Leukemia
- Most are asymptomatic, discovered on blood tests or exam
- Symptoms: fatigue, lethargy, loss of appetite, weight loss, reduced exercise tolerance
- Signs: enlarged, rubbery, mobile lymph nodes; may become matted; hepatosplenomegaly with advancing disease

4. DIAGNOSIS

Chronic Myelogenous Leukemia
- Patients have leukocytosis (average WBC at diagnosis is 125,000 and majority of cells are myelocytes)
- Peripheral blood smear demonstrates leukocytosis with a leftward shift and basophilia
- Leukocyte alkaline phosphatase is low
- Bone marrow is hypercellular with increased myeloid to erythroid ratio and all myeloid precursors seen; cytogenetics with the t9;22 translocation (Philadelphia chromosome)
- PCR of bone marrow aspirate or peripheral blood positive for the *bcr-abl* fusion protein

Chronic Lymphocytic Leukemia
- Flow cytometry of peripheral blood reveals a clonal lymphocytosis of 5,000 cells/mm³ or greater
- Peripheral blood smear with monomorphous small lymphocytes and "smudge cells"

5. <u>WORKUP</u>

Chronic Myelogenous Leukemia
- Evaluate spleen size
- Bone marrow biopsy for cytogenetics: t(9;22) translocation
- Accelerated phase if 10–19% blasts and blast crisis if 20% or more blasts in blood or bone marrow
- Labs: CBC, chemistry panel, LDH, and uric acid

Chronic Lymphocytic Leukemia
- Evaluate for autoimmune hemolytic anemia with direct Coomb's, haptoglobin, LDH, and reticulocyte count
- Evaluate for immune thrombocytopenia
- Bone marrow biopsy for cytogenetics by FISH to determine prognosis
  - 11q22–23 or 17p13 have poor prognosis; trisomy 12 is neutral; 13q14 is good
- Labs: CBC, chemistry panel, LDH, uric acid, B2 microglobulin, CD38, ZAP70
  - Poor prognosis if ZAP70 and CD38 greater than 30% unmutated type of CLL (life expectancy is 8–10 years versus 20–25 years)
- CT scan of the chest, abdomen, and pelvis

6. <u>STAGING OF CHRONIC LEUKEMIAS</u>

See **Tables 60.1** and **60.2**

TABLE 60.1.   Staging of Chronic Myelogenous Leukemias

	Blast %	Basophil %		
Chronic Phase				
Accelerated Phase	15–29%	More than 20%	Thrombocytosis or thrombocytopenia	Clonal cytogenetic evolution
Blastic Phase	More than 30%		Extramedullary blastic infiltration	
Blast Crisis	More than 30%			

TABLE 60.2.   Staging of Chronic Lymphocytic Leukemia

Rai Staging		Binet Classification	
Stage 0	Lymphocytosis alone (more than 5000/mL)	Stage A	Fewer than 3 lymph node areas of involvement
Stage 1	Lymphocytosis and LAD	Stage B	3 or more areas of lymph involvement, no anemia or thrombocytopenia
Stage 2	Lymphocytosis and HSM +/− LAD		
Stage 3	Lymphocytosis and anemia +/− HSM +/− LAD	Stage C	Anemia and/or thrombocytopenia
Stage 4	Lymphocytosis and thrombocytopenia +/− HSM, LAD, and/or anemia		

7. **TREATMENT**

Chronic Myelogenous Leukemia

- Curative treatment with allogeneic stem cell transplantation
- Tyrosine kinase inhibitors (imatinib, dasatinib, and nilotinib)
  - Imatinib mesylate induces a complete cytogenetic response of 85% at 5 years
  - Dasatinib and nilotinib indicated as 1st line for higher risk patients and/or intolerance of imatinib
- Leukapheresis for CNS or pulmonary symptoms of leukostasis
- Hydroxyurea 1–2 g PO bid if rapid cytoreduction is needed

Chronic Lymphocytic Leukemia

- No treatment for low-risk (Rai Stage 0/I/II) disease
  - Follow CBC every 3–6 months
- Systemic chemotherapy for Rai Stage III/IV, symptomatic, or refractory cytopenias due to bone marrow infiltration
  - Fludarabine plus rituximab with or without cyclophosphamide
  - Bendamustine and rituximab
  - Alemtuzumab can be used for relapsed CLL followed potentially with allogeneic stem cell transplantation
- Vaccinations: pneumococcal vaccine q 5 years, Hib vaccine, annual influenza vaccines
- AIHA or immune thrombocytopenia is treated with prednisone 1 mg/kg PO daily
  - Consider splenectomy for steroid-refractory autoimmune cytopenias

8. **COMPLICATIONS**

Chronic Myelogenous Leukemia

- Blast crisis leads to death from infection, hemorrhage, or thrombosis
- Splenomegaly, perisplenitis, or splenic infarction
- Gouty arthritis due to uric acid overproduction (from increased nucleic acid synthesis)

Chronic Lymphocytic Leukemia

- Immunocompromise due to bone marrow infiltration (particularly with encapsulated organisms, herpes reactivation)
- Hypogammaglobulinemia leads to infection
- Anemia (due to hypersplenism, marrow infiltration, hemolysis—AIHA, RBC aplasia)
- Thrombocytopenia (due to hypersplenism, infection/DIC, tumor burden leading to suppression of platelet production)
- 2–3-fold increased risk of secondary cancers
- Leukostasis
- Tumor lysis syndrome (due to large amount of uric acid and phosphate released from lysed blasts)

REFERENCES

Ann Oncol, 2011;22(Supp 6):vi50–4; *Ann Oncol*, 2009;20(Supp 4):105–7; *J Natl Compr Canc Netw*, 2009;7(9):984–1023; *J Clin Oncol*, 2011;29(5):544–50.

CHAPTER 61

LYMPHOMAS

1. **EPIDEMIOLOGY**

   Hodgkin's Lymphoma
   - Incidence of 7400 cases per year in the United States with age-adjusted yearly rate of 2.7 per 100,000 per year
   - 65,000 new cases of lymphoma per year in the United States
   - 12–15% of all lymphomas
   - Bimodal age distribution with first peak at 15–30 yo, then again around 60–70 yo
   - Reed-Sternberg cells are pathognomonic

   Non-Hodgkin's Lymphoma
   - 85% of all lymphomas with median age of diagnosis about 60–70 yo; 4% of all cancer diagnosis and more than 5 × more common than HL
   - 5-year relative survival is about 63% and improving with advances in medical therapy
   - AIDS-defining malignancy; it is related to significant immune suppression and poor prognosis

2. **PATHOPHYSIOLOGY**

   Hodgkin's Lymphoma
   - Polyclonal inflammatory infiltrate
   - B cells have rearranged immunoglobulin genes but do not express them
   - Proliferation of RS cells driven by NF-κB, which increases proliferation, decreases apoptosis
   - 20–40% of patients have proliferation of EBV-infected cells; EBV proteins can activate NF-κB

   Non-Hodgkin's Lymphoma
   - Clonal expansion of B, T, NK cells, or precursors of these cells
   - Multiple genetic and cytogenetic abnormalities, most commonly balanced translocations; immune cells particularly susceptible to mutation due to genetic processes involved in their maturation
   - B cells: immunoglobulin class switching and somatic hypermutation
   - T cells: receptor gene rearrangements
   - Associations with infections, including EBV (Burkitt lymphoma, non-Hodgkin's lymphoma in immunosuppressed patients, primary CNS lymphoma), HTLV-1 (adult T-cell lymphoma), HIV (diffuse large B-cell lymphoma), *Helicobacter pylori* (gastric MALT lymphoma), HHV-8 (primary effusion lymphoma, multicentric Castleman's disease), hepatitis C (lymphoplasmacytic lymphoma)

3. **CLINICAL PRESENTATION**

   Hodgkin's Lymphoma
   - Lymphadenopathy (cervical, axillary, or mediastinal), usually painless
   - 25% have constitutional ("B") symptoms: weight loss, night sweats, persistent fever

   Non-Hodgkin's Lymphoma
   - Lymphadenopathy (cervical, axillary, or inguinal): firm, nontender
   - Often associated with constitutional ("B") symptoms: weight loss, night sweats, persistent fever
   - Can involve any organ in the body: brain, lung, stomach, bowel, testicles, skin, bone marrow
   - Associated immunologic complications
     - Hematologic: autoimmune hemolytic anemia, immune thrombocytopenia
     - Neurological: demyelinating polyneuropathy, Guillain-Barre, peripheral neuropathy
     - Renal: glomerulonephritis
     - Skin: pemphigus

4. **DIAGNOSIS**
   - Excisional lymph node biopsy with immunohistochemistry or flow cytometry

5. **WORKUP**
   - Bone marrow biopsy
     - For Stages IIB, III, or IV Hodgkin's lymphoma
     - For Stage IV follicular lymphoma
     - Diffuse large B-cell lymphoma
   - Lumbar puncture
     - Any suspicion of CNS involvement
     - Diffuse large B-cell lymphoma with HIV infection; bone marrow, sinus, testicular, or paraspinous involvement
   - Labs: CBC, chemistry panel, ESR, LDH, uric acid, HBsAg, HBsAb, HCV Ab, HIV, pregnancy test, C-reactive protein, and B2-microglobulin
   - PET/CT scan of chest/abdomen/pelvis
     - Diffuse large B cell lymphoma
     - Hodgkin's lymphoma
   - CT/MRI of the head if neurological symptoms
   - Bone scan if bone pain or elevated alkaline phosphatase
   - MUGA (left ventricular function with nuclear gated imaging) scan or echocardiogram if anthracycline therapy is anticipated
   - Pulmonary function tests if bleomycin therapy is anticipated
   - Semen cryopreservation if chemotherapy is contemplated

6. **STAGING**

TABLE 61.1.   Staging of Non-Hodgkin Lymphomas

Ann Arbor Staging System for Non-Hodgkin Lymphomas	
Stage I	Involvement of a single nodal group or extranodal site (I$_E$)
Stage II	Involvement of 2 or more nodal groups on the same side of the diaphragm or localized involvement of an extranodal site or organ (II$_E$) and 1 or more nodal groups on the same side of the diaphragm
Stage III	Involvement of nodal groups on both sides of the diaphragm, which may be accompanied by localized involvement of an extranodal region or site (III$_E$), spleen (III$_S$), or both (III$_{SE}$)
Stage IV	Diffuse or disseminated involvement of 1 or more distant extranodal sites
B symptoms	Temperature higher than 38°C, night sweats, weight loss of more than 10% in past 6 months

7. **TREATMENT**

   Classical Hodgkin's Lymphoma
   - Stage I–II classically treated with ABVD chemotherapy (doxorubicin, bleomycin, vinblastine, and dacarbazine) × 2–4 cycles (depending on risk) with or without involved-field radiation therapy
   - Stage III–IV classically treated with ABVD or BEACOPP (bleomycin, etoposide, doxorubicin, cyclophosphamide, vincristine, procarbazine, and prednisone) × 4 cycles

   Nonclassical Hodgkin's Lymphoma
   - 60–70% are localized and do not involve the mediastinum
   - Stage IA/IIA: involved-field radiation therapy
   - Stage IB/IIB: rituximab with or without ABVD × 2–4 cycles with or without involved-field radiation therapy
   - Stage III/IV: ABVD with or without rituximab or ABVD with or without involved-field radiation therapy

Follicular Lymphoma

- Stage I/II disease: involved-field radiation therapy for localized disease
- Stage III/IV disease: R-CHOP vs R-bendamustine
  - Recommend CT scan after 2 cycles to assess response
  - Consider autologous or allogeneic stem cell transplantation for younger patients with early relapse or for refractory disease
  - Radioimmune (tositumomab injection [Bexxar] or ibritumomab tiuxetan [Zevalin]) therapy indicated for recurrent follicular lymphoma

Diffuse Large B-Cell Lymphoma (DLBCL)

- Stage I/II disease: R-CHOP × 3–4 cycles plus involved-field radiation therapy
  - CHOP-R (cyclophosphamide, doxorubicin, vincristine, prednisone, rituximab)
  - Radiation therapy for localized disease
  - Check PET scan after 3 cycles of chemotherapy
- Stage III/IV disease or bulky disease (10 cm or larger): R-CHOP × 6 cycles plus radiation therapy for bulky disease 10 cm or larger
  - PET scan after 3 cycles and after 6 cycles of chemotherapy
- Consider intrathecal or high-dose systemic methotrexate for CNS prophylaxis
  - Sinus, testicular, paravertebral, periorbital, or bone marrow involvement
- Allopurinol 300 mg PO daily and $NaHCO_3$ infusions to alkalinize urine (urine pH greater than 7) to prevent tumor lysis syndrome in bulky disease (1st cycle only)

8. COMPLICATIONS

Hodgkin's Lymphoma

- Superior vena cava syndrome due to mediastinal mass (uncommon)
- CNS paraneoplastic syndrome: cerebellar degeneration, neuropathy
- Nephrotic syndrome with hypoalbuminemia
- Hemophagocytic syndrome (pancytopenia, fever, hepatosplenomegaly, elevated ferritin and triglycerides, phagocytosis of hematopoietic lineage cells): associated with EBV infection
- Ichthyosis and pruritus
- Alcohol-induced node pain

Non-Hodgkin's Lymphoma

- Neurocognitive impairment/spinal cord compression due to CNS involvement
- Renal failure due to ureteral obstruction from enlarged retroperitoneal nodes
- Tumor lysis syndrome
- Higher risk infection
- Bleeding due to thrombocytopenia/DIC/vascular invasion of tumor
- Superior vena cava syndrome (especially primary mediastinal B-cell lymphomas)
- Respiratory problems/cardiac problems from pleural effusions
- GI obstruction, perforation, and bleeding in GI lymphoma

9. PROGNOSIS FOR HODGKIN'S LYMPHOMA

- The 5-year disease-specific survival rates for patients with Hodgkin's lymphoma are as follows
  - Stages I and II (nonbulky): more than 90%
  - Stage II (bulky) or III: 75–80%
  - Stage IV: 65%
  - In patients with Stage I or II disease, the following factors are poor prognostic findings: bulky disease, an ESR of 50 mm/h or higher, if the patient is otherwise asymptomatic, more than 3 sites of disease involvement, the presence of B symptoms, extranodal disease

REFERENCES

National Comprehensive Cancer Network. *NCCN Clinical Practice Guidelines in Oncology (NCCN Guidelines): Non-Hodgkin's Lymphomas.* Version 3.2012. Available at: www.nccn.org/professionals/physician_gls/pdf/nhl.pdf.

National Comprehensive Cancer Network. *NCCN Clinical Practice Guidelines in Oncology (NCCN Guidelines): Hodgkin's Lymphomas.* Version 2.2012. Available at: www.issuu.com/patients-_against-lymphoma/docs/nccn_hodgkin_treatment_guidelines.

CHAPTER 62

MULTIPLE MYELOMA

1. **EPIDEMIOLOGY**
   - 10% of all hematology cancers; age-adjusted annual incidence of 4.3/100,000/year in white men and 9.6/100,000/year for black men
   - Median age is 68–70 yo; 18% are younger than 50 yo, and 3% younger than 40 yo
   - Male to female ratio is 3:2

2. **PATHOPHYSIOLOGY**
   - Clonal proliferation of plasma cells (antibody-secreting mature B cells) secrete monoclonal (M) protein
   - Multiple myeloma (MM) cells interact with stromal cells and extracellular matrix of bone marrow; adhesion-mediated signaling leading to cytokine production, which promotes MM proliferation
   - MM cell proliferation, osteoclast activation, osteoblast suppression result in lytic bone lesions, hypercalcemia
   - Increased destruction and decreased production of normal antibodies result in bacterial infections (pneumonia: *Streptococcus pneumoniae, Staphylococcus aureus, Klebsiella pneumoniae*; pyelonephritis: *E. coli*)
   - Increased excretion of immunoglobulin light chains overwhelms secretory capacity of renal tubules leading to glycosuria, aminoaciduria, failure of urinary acidification, and concentration, which then leads to cast nephropathy and finally renal failure
   - MM cells replace normal marrow, resulting in normocytic anemia
   - M protein leads to hyperviscosity syndrome, Raynaud's phenomenon

3. **CLINICAL PRESENTATION**
   - Presenting symptoms
     - Bone pain (especially back) [58%]
     - Fatigue (due to anemia) [32%]
     - Pathologic fracture [26%]
     - Weight loss [24%]
     - Paresthesias [5%]
     - Fever [0.7%]
     - 34% are asymptomatic
   - Organ involvement: CRAB
     - **C**alcium (greater than 11 mg/dL)
     - **R**enal (Cr greater than 2 mg/dL)
     - **A**nemia (Hgb less than 10)
     - **B**one (lytic lesions, compression fractures, osteoporosis)

4. **DIAGNOSIS**
   - Serum M protein greater than 3 g/dL or presence of urine light chains (Bence-Jones proteins)
   - Clonal bone marrow plasma cells 15% or more
   - Myeloma-related organ dysfunction: lytic bone lesions; Ca greater than 11.5 g/dL; crt greater than 2 mg/dL; Hgb less than 10 g/dL
   - Biopsy-proven clonal plasmacytomas

5. **WORKUP**
   - SPEP (serum protein electrophoresis): detects 80% of MM
   - UPEP (urine protein electrophoresis): detects 20% of MM

- Serum immunofixation: determines monoclonal population and immunoglobulin type
- Free serum light chain ratio (will detect all light chain–only myeloma)
- Labs: β2-microglobulin, LDH, CBC, basic metabolic panel, Ca, albumin
- Skeletal survey (bone scan of no utility in MM)
- Bone marrow biopsy with classical cytogenetics and by FISH

6. **STAGING**

- Staging by the International Staging System has been shown to be most prognostic for survival and helps plan appropriate therapy for an individual with MM: β-2 microglobulin levels, albumin, bone survey for lytic lesions; PET shows many more areas of disease than radiographs
- Stage 1: both β2-microglobulin less than 3.5 mg/L and albumin greater than 3.5 g/dL
- Stage 2: β2-microglobulin between 3.5 and 5.5 and albumin less than 3.5
- Stage 3: β2-microglobulin greater than 5.5 mg/L

7. **TREATMENT**

- Asymptomatic Stage I disease: zoledronic acid for bone lesions; systemic therapy as dictated by clinical situation
- Transplant-eligible patients (younger than 65 yo and good performance status [Table 63.1])
  - Treated with lenalidomide-dexamethasone, bortezomib-dexamethasone, bortezomib-dexamethasone-cyclophosphamide, or lenalidomide-bortezomib-dexamethasone × 3–6 cycles and then autologous stem cell transplantation
  - Maintenance with lenalidomide or bortezomib
- Transplant-ineligible patients
  - Chemotherapy with melphalan, prednisone, and lenalidomide or bortezomib × 9 cycles
- Consider adjunctive bisphosphonate therapy (pamidronate or zoledronic acid)
- Erythropoietic agents to minimize anemia (use cautiously due to high risk of VTE)
- Localized radiation therapy for bone pain
- Vaccinations: pneumococcal vaccine, Hib vaccine, annual influenza vaccines
- Prophylactic trimethoprim-sulfamethoxazole during first 2 months of therapy and prophylactic acyclovir with bortezomib therapy
- Avoid NSAIDs
- Thalidomide and lenalidomide are thrombophilic, and prophylaxis is indicated: aspirin for low-risk patients and full-dose warfarin for high-risk patients

8. **COMPLICATIONS**

- Complications of hypercalcemia (see Chapter 18, Calcium Disorders)
- Increased risk of infection
- Renal failure/nephrotic syndrome/amyloidosis (i.e., due to light chain cast nephropathy/deposition)
- Bone pain/osteopenia due to skeletal lytic lesions
- Avascular necrosis of femoral/humeral head: rare, asymptomatic
- Decreased total lung capacity from vertebral compression fracture
- Spinal cord compression
- Anemia
- Hyperviscosity syndrome (i.e., oronasal bleeding, blurred vision neurologic symptoms, confusion, heart failure)
- Increased risk of venous and arterial thrombosis

9. **PROGNOSIS**

- Chromosome 13 or 17p deletions, and translocations of (4:14) or (14:16) carry worse prognosis

REFERENCES

Am Fam Physician, 2008;78(7):853–9 and *N Engl J Med*, 2011;364(11):1046–60.

CHAPTER 63

LUNG CANCER

1. **EPIDEMIOLOGY**
   - Most common cancer-related death in the United States
   - Brain is primary site of metastasis
   - 87% of lung cancer is related to smoking
   - 20% of people with lung cancer will have a normal CXR
   - Non-small cell lung cancer accounts for 80% of lung CAs; SCC is central and related to local recurrence, adenocarcinoma is peripheral and associated with distant metastases
   - Small cell lung cancer accounts for 13% of lung CA and is neuroendocrine in origin; usually unresectable at diagnosis; very poor prognosis if metastatic; 15% 5-year survival if limited to thorax
   - Paraneoplastic syndrome: SCC (PTHRP), small cell (SIADH [most common paraneoplastic syndromes]), or ACTH (secretion)
   - Asbestos exposure in a smoker increases lung cancer risk by 90-fold!
   - Metastasizes to lung: colon, renal cell, sarcoma, melanoma, ovarian, testicular, and endometrial

2. **PATHOPHYSIOLOGY**
   - Small cell carcinoma is a neuroendocrine tumor, classically associated with paraneoplastic syndromes due to secretion of ADH and/or ACTH
   - Multiple genetic and cytogenetic abnormalities: for example, EGFR oncogene in adenocarcinoma is a tyrosine kinase that initiates cell proliferation/inhibits apoptosis
   - Environmental carcinogens (tobacco smoke, asbestos, arsenic, polycyclic aromatic hydrocarbons) transform respiratory epithelium to malignant clones

3. **CLINICAL PRESENTATION**
   - 10% are asymptomatic
   - Nonspecific signs include weight loss, fatigue
   - Primary tumor causes chest discomfort, cough, dyspnea, hemoptysis
   - Intrathoracic spread
     - Chest wall invasion
     - Esophageal symptoms
     - Horner syndrome (ptosis, miosis, unilateral anhidrosis)
     - Pancoast tumor (thoracic inlet mass causing pain in distribution of C8, T1, T2)
     - Phrenic nerve paralysis
     - Pleural effusion
     - Recurrent laryngeal nerve paralysis
     - Superior vena cava obstruction
   - Extrathoracic spread
     - Bone
     - CNS
     - Lymph nodes
     - Liver
     - Adrenals
   - Paraneoplastic syndromes (in 10% of pts with lung cancer)
     - Hypercalcemia
     - SIADH
     - Cushing syndrome

4. <u>DIAGNOSIS</u>

- Tissue biopsy via bronchoscopy, CT-guided needle biopsy, or mediastinoscopy
- Cytology from pleural fluid or sputum cytology
- Pleural fluid to serum CEA ratio greater than or equal to 20 is lung cancer until proven otherwise

5. <u>WORKUP</u>

- Chest radiograph
- PET/CT scan of the chest and abdomen (for NSCLC); CT chest, abdomen, head for SCLC
- Bone scan for any bony pain and for SCLC
- MRI brain for new headache, AMS, or focal neurologic deficits, and for all SCLC and adenocarcinoma. Consider for Stage III squamous cell carcinoma of lung
- Bone marrow biopsy for small cell lung CA (SCLC) if peripheral blood smear abnormal
- Pulmonary functions tests if planned surgical resection
  - Patients are candidates for a pneumonectomy if FEV_1 is greater than 80% or greater than 2 L without undue dyspnea on exertion or interstitial lung disease; or lobectomy if FEV_1 is greater than 1.5 L
  - Increased risk of death or perioperative cardiopulmonary complications with lung resection surgery if: predicted postop FEV_1 is less than 40% or D_{LCO} is less than 40%; maximum oxygen uptake up to 10 mg/kg/min; PaO_2 less than 60 mmHg; or inability to walk up one flight of stairs
- Labs: CBC and chemistry panel

6. <u>STAGING</u>

- See **Table 63.1**

TABLE 63.1. TNM Staging for Non-Small Cell Lung Cancer

T0	No primary tumor
T1	Tumor up to 3 cm, surrounded by lung or visceral pleura, not more proximal than the lobar bronchus (1a up to 2cm, 1b 2–3 cm)
T2	Tumor larger than 3 but up to 7 cm or tumor with any of the following: invades visceral pleura, involves main bronchus 2 cm distal to the carina, atelectasis/obstructive pneumonia extending to hilum but not involving the entire lung (2a 3–5 cm, 2b 5–7 cm)
T3	Tumor larger than 7 cm: **or** directly invading chest wall, diaphragm, phrenic nerve, mediastinal pleura, **or** parietal pericardium **or** tumor in the main bronchus smaller than 2 cm distal to the carina **or** atelectasis/obstructive pneumonitis of entire lung **or** separate tumor nodules in the same lobe
T4	Tumor of any size with invasion of heart, great vessels, trachea, recurrent laryngeal nerve, esophagus, vertebral body, or carina **or** separate tumor nodules in a different ipsilateral lobe
N	Regional lymph nodes
N0	No regional node metastasis
N1	Metastasis in ipsilateral peribronchial and/or perihilar lymph nodes and intrapulmonary nodes, including involvement by direct extension
N2	Metastasis in ipsilateral mediastinal and/or subcarinal lymph nodes
N3	Metastasis in contralateral mediastinal, contralateral hilar, ipsilateral or contralateral scalene, or supraclavicular lymph nodes
M	Distant metastasis
M0	No distant metastasis
M1a	Separate tumor nodules in a contralateral lobe **or** tumor with pleural nodules or malignant pleural dissemination
M1b	Distant metastasis

(Continued)

TABLE 63.1. (*Continued*)

T/M Stage	N0	N1	N2	N3
T1	Ia	IIa	IIIa	IIIb
T2a	Ib	IIa	IIIa	IIIb
T2b	IIa	IIIb	IIIa	IIIb
T3	IIb	IIIa	IIIa	IIIb
T4	IIIa	IIIa	IIIb	IIIb
M1	IV	IV	IV	IV

Staging for Small Cell Lung Cancer
- Limited stage: single hemithorax, can use single port for radiation (including nodes and primary tumor)
- Extensive stage: malignant pericardial or pleural effusion or more than limited

7. TREATMENT

NSCLC
- Stage I/IIa: lobectomy with mediastinal lymph node sampling and adjuvant platinum-based chemotherapy in Stage II and III patients
- Stage III: platinum-based chemoradiation therapy and potential resection of Stage IIIa
- Stage IV: combination chemotherapy and palliative radiation therapy for symptom control
  - Adjunctive bevacizumab added to chemo for Stage IIIb/IV adenocarcinoma without treated brain metastases
  - EGFR inhibitors (gefitinib, erlotinib, or cetuximab) beneficial in nonsmokers with adenocarcinoma and who have cancers with EGFR mutations (exons 19 and 21)

Treatment of SCLC
- Chemotherapy with platinum plus etoposide × 4–6 cycles is foundation of therapy
- Thoracic radiation added concurrently to chemo in limited stage SCLC
- Prophylactic cranial irradiation indicated for limited stage or extensive SCLC, which has not progressed after induction therapy
- Relapsed or refractory SCLC can be treated with topotecan

REFERENCES

Am Fam Physician, 2007;75(1):56–63; *Chest,* 2007;132(Supp 3):29S–55S, *Chest,* 2007;132(Supp 3):131S–148S *Lancet,* 2011;378(9804):1741–55.

CHAPTER 64

PROSTATE CANCER

1. **EPIDEMIOLOGY**
   - Bone is most common site of metastases
   - Produces osteoblastic lesions on X-ray
   - Most common noncutaneous cancer
   - Second leading cause of cancer death in men in the United States
   - Incidence is 1 in 10,553 men younger than age 40 and 1 in 7 in men older than 70 yo
   - Only 1 in 30 will die from metastatic disease

2. **PATHOPHYSIOLOGY**
   - Progressive genetic mutations lead from normal prostate epithelium, resulting in prostatic intraepithelial neoplasia, which then leads to invasive cancer, then metastatic disease
   - Early lesion: hypermethylation of GSTP1 gene promoter results in loss of carcinogen detoxification
   - Lethality due to loss of androgen dependence; genetic abnormalities affecting androgen receptor have been identified
   - PSA is specific to prostate, not to prostate CA

3. **CLINICAL PRESENTATION**
   - Rarely symptomatic
   - Advanced disease can cause obstructive symptoms (hesitancy, intermittent stream, decreased force of stream), but BPH is far more common
   - Metastasizes first to bone; may cause pain, pathologic fractures, spinal cord compression

4. **DIAGNOSIS**
   - Transrectal ultrasound-guided core biopsies of prostate

5. **WORKUP**
   - Labs: CBC, basic metabolic panel, liver panel, and PSA (total PSA and add free PSA if total PSA is between 4 and 10)
   - CT or MRI of abdomen and pelvis
   - Chest X-ray
   - Bone scan for bone pain, elevated alkaline phosphatase, advanced stage, PSA greater than 10 ng/mL, or Gleason's score 8 or higher

6. **STAGING AND GRADING**
   - Gleason score
     - Grade of tumor: 1–5 with grade 1 closest to normal glandular appearance, grade 5 with no gland formation and sheets of cells. The two most common grades are reported as "4 + 3," most common grade reported first and second most common next. However, if a distinct nodule has higher grade this should also be reported. Used to prognose the cancer's aggressiveness.
     - See **Table 64.1**

TABLE 64.1.   TNM Staging of Prostate Cancer*

Group	T	N	M	Gleason	PSA	Recurrence Risk
I	1–2a (less than ½ of a single lobe)			6 or lower (well-differentiated, slight anaplasia)	10 or lower	Low (very low if T1, PSA density is less than 0.15/g, and fewer than 3 cores are positive with 50% or less tumor in each)
IIA	2b (more than ½ of a single lobe)			7 (moderately differentiated, moderate anaplasia)	10–20	Intermediate
IIB	2c (involving both lobes)			8 or higher (poorly differentiated, marked anaplasia)	20 or higher	High
III	3 (extracapsular, seminal vesicles)					Very high, already locally advanced
IV	4 (fixed or invading other structures or pelvic wall)	1 (any lymph node involvement)	1 (any distant metastasis)			

* The stage is determined based on whichever criterion gives the highest stage. Note that any nodal involvement or metastasis is Stage IV. Gleason score and PSA can increase the stage of T1 and T2 tumors.

7. **TREATMENT**

- Options for localized disease
  - Radical prostatectomy if life expectancy greater than 10 years
    - Pelvic lymph node dissection if risk of positive nodes greater than 7%
  - External beam radiotherapy
  - Brachytherapy
- Metastatic disease
  - Bilateral orchiectomy
  - LHRH agonists: goserelin or leuprolide
  - Addition of antiandrogens: bicalutamide or flutamide
  - External beam radiotherapy/sumariam[153] therapy
  - Chemotherapy with docetaxel and prednisone for refractory disease
  - Monthly zoledronic acid 2–4 mg IV monthly decreases skeletal complications in bone metastases or denosumab 120 mg SQ monthly
  - Abiraterone
  - Cabazitaxel: 2nd-line chemotherapy
  - Provenge vaccine (sipuleucel-T)

CHAPTER 65

ONCOLOGICAL EMERGENCIES

TABLE 65.1. Karnofsky/ECOG Performance Score

Karnofsky	ECOG	Description
100	0	Normal activity, no limitations on activity
90	1	Independent living with only minor effort
80		Cares for self, able to perform normal activities with some effort
70	2	Cares for self but unable to live independently without some assistance
60		Able to care for most needs, but needs occasional assistance
50	3	Requires considerable assistance and frequent medical care
40		Disabled, requires special assistance and frequent care
30	4	Severely disabled, could benefit from inpatient care
20		Very ill, requires urgent treatment and supportive care
10		Moribund
0	5	Dead

Source: Adapted from Karnofsky, Burchenal JH. The Clinical Evaluation of Chemotherapeutic Agents in Cancer. In MacLeod CM ed. *Evaluation of Chemotherapeutic Agents.* Columbia University Press. 1949: page 196.

1. ALTERED MENTAL STATUS IN KNOWN CANCER PATIENT

- Differential diagnosis: brain metastases, meningitis, stroke, paraneoplastic syndrome, hypoxia, hypercalcemia, hyponatremia (usually SIADH), sepsis, hyperviscosity, or medication effect

HYPERVISCOSITY SYNDROME

1. PATHOPHYSIOLOGY

- Blast count greater than 50,000/mL in AML leads to hyperviscosity and leukostasis, with invasion of leukemic cells through endothelium, resulting in ischemia and hemorrhage of brain and lung
- ALL with WBC greater than 300,000

2. CLINICAL PRESENTATION

- Mucosal bleeding, visual changes, headache, confusion, altered mental status, ataxia, vertigo, and seizures
- Visual disturbances, bleeding, neurologic manifestations
- "Sausage-link" or "boxcar" retinal veins
- Bleeding from mucosa, GI tract
- Neuro manifestations: HA, dizziness, vertigo, hearing loss, somnolence, seizures, stroke, coma

3. CAUSES

- Waldenström macroglobulinemia, myeloma, and leukemias

4. DIAGNOSIS

- Plasma viscosity greater than 2 is abnormal, and greater than 4 is usually symptomatic
- Whole blood viscosity greater than or equal to 55% is abnormal

5. **TREATMENT**
   - IV hydration
   - Urgent plasmapheresis or leukopheresis and hematology consultation
   - Do not transfuse if possible; Hgb is falsely low and transfusion increases viscosity

6. **COMPLICATIONS**
   - Visual loss
   - Confusion, stroke, dementia
   - Shortness of breath
   - CHF exacerbation
   - Mucous membrane bleeding (i.e., gum, rectal, menorrhagia)
   - Bing-Neal syndrome (neurologic symptoms: vertigo, hearing loss, paresthesias, ataxia, headaches, seizures, coma)

MALIGNANT SPINAL CORD COMPRESSION

1. **PATHOPHYSIOLOGY**
   - Metastases (from breast, lung, prostate more than in kidney, lymphoma, and myeloma) to epidural space, causing edema, compression, and ischemia of spinal cord
   - Focal pain at lesion (direct vertebral damage) results in sensory deficit (contralateral spinothalamic tract, 1–2 segments higher than lesion), motor deficit (ipsilateral corticospinal tract), incontinence (autonomic tracts), ataxia (ipsilateral spinocerebellar tract)

2. **CLINICAL PRESENTATION**
   - Patients with known cancer who develop acute lower extremity neurologic deficits or fecal incontinence have cord compression until proven otherwise
   - Pain, worse when lying down, increases with Valsalva
   - Muscle weakness (usually symmetric), radicular symptoms
   - Bowel/bladder dysfunction is a late finding

3. **EVALUATION**
   - Emergent MRI with gadolinium of *entire spine;* rule out vertebral metastases
   - Thoracic (70%), lumbar (20%), cervical spine (10%), and 30% with multiple sites
   - CT myelogram for patients unable to have an MRI

4. **MANAGEMENT**
   - Strict spine precautions with patient in neutral position for any spinal instability
   - Dexamethasone 20 mg IV × 1, then 8 mg IV q 6 h
   - Emergent neurosurgical decompression and spine stabilization for unstable vertebral fractures or epidural metastases
   - Postop radiation after surgical healing
   - Immediate radiation to spine if patient not a surgical candidate or has no epidural metastases

5. **PROGNOSIS**
   - The median survival is approximately 6 months for solid tumors
   - Outcomes are better for those who are ambulatory at the beginning of therapy
   - If nonambulatory at the conclusion of RT, the median survival is only 1 month
   - Multiple metastases and patients with lung CA have worse prognosis than breast or prostate CA

SUPERIOR VENA CAVA SYNDROME

1. **PATHOPHYSIOLOGY**
   - Obstruction of SVC by malignancy (lung CA, lymphoma) or thrombosed central venous catheter, which leads to dilated neck veins, facial swelling and cyanosis, laryngeal edema, airway obstruction

2. **CLINICAL PRESENTATION**

   - Dyspnea (75%), cough, facial swelling and plethora, and venous distension of neck and chest wall (70%)
   - Edema of face, trunk, or extremities
   - Facial plethora
   - Distention of jugular or thoracic veins

3. **CAUSES**

   - Lung cancer, lymphoma, and mediastinal germ cell tumor or a venous clot around a central vascular access device (10% of all cases)
   - Must also rule out malignant pericardial effusion with tamponade

4. **DIAGNOSIS**

   - CT scan of chest with IV contrast to diagnosis SVC syndrome

5. **EVALUATION**

   - Tissue diagnosis of cancer via lymph node biopsy, bronchoscopy, mediastinoscopy, thoracotomy, pleural fluid cytology, or possibly bone marrow biopsy in lymphoma before beginning treatment

6. **TREATMENT**

   - Dexamethasone 4–6 mg IV q 6 h
   - Head of bed elevation and supplemental oxygen
   - Urgent radiation or chemotherapy depending on cancer type
   - Endovascular stent placement should be considered in symptomatic patients while diagnosis of malignancy is made

7. **PROGNOSIS**

   - The average life expectancy among patients who present with lung cancer–associated SVC syndrome is approximately 6 months

TUMOR LYSIS SYNDROME (TLS)

1. **PATHOPHYSIOLOGY**

   - Destruction of rapidly growing tumor cells (usually leukemias and lymphomas undergoing treatment)
     - Increased uric acid leads to precipitation in renal tubules causing AKI
     - Increased PO_4 decreases Ca resulting in tetany, seizures; Ca phosphate precipitation in kidneys causes AKI
     - Increased K results in ventricular arrhythmia

2. **CLINICAL PRESENTATION**

   - Nausea, weakness, myalgias, dark urine, and arrhythmias

3. **CAUSES**

   - Cell lysis from chemo- or radiation therapy (usually with high-grade lymphomas; acute leukemias; CML in blast crisis; bulky, metastatic germ cell tumor of testis)
   - Markedly elevated LDH correlates with risk of TLS; if LDH is less than 1000, TLS is unlikely

4. **DIAGNOSIS OF TLS IN ADULTS**

   - Lab diagnosis: uric acid greater than 8 mg/dL; phosphorus greater than 4.5 mg/dL; potassium greater than 6 mmol/L; corrected calcium less than 7 mg/dL or ionized calcium less than 1.12 mmol/L
   - Clinical diagnosis: AKI with a serum creatinine greater than 1.5 mg/dL, an increase in 0.3 mg/dL or more above baseline, or a decrease in urine output less than 0.5 mL/kg/h; or **electrolyte-induced** cardiac dysrhythmias, seizure, tetany, hypotension, or heart failure

5. **TREATMENT**

   - IV hydration, allopurinol 300 mg PO bid, and keep urine pH 7 or higher
   - Rasburicase 0.2 mg/kg/day IV if uric acid greater than 8 or creatinine greater than 1.6 after 2 days, standard therapy
   - May need temporary hemodialysis for severe, refractory tumor lysis syndrome

6. COMPLICATIONS

- Death most commonly due to hemorrhage and renal failure
- Hypophosphatemia leads to renal failure
- Hyperuricemia leads to uric acid nephropathy
- Hyperkalemia leads to cardiac arrhythmias
- Hypocalcemia leads to tetany/cardiac arrhythmias
- See **Table 65.2** and **Figure 65.1**

TABLE 65.2. Risk of Tumor Lysis Syndrome by Cancer Type

Low-Risk Cancers	Indolent NHL, ALL with WBC less than 50 K, AML with WBC less than 10 K, CLL with WBC less than 10K, solid organ malignancies
Intermediate-Risk Cancers	DLBCL, ALL with WBC 50–100 K, AML with WBC 10–50 K, treated CLL with WBC 10–50 K
High-Risk Cancers	Burkitt's lymphoma, lymphoblastic lymphoma, B cell ALL, ALL with WBC greater than 100 K, AML with WBC greater than 50 K, monoblastic AML, or CLL with WBC greater than 50 K

NHL = Non-Hodgkin's lymphoma, ALL = acute lymphocytic leukemia, WBC = white blood cells, AML = acute myelogenous leukemia, CLL = chronic lymphocytic leukemia, DLBCL = diffuse large B cell lymphoma

Source: Adapted from *J Clin Oncology,* 2008; 28: 2767.

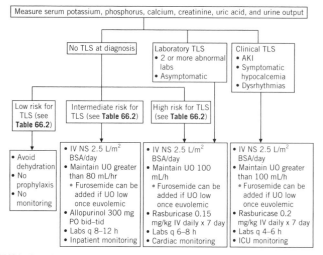

FIGURE 65.1. Evaluation and Management of Tumor Lysis Syndrome (TLS)

Source: Adapted from *NEJM,* 2011; 364: 1844–54.

HYPERCALCEMIA OF MALIGNANCY

1. PATHOPHYSIOLOGY

- Humorally mediated via parathyroid hormone–related peptide (squamous cell, renal CA) or 1,25-OH Vitamin D (lymphoma) mimics primary hyperparathyroidism
- Direct bony invasion by metastatic disease (leukemia, lymphoma, myeloma)

2. CLINICAL PRESENTATION

- See Chapter 18, Calcium Disorders

3. DIAGNOSIS

- Low iPTH and often an elevated level of PTH-related peptide

4. TREATMENT OF HYPERCALCEMIC CRISES

- Aggressive isotonic saline hydration
- Bisphosphonates: pamidronate 90 mg IV or zoledronic acid 4 mg IV
- Calcitonin 4–8 international units/kg SQ q 6–12 h
- Prednisone 40 mg/day, or its equivalent, is effective for hematologic malignancies
- Consider addition of IV furosemide *once euvolemic* to enhance calciuresis
- Options for refractory hypercalcemia
  - Gallium nitrate 200 mg/m^2 IV daily × 5 days

BRAIN METASTASES

1. PATHOPHYSIOLOGY

- Hematogenous spread to brain, most frequently from lung primary, metastases (from breast primary, colon, melanoma, or renal cell cancer); classically found at grey-white matter junction—the vascular watershed (terminal arterioles)
- Hematologic malignancies and breast and lung CA may spread to subarachnoid space through arterial circulation, leading to leptomeningeal metastases

2. CLINICAL PRESENTATION

- Headache (50%), focal weakness (40%), cognitive impairment (75%), gait disturbance (25%), seizure (15%), and behavioral changes (30%)
- Headache (especially in the early morning), focal weakness, sensory loss, gait instability, seizures, intractable nausea and vomiting

3. CAUSES

- From most common CA to least: lung, breast, melanoma, colon, leukemia/lymphoma, renal cell, germ cell
- Percentage of melanomas metastatic to the brain is about 50%

4. DIAGNOSIS

- MRI of brain with gadolinium

5. TREATMENT

- Dexamethasone 20 mg IV × 1, then 10 mg IV q 6 h
- Anticonvulsants only indicated if a seizure occurs; no role for prophylaxis
- Radiation oncology and neurosurgery consultations

6. PROGNOSIS

- Median survival of patients who receive supportive care and corticosteroids is approximately 1–2 months; the use of WBRT in large series increased the average survival to 3–6 months

Pericardial Tamponade

- Clinical presentation: dyspnea, fatigue, distant heart sounds, distended neck veins, tachycardia, hypotension, narrow pulse pressure, and pulsus paradoxus
- Causes: metastatic lung or breast CA, melanoma, leukemia or lymphoma
- Treatment: pericardiocentesis followed by a subxiphoid pericardiotomy

Neutropenic Fever
- Neutropenia (ANC less than 500) plus a fever (38°C or higher × 2 or 38.3°C or higher × 1)
- Evaluation: CBCD, urinalysis with micro, chest X-ray, urine culture, blood cultures drawn peripherally and through all ports if indwelling catheter is present
  - Stool culture and *C. difficile* toxin only if diarrhea present
  - Avoid rectal examinations
- Empiric therapy
  - Monotherapy with ceftazidime, cefepime, or imipenem-cilastatin for hemodynamically stable patients with no significant comorbidities and no clear source of fever
  - Add vancomycin if hypotensive, severe mucositis, obvious tunnel infection, a history of fluoroquinolone prophylaxis, or a high prevalence of MRSA
  - Add filgrastim 5 mcg/kg/day SQ for high-risk patients (hypotension, pneumonia, sepsis, systemic fungal infections, or severe cellulitis) with prolonged neutropenia
  - Add antifungal therapy for persistent fevers longer than 5 days or decompensation on antibiotics: amphotericin B, caspofungin, or micafungin
  - Duration of therapy
    - 14 days for any bacteremia
    - If cultures negative, continue therapy at least 7 days and until patient afebrile × 24 h and ANC is greater than 500 cells/μL
    - If pt remains febrile, continue antibiotics for 4–5 days after ANC is greater than 500 cells/μL
    - If cultures are positive, continue broad-spectrum antibiotics until ANC is greater than 500 cells/μL, then can narrow based on sensitivities of cultured organism

PARANEOPLASTIC SYNDROMES

1. **PATHOPHYSIOLOGY**

- Endocrine: ectopic hormone production with loss of normal feedback
  - Parathyroid hormone-related protein (PTHrP) results in hypercalcemia (squamous cell, renal CA)
  - 1,25-OH Vitamin D results in hypercalcemia (lymphoma)
  - ADH results in SIADH leading to hyponatremia (lung CA)
  - ACTH results in Cushing's syndrome (lung CA)
- Hematologic
  - Ectopic growth factors promote erythrocytosis, granulocytosis, thrombocytosis, eosinophilia
  - Immobilization, obstruction of blood flow by tumors, indwelling catheters, procoagulant factors from cells increase risk for DVT
- Neurologic: tumors produce onconeuronal antigens; reacting antibodies cross-react with CNS antigens (molecular mimicry)
  - Anti-Hu associated with encephalomyelitis (SCLC)
  - Anti-Yo associated with cerebellar degeneration (ovarian, breast CA)
  - Anti-Ma associated with limbic encephalitis (testicular CA)

SIADH

1. **DIAGNOSIS**

- Euvolemic
- Urine Na greater than 30 mEq/L and Urine Osm greater than 100 mOsm/L
- Hypothyroidism and adrenal insufficiency have been excluded

2. **TREATMENT**

- Fluid restriction 800–1500 mL/day
- Demeclocycline 300–600 mg PO bid
- Conivaptan 20 mg IV load, then continuous drip 40 mg/day × 4 days for refractory cases

PARANEOPLASTIC NEUROLOGICAL SYNDROMES

1. DIAGNOSIS
- Exclude other causes of neurological syndromes

2. EVALUATION
- Labs: ANA, SPEP, UPEP, α-fetoprotein, β-hCG
- MRI of brain with gadolinium
- Lumbar puncture with CSF analysis
- CT scan of chest, abdomen, and pelvis
- Testicular exam in men and breast exam in women
- Mammogram
- Consider paraneoplastic autoantibodies
  - Anti-Hu: small cell lung cancer
  - Anti-Yo: gynecological cancers
  - Anti-Ri: gynecological cancers and small cell lung cancer
  - Anti-Tr and Anti-CV2: Hodgkin's lymphoma
  - Anti-Ma: small cell lung cancer
  - Antiamphiphysin: germ cell tumors of testis and breast cancer

3. TREATMENT
- Cornerstone of care is treatment of underlying cancer
- Immunotherapy: IVIG, plasmapheresis, or corticosteroids
- Physical, occupational, and speech therapy

Other General Rules of Thumb for Clinical Oncology
- Dyspnea in a cancer patient: consider pulmonary embolus, malignant pleural effusion or postobstructive pneumonia, lymphatic spread of cancer
- Never use granulocyte colony–stimulating factors and chemotherapy concurrently
  - Must have at least a 24-hour window before or after chemotherapy

MANAGEMENT OF COMMON CHEMOTHERAPY- OR RADIATION-ASSOCIATED PROBLEMS

1. NAUSEA AND VOMITING—ACUTE
- Mild–moderate: metoclopramide or prochlorperazine with or without lorazepam
- Severe: ondansetron, granisetron, or dolasetron with or without dexamethasone

2. NAUSEA AND VOMITING—DELAYED
- Dexamethasone 8 mg IV bid × 48 h plus metoclopramide
- Aprepitant PO or fosaprepitant IV (neurokinin inhibitors)

3. ANOREXIA AND WEIGHT LOSS
- Trial of megestrol 80–160 mg PO qid or dronabinol 2.5–10 mg PO bid
- Screen for depression and start antidepressants if present

4. **BONE PAIN**
   - Focal bone pain: external beam radiation therapy with or without opioids
   - Diffuse bone pain: bisphosphonates (if breast or prostate CA, or multiple myeloma), hormonal therapy, Samarium[153] with opioids, NSAIDs, or corticosteroids

5. **NEUROPATHIC PAIN (WITHOUT NEUROLOGICAL DEFICITS)**
   - Tricyclic antidepressants, gabapentin, SSRIs, opioids, pregabalin, and venlafaxine
   - Refractory pain: consider nerve blocks, intrathecal opioids, or epidural steroids

6. **FATIGUE**
   - Assess for anemia, depression, malnutrition, premature menopause; side effect of chemotherapy, radiation therapy, or underlying sleep disorders
   - Regular exercise program essential with or without methylphenidate 5 mg PO bid–tid

7. **DIARRHEA**
   - Rule out *Clostridium difficile* colitis by checking stool for *C. difficile* toxin × 3
   - If *C. difficile* negative, use loperamide or diphenoxylate/atropine as needed

8. **CHRONIC CONSTIPATION ORAL THERAPY**
   - Senna 1–2 tabs daily–bid, colace 100 mg bid with or without lactulose 30 mL daily–bid

9. **ALOPECIA**
   - Shave remaining hair from head; consider using a wig or scarves

10. **CHEMOTHERAPY-INDUCED ANEMIA IN INCURABLE CANCERS**
    - Epoetin-α or darbepoetin-α with iron to keep hemoglobin 10–11 g/dL
    - Avoid use of erythropoietic agents in cancer patients **not** receiving chemotherapy

11. **MUCOSITIS OR STOMATITIS**
    - Compounded mixture of viscous lidocaine/diphenhydramine/sucralfate as needed
    - Gelclair: rinse mouth with 1 packet tid as needed

12. **RADIATION-INDUCED THRUSH OR ODYNOPHAGIA (POSSIBLY CANDIDAL ESOPHAGITIS)**
    - Oral fluconazole 200 mg × 1, then 100 mg daily × 7 days (thrush) or × 3 weeks (esophagitis)

13. **DRY MOUTH (SECONDARY TO HEAD AND NECK RADIATION THERAPY)**
    - Pilocarpine 5 mg PO qid prn

14. **RADIATION-INDUCED PNEUMONITIS**
    - Consider prednisone 30–60 mg PO daily × 2–3 weeks, then taper

15. OBSTRUCTIVE UROPATHY WITH URINARY RETENTION

- α_1-blockers: alfuzosin, doxazosin*, tamsulosin, and terazosin*

16. RADIATION-INDUCED PROCTITIS

- Hydrocortisone creams, steroid enemas, or mesalamine suppositories
- Hyperbaric oxygen therapy may be helpful for refractory cases

REFERENCES

Am Fam Physician, 2006;74(11):1873–80; *Am Fam Physician,* 2007;75(8):1207–14; *Am J Med Sci,* 2010;340(4):301–8; *N Engl J Med,* 2011;364(19):1844–54; *Neurosurg Clin N Am,* 2011;22(1):97–104.

SECTION 8

PULMONARY MEDICINE

CHAPTER 66

EVALUATION OF CHRONIC COUGH

1. **EPIDEMIOLOGY**
   - Nearly all adult cases of chronic cough in nonsmokers who are not taking an ACEI can be attributed to the "Pathologic Triad of Chronic Cough" (asthma, GERD, upper airway cough syndrome [UACS; previously known as postnasal drip syndrome]).
   - ACEI cough is idiosyncratic, occurrence is higher in female than males

2. **PATHOPHYSIOLOGY**
   - Afferent (sensory) limb: chemical or mechanical stimulation of receptors on pharynx, larynx, airways, external auditory meatus, esophagus stimulates vagus and superior laryngeal nerves
   - Receptors upregulated in chronic cough
   - CNS: cough center in nucleus tractus solitarius
   - Efferent (motor) limb: expiratory and bronchial muscle contraction against adducted vocal cords increases positive intrathoracic pressure

3. **DEFINITION**
   - Subacute cough lasts between 3 and 8 weeks
   - Chronic cough duration is at least 8 weeks

4. **DIFFERENTIAL DIAGNOSIS**
   - Respiratory tract infection (viral or bacterial)
   - Asthma
   - Upper airway cough syndrome (postnasal drip syndrome)
   - CHF
   - Pertussis
   - COPD
   - GERD
   - Bronchiectasis
   - Eosinophilic bronchitis
   - Pulmonary tuberculosis
   - Interstitial lung disease
   - Bronchogenic carcinoma
   - Medication-induced cough

5. **EVALUATION AND TREATMENT OF THE COMMON CAUSES OF CHRONIC COUGH**
   - Upper airway cough syndrome: rhinitis, sinusitis, or postnasal drip syndrome
   - Presentation: symptoms of rhinitis, frequent throat clearing, itchy throat or palate, although some are asymptomatic; exam may reveal edematous nasal turbinates and a glistening "cobblestone" appearance of the oropharynx
     - Empiric trial of an oral antihistamine
     - Nasal corticosteroids × 3–4 weeks
     - Ipratropium nasal spray can be added for refractory cough
     - Consider empiric antibiotics if coronal CT scan of sinuses suggests sinusitis

- Cough-variant asthma: atopic history or family history of eczema, allergies, or asthma; history of cough triggers (e.g., exercise, cold exposure, environmental allergens, or animal dander); only manifestation of asthma in up to 55% of pts
  - Test with routine spirometry, and, if normal, a methacholine challenge test; if both are normal, they effectively rule out cough-variant asthma
  - Consider an empiric trial of inhaled steroids and albuterol for 6–8 weeks
  - Leukotriene receptor antagonists can be added for refractory symptoms
- Gastroesophageal reflux (GERD): history of heartburn, dyspepsia, or sour taste in the mouth exacerbated by meals and supine position; also, may have frequent throat clearing, morning hoarseness, and a globus sensation
- Up to 75% of patients with GERD-induced cough have no reflux symptoms
  - Nonpharmacologic interventions: diet high in protein; avoid bedtime snacks, fatty foods, chocolate, excess alcohol, caffeine, mints, and citrus fruits; smoking cessation and elevate head of the bed 6 inches
  - Empiric trial of proton pump inhibitor or moderate–high dose H_2-blockers for 4–6 months; extend therapy for 3 months past resolution of symptoms
  - Metoclopramide 10 mg PO after meals and at bedtime can be added for refractory cough
  - Insufficient data to support Nissen fundoplication for refractory cases
  - Esophageal pH probe testing usually not necessary but solidifies diagnosis

6. <u>EVALUATION OF LESS COMMON CAUSES OF CHRONIC COUGH</u>

- Initial studies and interventions to consider
  - Chest X-ray, place a PPD test, and stop ACEI therapy
  - Investigate for toxic occupational exposures and counsel to stop smoking
  - Pulmonary function tests to assess for chronic bronchitis or cough asthma
  - Coronal CT scan of paranasal sinuses to rule out chronic sinusitis
  - Induced sputum for eosinophils greater than 3% and normal methacholine challenge test indicate eosinophilic bronchitis; treat with inhaled steroids × 14 days
- Second-tier diagnostic studies
  - High-resolution CT scan of chest to evaluate for interstitial lung disease or bronchiectasis if chest X-ray abnormal and high clinical suspicion
  - Bronchoscopy indicated if high suspicion for lung cancer or foreign body
- See **Figure 66.1**

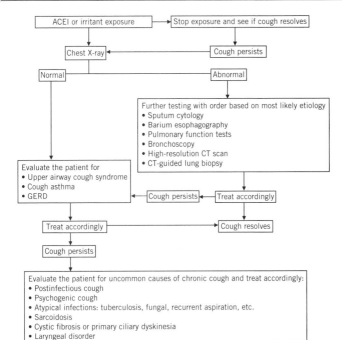

FIGURE 66.1.   Evaluation of Chronic Cough in Immunocompetent Patients

Source: Adapted from Chest, 1998; 114 (Suppl 2 Managing): 166S.

REFERENCES

Am Fam Physician, 2011;84(8):887–92; Chest, 1998;114(2 Suppl Managing):133S–81S; Eur Respir J, 2004; 24(3):481–92; Otolaryngol Head Neck Surg, 2006;134(4):693–700; Ann Allergy Asthma Immunol, 2007;98(4):305–13; Chest, 2006;129:59–94; Thorax, 2004;59(4):342–6; Am Fam Physician, 2004;69(9):2159–66; Am J Respir Crit Care Med, 2011;183(6):708–15.

CHAPTER 67

EVALUATION OF DYSPNEA

1. **PATHOPHYSIOLOGY**
   - Afferent (sensory) limb: feedback from peripheral receptors to sensory cortex
     - Decreased PaO_2, increased $PaCO_2$, decreased pH all stimulate chemoreceptors in carotid bodies and medulla
     - Bronchospasm stimulates mechanoreceptors in lung
     - Interstitial fluid, increased PA pressure triggers pressure receptors in pulmonary vasculature
     - Exercise stimulates metaboreceptors in skeletal muscle
   - Efferent (motor) limb: feed-forward from motor cortex to ventilatory muscles
   - CNS: respiratory center in medulla
   - Mismatch between feedback and feed-forward signals increase dyspnea

2. **ETIOLOGIES**
   - Common etiologies
     - Asthma: intermittent breathlessness, certain triggers, allergic rhinitis, prolonged expiration, wheezing
     - COPD: history of smoking, barrel chest, prolonged expiration, wheezing
     - CHF: history of HTN, CAD, or DM; orthopnea, paroxysmal nocturnal dyspnea, pedal edema, JVD, bibasilar rales, wheezing, S3 gallop
     - Anxiety: history of anxiety, PTSD, OCD, panic disorder; sighing breathing
     - GERD: postprandial dyspnea
   - Hemoptysis suggests cancer, pneumonia, bronchiectasis, arteriovenous malformation
   - Recurrent pneumonia suggests lung cancer, bronchiectasis, aspiration
   - Drug exposure: β blockers can exacerbate reactive airway disease; amiodarone and nitrofurantoin can cause pneumonitis; methotrexate can cause lung fibrosis
   - Immunosuppression: consider opportunistic infections including PCP, tuberculosis, legionella, cytomegalovirus, aspergillus, and coccidiomycosis

3. **DIFFERENTIAL DIAGNOSIS**
   - Panic attack
   - Pneumonia
   - COPD
   - Interstitial lung disease
   - Asthma
   - Pneumothorax
   - Pulmonary embolus
   - CHF
   - Acute myocardial infarction
   - Arrhythmia
   - Metabolic acidosis
   - Cyanide toxicity
   - Methemoglobinemia
   - Carbon monoxide poisoning
   - Conversion disorders
   - Malingering

4. **WORKUP**

- Initial testing
  - CBC, chemistry panel, chest radiograph, ECG, spirometry, pulse oximetry
  - Treat common causes (asthma, COPD, CHF, pleural effusion, anemia) accordingly
- Secondary testing
  - Echocardiogram, BNP, pulmonary function testing, arterial blood gas, Holter monitor, ventilation-perfusion scan, high-resolution CT scan, myocardial perfusion cardiac study
  - Treat cause accordingly (pericardial disease, CHF, valvular heart disease, CAD, arrhythmia, restrictive lung disease, interstitial lung disease, chronic PE)
- Tertiary testing
  - Cardiac catheterization, cardiopulmonary exercise testing, bronchoscopy, esophageal pH testing, open lung biopsy
  - Treat cause accordingly (GERD, CAD, deconditioning, pulmonary hypertension, psychogenic dyspnea)

5. **TREATMENT**

- Treat accordingly based on etiology of dyspnea

REFERENCE

Am Fam Physician, 2005;71(8):1529–37.

CHAPTER 68

EVALUATION OF HEMOPTYSIS

1. **EPIDEMIOLOGY**
   - United States: bronchitis 50%, primary lung cancer 23%, bronchogenic carcinoma 5–44% (20% develop hemoptysis at some point, but only 7% at initial diagnosis), idiopathic 7–34%
   - Worldwide: Tb is the most common cause with prevalence of 2 billion people
   - Massive hemoptysis, whether in developed or developing countries, is attributed to Tb, mycetoma, or lung abscess

2. **PATHOPHYSIOLOGY**
   - Anatomic approach
   - Alveolar (diffuse alveolar hemorrhage): capillaries overloaded by pulmonary circulation (low pressure)
   - Inflammatory: small-vessel vasculitis (granulomatosis with polyangiitis [formerly known as Wegener's granulomatosis], microscopic polyangiitis, SLE, Goodpasture's syndrome, post-BMT)
   - Noninflammatory: inhalational injury (burns, cocaine, toxins)
   - Small and medium airways: bronchial vessels from systemic circulation (high pressure)
   - Infectious: bronchitis, bronchiectasis, pneumonia (especially cavitary), tuberculosis, lung abscess, paragonimiasis
   - Noninfectious: inhalation, trauma, foreign body, lung cancer (especially in proximal airways, which leads to erosion into hilar vessels), metastases
   - Pulmonary vessels: increased LA pressure from CHF, MR with focal regurgitant jet, AVMs, PE
   - Pulmonary hypertension

3. **CLINICAL PRESENTATION**
   - Hemoptysis: spitting of blood from lungs or bronchi
   - Historical clues
     - Fever, productive cough suggests upper respiratory infection, pneumonia
     - Dyspnea on exertion with orthopnea suggests CHF
     - Pleuritic chest pain suggests pulmonary embolus
     - Anticoagulant use suggests medication effect
     - History of breast, colon, or renal cancer suggests metastatic disease
     - History of chronic lung disease suggests bronchiectasis or lung abscess
     - HIV or immunosuppression suggests neoplasia, TB, or Kaposi's sarcoma
     - Tobacco use suggests bronchitis, lung cancer, or pneumonia
     - Weight loss suggests emphysema, lung cancer, tuberculosis, bronchiectasis, lung abscess, or HIV

- See **Table 68.1**

TABLE 68.1. Causes of Hemoptysis

Category	Causes
Infectious	Bronchitis, pneumonia (viral, bacterial, fungal), bronchiectasis, aspergillosis, tuberculosis
Malignancy	Primary lung cancer or lung metastases
Cardiovascular	PE, pulmonary artery rupture, CHF, mitral stenosis
Vasculitis	Granulomatosis with polyangiitis (formerly known as Wegener's granulomatosis) or Goodpasture's syndrome
Miscellaneous	Chest trauma, foreign body, anticoagulation, epistaxis, bronchovascular fistula, pulmonary arteriovenous malformation

Source: Information from *Arch Intern Med*, 1991; 151(12): 2449–51 and *Chest*, 1997; 112(2): 440–4.

EVALUATION OF HEMOPTYSIS

- Labs: CBC, chemistry panel, PT, PTT, urinalysis, and oximetry
- Chest X-ray and high-resolution CT scan of the chest (tracheal or proximal bronchial lesions missed by CXR)
- Tests to consider: sputum culture, PPD, sputum for AFB, coccidioidomycosis titer, and antineutrophil cytoplasmic and antiglomerular basement membrane antibodies
- Fiberoptic bronchoscopy indicated for unexplained hemoptysis

MANAGEMENT OF MASSIVE HEMOPTYSIS

- See **Figure 68.1**
- Intubation (preferably selective intubation of normal lung) and mechanical ventilation with the affected lung kept dependent in the lateral decubitus position
- Transfuse platelets or fresh frozen plasma for thrombocytopenia or a coagulopathy
- Pulmonary angiogram and selective embolization of the bronchial artery
- Lobectomy or pneumonectomy in refractory cases

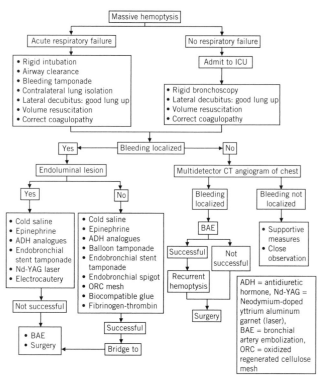

FIGURE 68.1. **Management of Massive Hemoptysis**

Source: Adapted from Respiration, 2010; 80(1): 38–58.

6. COMPLICATIONS

- Exsanguination
- Hemorrhagic shock
- Asphyxiation
- Respiratory failure

REFERENCES

Respiration, 2010;80(1):38–58; *Am Fam Physician*, 2005;72(7):1253–60; *Chest*, 2008;133(1):212–9; *Curr Opin Pulm Med*, 2008;14(3):195–202; *Clin Chest Med*, 1994;15(1):147–67.

CHAPTER 69

EVALUATION OF PLEURAL EFFUSIONS

1. **EPIDEMIOLOGY**
   - United States: 1.5 million cases annually; mostly due to CHF, bacterial PNA, malignancy, and PE
   - Worldwide: 320/100,000

2. **PATHOPHYSIOLOGY**
   - Increased fluid entering pleural space (from interstitium, capillaries in parietal pleura, or holes in diaphragm) or decreased drainage of pleural space by lymphatics in parietal pleura leads to effusion
   - Transudate: due to systemic process
     - Left-sided CHF: fluid accumulates in lung interstitium faster than the ability of lymphatics to drain pleural space, leading to bilateral effusion
     - Hepatic hydrothorax: cirrhotic ascites enter pleural space via holes in diaphragm, which leads to right-sided (90%) or bilateral (10%) effusion
   - Exudate: due to local process
     - Bacterial pneumonia: parapneumonic effusion or empyema (frankly purulent)
     - Cancer: most commonly lung, breast, lymphoma; also mesothelioma
     - Pulmonary embolism
     - Viral infection
     - Tuberculosis: hypersensitivity reaction to TB antigen
     - Chylothorax: damaged thoracic duct from trauma or mediastinal tumors
     - Hemothorax: trauma or malignancy

3. **CLINICAL PRESENTATION**
   - Dyspnea, cough, and pleuritic chest pain are common
   - Historical clues
     - Trauma history suggests hemothorax
     - Cancer history suggests malignant effusion
     - Recent abdominal surgical procedures suggest postoperative effusion, subphrenic abscess, pulmonary embolism
     - Alcohol abuse or pancreatic disease suggests pancreatic effusion
     - Chronic hemodialysis suggests heart failure or uremic pleuritis
     - Cirrhosis suggests hepatic hydrothorax, spontaneous bacterial empyema
     - Cardiac surgery suggests Dressler's syndrome
     - Esophageal procedure suggests esophageal perforation
     - Asbestos exposure suggests mesothelioma, benign asbestos effusion
     - Childbirth suggests postpartum pleural effusion
     - HIV infection suggests pneumonia, TB, lymphoma, Kaposi's sarcoma
     - Rheumatoid arthritis suggests rheumatoid pleuritis
     - Lupus suggests lupus pleuritis, pneumonia, pulmonary embolism
   - Signs
     - Ascites: hepatic hydrothorax, ovarian cancer, Meigs' syndrome
     - Dyspnea on exertion, orthopnea, peripheral edema: CHF
     - Pericardial friction rub, pericarditis
     - Unilateral leg swelling: PE
     - Yellowish nails, lymphedema: yellow nail syndrome
     - Fever: pneumonia, empyema, tuberculosis

- See **Tables 69.1** through **69.3**

TABLE 69.1. Classification of Pleural Effusions

Test	Transudate	Exudate*
PF NT-proBNP[†]	1300 pg/mL or greater	Less than 1300 pg/mL
Serum-PF albumin gradient[†]	Greater than 1.2 g/dL	Up to 1.2 g/dL
Serum-PF protein gradient[†]	3.1 mg/dL or greater	Less than 3.1 mg/dL
PF protein/serum protein	Up to 0.5	Greater than 0.5
PF LDH (international units)	Up to 200	Greater than ⅔ upper limit of labs normal range (or greater than 200)
PF LDH/serum LDH	Up to 0.6	Greater than 0.6

PF = pleural fluid, NT = N-terminal (as in NT-pro-BNP), BNP = B-type natriuretic peptide, LDH = lactate dehydrogenase

* Light's criteria: only one test needs to be abnormal to classify effusion as an exudate; 80–85% accurate for exudates:
  • PF glucose less than 60 suggests cancer, tuberculosis, empyema, or effusion from lupus or RA
  • Bloody effusion suggests CA, tuberculosis, PE, or trauma
  • PF lymphocytosis greater than 50%: 90–96% from CA or tuberculosis
  • PF pH less than 7.2: empyema, malignancy, RA, or SLE

† Useful to diagnose transudative effusions after patient has received diuretics

Source: Adapted from *NEJM*, 2002; 346(25): 1971–7, *Curr Opin Pulm Med*, 2011; 17(4): 215–9, and *Med Clin N Amer*, 2011; 95(6): 1055–70.

TABLE 69.2. Causes of Transudative Effusions

• Constrictive pericarditis • Urinothorax	• Hepatic hydrothorax • Heart failure*	• Nephrotic syndrome • Peritoneal dialysis	• Severe hypoalbuminemia* • Superior vena cava syndrome

* Most common causes of transudative pleural effusions

Source: Adapted from *NEJM*, 2002; 346(25): 1971–7.

ABLE 69.3.   Evaluation of Exudative Effusions

Diagnosis	PF Appearance	Diagnostic PF Testing
Empyema	Purulent	PF pH less than 7.2*, increased WBC†, glc less than 40 mg/dL, positive culture
Malignant	+/- Bloody	Positive pleural fluid cytology (60% of time)
Chylothorax	Milky	Triglycerides greater than 110 mg/dL
Pancreatitis	–	High amylase
Uremia	–	Blood urea nitrogen (usually greater than 100 mg/dL)
Sarcoidosis	–	High angiotensin converting enzyme level
Lupus pleuritis	–	PF antinuclear antibody (ANA) greater than or equal to 1:160
Rheumatoid lung	Yellow-green	Characteristic cytology, glucose less than 30 mg/dL
Ovarian hyper-stimulation syn.		Fertility medication use
Meigs' syndrome	–	Ascites and ovarian fibroma present
Amebic abscess	Anchovy paste	Elevated amebic titers and liver abscess present
Pulmonary embolus	Bloody	Positive CT pulmonary angiogram or V/Q scan
Tuberculosis	Bloody	Positive AFB on pleural biopsy and less than 5% mesothelial cells in pleural fluid AFB RNA by PCR (40–80% sensitive); adenosine deaminase greater than 40 units/L (93% sensitive/90% specific)
Mesothelioma	–	PF mesothelin greater than 20 nmol/L (+LR = 7.1/–LR = 0.32)

F = pleural fluid, glc = glucose, ANA = antinuclear antibody, CT = computed tomography, V/Q = ventilation/perfusion, AFB = acid fast bacili,
R = likelihood ratio
Fluid for pleural fluid pH should be collected in a lithium heparin tube and kept on ice
Increased WBC = pleural fluid white blood count greater than 25,000 cell/µL (collect in a purple top tube)
• Pleural fluid lymphocytosis greater than 50%: 90–96% secondary to either malignancy or tuberculosis
• Pleural fluid pH less than 7.2: empyema, malignancy, tuberculosis, ruptured esophagus, urinothorax, lupus pleuritis, or rheumatoid lung
• Bloody effusion: trauma, malignancy, pulmonary embolus, tuberculosis, or traumatic tap
• **Any significant parapneumonic effusion should be aspirated and analyzed.**

Source: Adapted from *AFP*, 2006; 73(7): 1211–20.

COMPLICATIONS

- Trapped lung (formation of a restrictive, fibrous pleural peel around the visceral pleura)
- Empyema
- Severe sepsis

REFERENCES

Am Fam Physician, 2006;73(7):1211–20; *N Engl J Med*, 2002;346(25):1971–7; *Curr Opin Pulm Med*, 2011;17(4):215–9; *Med Clin North Am*, 2011;95(6):1055–70.

CHAPTER 70

ASTHMA EXACERBATION

1. **EPIDEMIOLOGY**
   - Prevalence in United States is around 8% of population (9% for kids younger than 18 yo)
   - Mortality is 2/100,000/year
   - Most common reason for exacerbation is inadequate medical therapy combined with noncompliance
   - Predominantly in boys during childhood: male-to-female ratio of 2:1 until puberty, then it becomes 1:1; 50% of these children have symptom resolution by early adulthood; boys are more likely to have symptom resolution than girls
   - Most adult-onset asthma is diagnosed over age 40 yo in women
   - United States spends about 14 billion dollars per year on asthma, about 25% of which is on asthma exacerbations

2. **PATHOPHYSIOLOGY**
   - Exposure to allergens causes inflammation driven by mast cells, dendritic cells, and eosinophils, which activate inflammatory mediators leading to simultaneous inflammation and repair in airways
   - Epithelial damage
   - Subepithelial fibrosis results in basement membrane thickening
   - Smooth muscle hypertrophy results in airway hyperresponsiveness, which enables reversible obstruction
   - Increased vascular flow leads to airway edema
   - Goblet cell and submucosal gland hypertrophy → mucus hypersecretion

3. **CLINICAL PRESENTATION**
   - Signs: use of accessory muscles, chest wall retractions, tachypnea, cyanosis, hypoxia
   - Mild: dyspnea with activity
   - Moderate: dyspnea that prevents usual activity
   - Severe: dyspnea at rest, interferes with conversation

4. **DIAGNOSIS**
   - Reversible airflow obstruction on spirometry confirms asthma diagnosis
     - FEV_1 less than 80% predicted or FEV_1/FVC less than 70%
     - FEV_1 increases to 12% or more and 200 mL or FVC increases to 12% or more after inhaled β_2-agonist
     - Bronchoprovocation test with inhaled methacholine can diagnose hyperbronchial responsiveness, which is suggestive of asthma
       - Consider this test if spirometry is normal and clinical history very suggestive of asthma

5. **DIFFERENTIAL DIAGNOSIS**
   - COPD
   - Churg-Strauss syndrome
   - Eosinophilic pneumonia
   - CHF
   - Vocal cord paralysis
   - Vocal cord dysfunction
   - Foreign body aspiration
   - Laryngotracheal masses

- Tracheomalacia
- Angioedema
- Bronchiectasis
- Allergic bronchopulmonary aspergillosis
- Cystic fibrosis
- Bronchiolitis obliterans
- Conversion disorders
- Munchausen syndrome
- Malingering

5. **EVALUATION**
   - Pulmonary function testing
   - Consider allergen skin testing if exogenous trigger suspected
   - See **Tables 70.1** through **70.3**

TABLE 70.1.   Classification of Asthma Severity*

Class	Days with Symptoms	Nights with Symptoms	PEF or FEV₁††	SABA Use for Symptoms
Mild intermittent	2 or fewer/week	2 or fewer/month	80% or more	2 days or fewer/week
Mild persistent	3–6/week	3–4/month	80% or more	More than 2 days/week
Moderate persistent	Daily	More than 1/week	More than 60% up to 80%	Daily
Severe persistent	Daily	Most nights	Up to 60%	Several times/day

PEF = peak expiratory flow, variability = daily variability over 1–2 weeks, FEV1 = Forced expiratory volume in 1 second, SABA = short-acting β_2-agonist
* Same criteria used for children under 5 although spirometry not possible
† % personal best for PEF, % predicted for FEV¹; may not correlate with symptoms

Source: Adapted from National Heart, Lung, and Blood Institute, National Asthma Education and Prevention Program. *Expert Panel Report 3: guidelines for the diagnosis and management of asthma.* Summary report 2007: 344 available at www.nhlbi.nih.gov/guidelines/asthma/asthgdln.htm.

TABLE 70.2.   Predicted PEF (Liters/Min) for Nonsmoking Patients

Age (years)	Women (height in inches)					Men (height in inches)					Children	
	55	60	65	70	75	60	65	70	75	80	Height (inches)	PEF (L/min)
20	390	423	460	496	529	554	602	649	693	740	44	160
30	380	413	448	483	516	532	577	622	664	710	48	214
40	370	402	436	470	502	509	552	596	636	680	52	267
50	360	391	424	457	488	486	527	569	607	649	56	320
60	350	380	412	445	475	463	502	542	578	618	60	373
70	340	369	400	432	461	440	477	515	550	587	64	427

Source: Adapted from *Am Rev Resp Dis,* 1963; 88: 644–51.

TABLE 70.3. Risk Factors for Death in Asthmatics

Sudden, severe attacks	Prior intubation/ICU stay	2 or more ER/hospitalizations/year
Hospital/ER in last month	Recent systemic steroids	More than 2 albuterol canisters/ month
Cardiac problems	Illicit drug use	Low socioeconomic class
Psychosocial problems	Lack of asthma action plan	Denial of asthma diagnosis

Source: Adapted from *Proc Amer Thor Society,* 2009; 6(4): 357–66.

7. TREATMENT

Trigger Avoidance/Control
- Possible triggers: smoke, allergens, medications (β blocker, aspirin, NSAIDs)
- Exercise-induced: starts during and peaks 5–10 minutes after exercise
  - Inhaled β_2 agonist or mast cell stabilizer for prophylaxis
- Allergic rhinitis: control with intranasal steroids, allergen avoidance
- Gastroesophageal reflux: raise head of bed, avoid bedtime snack, medications

Stepwise Approach to Stable Asthma Management
- Gain control early with oral steroids or high-dose inhaled steroids
- Step down therapy every 1–2 months to least medications necessary
- Never use salmeterol or formoterol **alone without** an inhaled steroid
- Consider anti-IgE therapy if severe allergic asthma with elevated serum IgE
- See **Tables 70.4** and **70.5** and **Figure 70.1**

TABLE 70.4. Management of Stable Asthma

Class	Preferred Meds	Additional Medications
Mild intermittent	SA β_2-agonist* prn	—
Mild persistent	Low-dose inhaled steroids (see Table 70.5) and SA β_2-agonist* prn	Mast cell stabilizers (children) or leukotriene receptor blockers
Moderate persistent	LA β_2-agonists **and** low–medium dose inhaled steroids	Leukotriene receptor blockers or zileuton with or without theophylline SR‡
Severe persistent	High dose inhaled steroids (See Table 70.5) **AND** LA β_2-agonists†	Oral steroids with or without omalizumab if elevated serum IgE level

* SA = short-acting β_2-agonists: albuterol and levalbuterol used for breakthrough symptoms in all classes
† LA = long-acting β_2-agonists: salmeterol and formoterol
‡ Theophylline SR titrated to level 5–15 mcg/mL

TABLE 70.5. Inhaled Steroids: Recommended Daily Doses for Adults*

Drug	Form	Adult Daily Doses		
		Low	Medium	High
Beclomethasone MDI	40 mcg/puff	2–6	6–12	More than 12
	80 mcg/puff	1–3	3–6	More than 6
Budesonide DPI	180 mcg/dose	1–3	3–7	More than 7
	Soln for nebs	–	–	–
Ciclesonide MDI	80 mcg/puff	1–3	4–6	More than 7
	160 mcg/puff	1–2	3–4	More than 6
Flunisolide MDI	250 mcg/puff	2–4	4–8	More than 8
	80 mcg/puff	2–6	6–15	More than 15
Fluticasone MDI	110 mcg/puff	1–2	2–4	More than 4
	220 mcg/puff	1	2	More than 2
	44 mcg/dose	2–6	6–12	More than 12
Fluticasone DPI	100 mcg/dose	1–3	3–6	More than 6
	250 mcg/dose	1	2	More than 2
Mometasone DPI	220 mcg/dose	1	2	More than 2
	110 mcg/dose	1–2	3–4	More than 4
Triamcinolone MDI	75 mcg/puff	4–8	8–12	More than 12

MDI = metered dose inhaler, DPI = dry powder inhaler; all doses in puffs (MDI) or inhalations (DPI)

Sources: Adapted from Hamilton RJ, ed. *Tarascon Pocket Pharmacopoeia, 2012.* Burlington, MA: Jones and Bartlett Publishing.

Initial Assessment of Severity in Acute Asthma Exacerbations in Adults			
Symptoms	Mild	Moderate	Severe
Speaking in	Sentences	Phrases	Words
Heart rate	Less than 100 beats/min	100–120 beats/min	More than 120 beats/min
PEF/FEV$_1$ (% predicted)	Greater than 70%	40–70%	Less than 40% (esp. Less than 25%)
Room air pulse oximetry	Greater than 95%	91–95%	or less 90%
Mental status	Alert	Drowsy	Lethargic/obtunded
PaCO$_2$ (mmHg)	Less than 40	40–50	Greater than 50t

Inpatient treatment of moderate–severe asthma exacerbations
- Oxygen to keep SaO$_2$ above 90%
- Albuterol 2.5 mg Neb q1 h until stable, then q 2 h/q 1 h prn x 24 h, then q 4 h/q 2 h prn
  - Consider 2.5 mg Neb q 20 min x 3 **or** 10 mg continuous over 1 h for severe asthma
  - Albuterol and levalbuterol are equally efficacious
- Ipratropium 0.5 mg Neb q 20 min x 3 for severe asthma, then q 4 h/q 2 h prn, then q 6 h
- Methylprednisolone 60 mg IV q 6 h until bronchospasm controlled, then prednisone 1 mg/kg PO daily to complete 10–14 days of therapy, then taper
- Consider magnesium 2 g IV over 20 minutes for severe asthma exacerbations
- Empiric antibiotics for pneumonia or bronchitis **only** if purulent sputum production

---

Good response after 1–2 h
- Continue current therapy on wards
- Serial PEF and oximetry monitoring
- Smoking cessation counseling, if applicable, and patient education

Partial/poor response after 1–2 h
- Consider noninvasive positive pressure ventilation in ICU
- Continue q 1 h nebulizer treatments

PEF = peak expiratory flow rate, FEV$_1$ = forced expiratory volume at 1 second, PaCO$_2$ = partial pressure of carbon dioxide, SaO$_2$ = arterial oxygen saturation, ICU = intensive care unit, ABG = arterial blood gas, cmH$_2$O = centimeters of water.

Reassess after 1–2 h
- ABG
- Serial PEF and oximetry monitoring
- Consider IV aminophylline only for severe, refractory asthma (high risk of toxicity)
- Consider intubation for: persistent PaCO$_2$ Greater than 50 with respiratory acidosis, worsening mental status, hemodynamic instability, or progressive deterioration despite maximal medical therapy
  - Propofol and ketamine will bronchodilate
  - Maximize expiratory time
  - Keep plateau at 30 cmH$_2$O

FIGURE 70.1.   Management of Acute Asthma Exacerbations

Source: Information from: *Allergy,* 2008; 63(8): 997–1004, *Curr Opin Pulm Med,* 2008; 14(1): 13–23, *Curr Opin Crit Care,* 2011; 17(4): 335–41, and *Proc Am* Thor Soc, 2009; 6(4): 357–66.

8. COMPLICATIONS

- Pneumothorax
- Respiratory failure

REFERENCES

Allergy, 2008;63(8):997–1004; *Curr Opin Pulm Med,* 2008;14(1):13–23; *Curr Opin Crit Care,* 2011;17(4):335–4 *Proc Am Thorac Soc,* 2009;6(4):357–66; *Am Fam Physician,* 2005;71(8):1529–37; *Am Fam Physician,* 2011;84(1):40–7; *Am Fam Physician,* 2009;79(9):761–7; *Curr Opin Crit Care,* 2011;17(4):335–41.

CHAPTER 71

CHRONIC OBSTRUCTIVE PULMONARY DISEASE EXACERBATION

1. EPIDEMIOLOGY

- Fourth leading cause of death in the United States
- Prevalence is 20% in the United States
- Cigarette smoking is implicated in 90% of cases
- 75% of patients have serious chronic dyspnea and nearly 25% have profound total body pain
- 60 yo smoker with chronic bronchitis has a 10-year mortality of 60%, which is 4 times higher than age-matched nonsmoking asthmatics
- Inpatient mortality is 11%, 6-month mortality is 33%, and 1-year mortality is 43%
- Those who survived first hospitalization have a 50% chance of rehospitalization within 6 months
- Initial hospitalization: 93% are male, mean age is 63.5 yo, less than 1% never smoked, mean FEV_1 is 47%, and 50% are admitted to the ICU

2. PATHOPHYSIOLOGY

- Large airways: mucus and goblet cell hyperplasia increase mucus, which leads to cough then chronic bronchitis
- Small airways: irreversible airway obstruction (decreased FEV_1) with compensatory hyperinflation (increased residual volume)
- Initially, air trapping maintains airflow (increased lung volume increases elastic recoil, increased airway diameter decreases airway resistance)
- Hyperinflation flattens diaphragm decreases inspiratory capacity
- Decreased abdominal pressure transmitted to diaphragm
- Shorter, less effective diaphragmatic muscle fibers
- Due to Laplace's law, need to increase tension to produce a given pressure
- Lung parenchyma: with chronic inflammation, elastase activity exceeds antielastase activity, leading to degradation of extracellular matrix, cell death, and patchy enlarged air spaces (i.e., emphysema)
- FEV_1 less than 50% predicted associated with hypoxemia
- FEV_1 less than 25% predicted associated with hypercapnia

3. CLINICAL PRESENTATION

- Acute change from baseline dyspnea, cough, or sputum production
- Other symptoms: chest tightness; tachycardia; decreased exercise tolerance; confusion; depression; insomnia; change to color, volume, or tenacity of sputum; dyspnea; tachypnea; wheezing; fever; fatigue; malaise
- Physical findings
  - Cardiac impulse palpable below the xiphoid [LR+ 7.4, LR− NS]
  - Hoover sign: hands placed on costal margin, with fingers touching at xiphoid process—with normal respiration, the hands will separate; in COPD, the hyperexpansion prevents further excursion and the hands come closer together [LR+ 4.2, LR− 0.5]
  - Accessory (scalene/sternocleidomastoid) muscle use [LR+ 3.3, LR− 0.7]
  - Decreased breath sounds [LR+ 3.2, LR− 0.5]
  - Wheeze [LR+ 2.8, LR− 0.8]
  - Barrel chest [LR+ 1.5, LR− 0.6]

4. DIAGNOSIS

- **Spirometry**: airflow obstruction that is not fully reversible
  - FEV_1/FVC less than 70% predicted and postbronchodilator FEV_1 less than 80%
- **Diagnosis of COPD exacerbations**: increase in dyspnea, cough, sputum volume, or purulence

5. DIFFERENTIAL DIAGNOSIS

- Asthma
- CHF
- Angioedema
- Bronchiectasis
- Allergic bronchopulmonary aspergillosis
- Cystic fibrosis
- Bronchiolitis obliterans
- Conversion disorders
- Munchausen syndrome
- Malingering
- Interstitial lung disease

6. EVALUATION

- Baseline pulmonary function test, pulse oximetry, chest X-ray
- Labs: α-1 antitrypsin

Evaluation of COPD Exacerbations

- Assess with chest X-ray, sputum culture, oximetry, or arterial blood gas
- Admit for moderate–severe exacerbations: respiratory acidosis, need for ventilation, PEF less than 100 L/min, FEV_1 less than 1 L or less than 40% predicted, or serious comorbidities
- See **Table 71.1**

TABLE 71.1.   Management of Stable COPD by Stage

Stage*	Spirometry	Therapy
All	No smoking! Influenza, pneumococcal vaccines, and exercise	
0 (at risk)	Normal	
I (mild)	$FEV_1/FVC<70\%$ $FEV_1 \geq 80\%$ predicted	Short-acting or long-acting β_2-agonist or anticholinergic (AC) agent[†] prn
II (moderate)	$FEV_1/FVC<70\%$ $50\% \leq FEV_1<80\%$	Scheduled long-acting β_2-agonist or AC agent[†] and pulmonary rehabilitation[‡]
III (severe)	$FEV_1/FVC<70\%$ $30\% \leq FEV_1 <50\%$	Add inhaled steroids to scheduled long-acting bronchodilators (especially if greater than or equal to 1 exac./yr)
IV (very severe)	$FEV_1 <30\%$ or $<50\%$ + chronic respiratory failure	As for Stage III; oxygen[§] (improves survival!); consider bullectomy/transplant[‖]; Consider roflumilast[¶]

* FEV_1 used to stratify severity
BODE index (body mass index, airway obstruction, dyspnea, exercise capacity on 6 min. walk) better to assess risk of death: see http://content.nejm.org/[§]/cgi/reprint/350/10/1005.pdf
† Bronchodilators (anticholinergics >β_2-agonists » methylxanthines): use combination therapy if monotherapy inadequate; long-acting anticholinergic (tiotropium) and β_2-agonist (e.g., salmeterol or formoterol) are preferred over short-acting anticholinergic (ipratropium) or β_2-agonist (e.g., albuterol)
‡ Aerobic exercise, good nutrition and education
§ $PaO_2 \leq 55$ mmHg/O_2 sat ≤88% ($PaO_2 \leq 60$ mmHg if pulmonary hypertension, polycythemia, or cor pulmonale)
‖ Bullectomy or lung-volume reduction surgery best for upper lobe emphysema and low exercise capacity; lung transplantation indicated for idiopathic emphysema or α-1 antitrypsin deficiency
¶ Roflumilast 500 mcg PO daily (PDE₄ inhibitor) decreases COPD exacerbations

Source: Adapted from the GOLD initiative 2010 executive summary available at www.goldcopd.org/uploads/users/files/GOLDReport_April112011.pdf

TREATMENT OF ACUTE COPD EXACERBATIONS

- Albuterol 2.5 mg and ipratropium 0.5 mg nebulized q 2–4 h
- Antibiotics × 5–10 days for severe exacerbations or presence of purulent sputum
  - Uncomplicated exacerbation if age 65 yo or younger, FEV_1 50% or more, and fewer than 4 exacerbations/year
    - New macrolide, doxycycline, or 2nd–3rd generation cephalosporin
  - Complicated exacerbation if age older than 65 yo, FEV_1 less than 50%, more than 4 exacerbations/year, or use of antibiotics in the last 3 months
    - Use amoxicillin-clavulanate or a respiratory quinolone
  - Risk for pseudomonas if recurrent antibiotic use, recurrent steroid courses, or if bronchiectasis is present; use an antipseudomonal quinolone
- Systemic steroids with methylprednisolone 30–40 mg/day (or prednisone 40–60 mg PO daily) × 7–10 days if FEV_1 is less than 50% predicted, **or** if $PaCO_2$ is greater than 45 and pH is less than 7.35 with or without steroid taper
- Oxygen if hypoxia to maintain SaO_2 is 88–90% or PaO_2 is 55 mmHg or higher
- Noninvasive positive-pressure ventilation if acute respiratory acidosis (pH 7.35 or less, $PaCO_2$ 45 mmHg or higher) and no contraindications to its use
- Indications for ICU admission: $PaCO_2$ greater than 60 mmHg and pH less than 7.25, depressed level of consciousness, unstable medical comorbidities, hemodynamic or rhythm instability, and need for invasive mechanical ventilation
- Indications for mechanical ventilation: severe respiratory acidosis refractory to noninvasive ventilation, respiratory arrest, hemodynamic instability, or obtundation

COMPLICATIONS

- Progressive dyspnea
- Respiratory failure
- Frequent/recurrent pulmonary infections
- Pulmonary hypertension results in cor pulmonale
- Depression

REFERENCES

)LD initiative at www.goldcopd.com; *Am J Med*, 2006;119:S46; *Am J Med*, 2007;120(8 Suppl 1):S4–13; *n Fam Med*, 2006;4(3):253–62; *Lancet*, 2004;364(9437):883–95; *Chest*, 2008;133(3):756–66; *Am Fam 'ysician*, 2010;81(5):607–13.

CHAPTER 72

PERIOPERATIVE PULMONARY EVALUATION AND MANAGEMENT

1. PREOPERATIVE RISK STRATIFICATION

- Few patients have an absolute pulmonary contraindication to surgery
- Preoperative spirometry should *not* be used to prevent surgery but rather as a tool to optimize preoperative lung function; appropriate if the patient has
  - Asthma or COPD and airflow obstruction that has not been optimized
  - Unexplained dyspnea or cough and will undergo major surgery (as below)
  - Patient will be undergoing lung resection surgery
- Indications for an arterial blood gas: resting hypoxia, risk for chronic hypercapnia, or anticipated lung resection surgery

2. PERIOPERATIVE PULMONARY MANAGEMENT TABLES

TABLE 72.1. Risk Factors for Perioperative Pulmonary Complications*

• Age older than 60 years	• COPD
• Smoking within 8 weeks of surgery	• CHF
• Poor general health (ASA 3 or more)†	• Elevated arterial carbon dioxide pressure ($PaCO_2$ 45 mmHg)
• Emergency surgery	• Functional dependence for ADLs
• Thoracic, abdominal aortic aneurysm, neurosurgery, head and neck or upper abdominal surgery	• Impaired sensorium
• Surgery lasting more than 3 hours	• Malnourished (albumin less than 3.5 g/dL)
• General anesthesia	• Renal failure (blood urea nitrogen [BUN] 21 mg/dL or higher)
• Long-acting neuromuscular blockade	• Transfusion more than 4 units of blood

Note: Obesity alone or asthma does not appear to increase risk

ASA = aspirin, COPD = chronic obstructive pulmonary disease, CHF = congestive heart failure, ADL = activities of daily living, BUN = blood urea nitrogen
* Perioperative pulmonary complications include atelectasis, pneumonia, or respiratory failure
† American Society of Anesthesiologists Classification at www.asahq.org/clinical/physicalstatus.htm

Source: Adapted from *Ann Intern Med*, 2006; 144(8): 575–80.

TABLE 72.2. Postoperative Respiratory Failure Index

Factor	Score	Factor	Score
Type of surgery		Albumin less than 3 g/dL	9
AAA repair	27	BUN greater than 30 mg/dL	8
Thoracic surgery	21	History of COPD	6
Neurosurgery, upper abdomen, or peripheral vascular surgery	14	Partially or fully dependent functional status	7
Neck surgery	11	Age 70 yo or older	6
Emergency surgery	11	Age 60–69 yo	4

Class	Points	Incidence of Postoperative Respiratory Failure
1	10 or fewer	0.5%
2	11–19	1.8%
3	20–27	4.2%
4	28–40	10.1%
5	More than 40	26.6%

Source: Adapted from *Ann Intern Med*, 2006;144:575.

INTERVENTIONS TO REDUCE PERIOPERATIVE RISK

- Smoking cessation: beneficial if patient quits 8 or more weeks prior to surgery
- Inhaled tiotropium 1 puff daily for COPD with or without β_2 agonists for wheezing
- Oral or inhaled steroids and inhaled tiotropium if COPD or asthma and pulmonary function not optimal (no increase in risk of infections, but potential for adrenal suppression if 20 mg/day or more of prednisone for at least 3 weeks)
- Defer elective surgery for acute exacerbations of pulmonary disease
- Consider shorter procedures (under 3 hours), laparoscopic approach, and spinal/epidural or regional anesthesia rather than general anesthesia for high-risk patients
- Avoid long-acting neuromuscular blockers (e.g., pancuronium)
- Postoperative lung expansion maneuvers and early mobilization recommended
- Consider postoperative epidural analgesia for thoracic or upper abdominal surgery

REFERENCES

Ann Intern Med, 2006;144(8):575–80; *Anesth Clin N Amer*, 2004;22:77; *Ann Surg*, 2000;232(2):242–53.

CHAPTER 73

DIFFUSE INTERSTITIAL LUNG DISEASE

1. **EPIDEMIOLOGY**
   - 75% of IPF are older than 60 yo at diagnosis
   - Almost all patients with lymphangioleiomyomatosis (LAM) are women

2. **PATHOPHYSIOLOGY**
   - Predominant histopathological patterns
     - Granulomatous: T cells, macrophages, and epitheloid cells organized into granulomas
       - Known cause: hypersensitivity pneumonitis
       - Unknown cause: sarcoidosis, granulomatosis with polyangiitis (formerly known as Wegener's granulomatosis), Churg-Strauss
     - Inflammatory/fibrotic: epithelial injury induces alveolar inflammation; interstitial and vascular inflammation leads to interstitial fibrosis, irreversible scarring, and impaired gas exchange
     - Known cause: asbestos, inhalation, medications (nitrofurantoin, amiodarone), chemotherapy (bleomycin), radiation, aspiration, post-ARDS, desquamative interstitial pneumonia, Langerhans cell granulomatosis
     - Unknown cause: idiopathic pulmonary fibrosis (usual interstitial pneumonia), diffuse alveolar damage, cryptogenic organizing pneumonia, nonspecific interstitial pneumonia, rheumatologic diseases, Goodpasture's syndrome, pulmonary alveolar proteinosis, eosinophilic pneumonia, lymphangioleiomyomatosis, amyloidosis, genetic diseases, graft-versus-host, etc.

3. **CLINICAL PRESENTATION**
   - Progressive dyspnea and cough
   - Acuity of onset ranges from years (UIP) to days/weeks (AIP)
   - Signs: crackles, inspiratory squeaks; rarely cor pulmonale

4. **DIAGNOSIS**
   - Definitive diagnosis is via a tissue biopsy
   - History: occupational/environmental exposures, travel, meds, medical comorbidities

5. **DIFFERENTIAL DIAGNOSIS**
   - CHF
   - Fungal pneumonia
   - Miliary tuberculosis
   - Pulmonary hypertension
   - Interstitial spread of cancer

6. **EVALUATION**
   - Chest X-ray and arterial blood gas
   - High-resolution chest CT: reticulonodular infiltrates, interstitial infiltrates, "ground glass" opacities, or honeycombing
   - Pulmonary function testing reveals a pattern of restrictive lung disease with a decline in lung volumes and diffusion capacity
   - Labs: CBCD, chemistry panel, angiotensin converting enzyme, ANA, RF, antineutrophil cytoplasmic antibody, antiglomerular basement membrane antibody, anti-ScL-70, HIV, ESR, CK, HLA-B27, aldolase levels, and coccidioidomycosis titers
   - Induced sputa or bronchoalveolar lavage for cytology and AFB or fungi
   - Open lung biopsy
   - See **Figure 73.1**

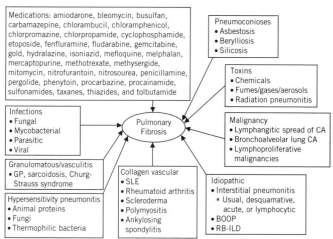

Medications: amiodarone, bleomycin, busulfan, carbamazepine, chlorambucil, chloramphenicol, chlorpromazine, chlorpropamide, cyclophosphamide, etoposide, fenfluramine, fludarabine, gemcitabine, gold, hydralazine, isoniazid, mefloquine, melphalan, mercaptopurine, methotrexate, methysergide, mitomycin, nitrofurantoin, nitrosourea, penicillamine, pergolide, phenytoin, procarbazine, procainamide, sulfonamides, taxanes, thiazides, and tolbutamide

Pneumoconioses
• Asbestosis
• Berylliosis
• Silicosis

Toxins
• Chemicals
• Fumes/gases/aerosols
• Radiation pneumonitis

Infections
• Fungal
• Mycobacterial
• Parasitic
• Viral

Pulmonary Fibrosis

Malignancy
• Lymphangitic spread of CA
• Bronchoalveolar lung CA
• Lymphoproliferative malignancies

Granulomatous/vasculitis
• GP, sarcoidosis, Churg-Strauss syndrome

Collagen vascular
• SLE
• Rheumatoid arthritis
• Scleroderma
• Polymyositis
• Ankylosing spondylitis

Idiopathic
• Interstitial pneumonitis
  • Usual, desquamative, acute, or lymphocytic
• BOOP
• RB-ILD

Hypersensitivity pneumonitis
• Animal proteins
• Fungi
• Thermophilic bacteria

GP = granulomatosis with polyangiitis (formerly known as Wegener's granulomatosis), SLE = systemic lupus erythematosus, BOOP = bronchiolitis obliterans with organizing pneumonia, RB-ILD = respiratory bronchiolitis-interstitial lung disease, CA = cancer

FIGURE 73.1. Causes of Diffuse Interstitial Lung Disease

Source: Adapted from *South Med J*, 2007; 100(6): 579–87.

TREATMENT OF DIFFUSE INTERSTITIAL LUNG DISEASE (DILD)

• Targeted therapy of any underlying disease that has been identified
• Avoidance of offending medication(s) or occupational exposures if relevant
• Supplemental O_2 to keep PaO_2 above 55 mmHg; pneumococcal and influenza vaccines
• Idiopathic interstitial pneumonitis: prednisone 0.5–1 mg/kg/day often, with cyclophosphamide 2 mg/kg PO daily OR azathioprine 2 mg/kg PO daily
• Refer appropriate patients for lung transplantation

COMPLICATIONS

• Pulmonary hypertension
• Cor pulmonale
• Respiratory failure

REFERENCES

South Med J, 2007;100(6):579–87; *Chest*, 2006;129(Suppl 1):180S–5S; *Curr Opin Pulm Med*, 2008;14(5):427–33; *Thorax*, 2008;63(Suppl 5):v1–58.

CHAPTER 74

PULMONARY HYPERTENSION

1. **EPIDEMIOLOGY**
   - Uncommon; incidence 2.4–7.6 cases per million, prevalence of 15–50 cases per million
   - Poor prognosis with 15% mortality within 1 year
   - Male to female ratio is 1:2; mean age of onset is around 37 yo; idiopathic type is most common at 39%; 70% arise from a germline mutation in BMPR2 gene
   - Drug-induced PAH is primarily related to anorexigen (diet pill), 10%; other drugs such as amphetamine and L tryptophan are also associated with its development
   - 25–50% of patients suffer from Eisenmenger syndrome
   - 4% or patients with PE go on to develop PAH
   - 4% PE patients go on to develop PAH

2. **CLINICAL PRESENTATION**
   - Early phases are asymptomatic
   - Presenting symptoms are dyspnea on exertion, fatigue, chest pain, palpitations, and edema
   - Signs: R parasternal lift, accentuated second heart sound, pansystolic murmur (tricuspid regurgitation), third heart sound, diastolic murmur (pulmonary valve insufficiency), peripheral edema
   - Risk factors are congenital heart disease, connective tissue disease, portal hypertension, sickle cell disease, thyroid disease, and HIV

3. **DEFINITION**
   - Mean pulmonary artery pressure is greater than 25 mmHg (rest)
   - Pulmonary arterial hypertension (PAH): above and normal PCWP or normal LVEDP
   - See **Table 74.1**

TABLE 74.1. Classification of Pulmonary Hypertension (PHTN)

Subtypes of PHTN	Causes
Pulmonary arterial hypertension (PAH)	• Idiopathic • Familial • Associated with a connective tissue disease • Associated with HIV infection • Portopulmonary hypertension • Drug-induced or toxin-induced • Pulmonary veno-occlusive disease • Pulmonary capillary hemangiomatosis
PHTN with left heart disease	• Chronic CHF, moderate–severe MS or MR
Secondary to chronic hypoxia	• COPD, DILD, OSA, obesity-hypoventilation syncope, neuromuscular disorders, intracardiac right-to-left shunts
Recurrent pulmonary emboli	• Recurrent PE or tumor emboli
Miscellaneous	• Sarcoidosis, Langerhans cell histiocytosis, schistosomiasis, and lymphangiomatosis

Source: Adapted from *J Am Coll Cardiol*, 2004(12 Suppl S); 43: 5S–12S.

EVALUATION OF PULMONARY HYPERTENSION

- ECG: right axis deviation, right atrial abnormality, and right ventricular hypertrophy
- Chest X-ray: enlarged right atrium and ventricle, dilated pulmonary arteries, and "pruning" of the peripheral pulmonary vasculature
- Pulmonary function test: screen for underlying obstructive or restrictive lung disease
- Nocturnal polysomnogram: evaluate for obstructive or central sleep apnea
- Arterial blood gas: screen for resting hypoxia or hypercarbia
- V/Q scan superior to CT pulmonary angiogram to screen for recurrent PE
- Echocardiogram: evaluate left ventricular systolic and diastolic function, valve abnormalities, chamber sizes, and noninvasive estimate of pulmonary pressures
- Right heart catheterization: confirms diagnosis of pulmonary arterial hypertension
- Labs: CBCD, chemistry panel, ANA, RF, anti-Scl-70, anticentromere, HIV, and ESR
- 6-minute walk test to determine functional capacity

TREATMENT

- Supplemental oxygen to keep SaO_2 90% or more
- Interventions: influenza and pneumococcal vaccinations; smoking cessation; chronic anticoagulation; and *avoid* decongestants, pregnancy, NSAIDs, and air travel
- Consider cautious diuresis and/or digoxin therapy for right ventricular dysfunction
- Pulmonary vasoreactivity as determined by inhaled nitric oxide testing during right heart catheterization can benefit from nifedipine ER, amlodipine, or diltiazem therapy
- Initial medication therapy for functional classes 2–3 and good hemodynamic profile
  - Endothelin receptor antagonists: bosentan or ambrisentan
  - Phosphodiesterase-5 inhibitors: sildenafil
- Initial medication therapy for functional classes 3–4 with poor hemodynamic profile
  - Prostanoid therapy: epoprostenol IV or inhaled iloprost or treprostinil SQ or IV

COMPLICATIONS

- Cor pulmonale
- Hypoxemia
- Cardiac arrhythmias
- Hemoptysis

EFERENCES

m J Med Sci, 2008;335(1):40–5; *Circulation,* 2008;118(21):2190–9; *Crit Care Med,* 2007;35(9):2037–50; xpert Opin Pharmacother, 2008;9(1):65–81.

SECTION 9

RENAL

CHAPTER 75

EVALUATION OF ACID-BASE DISORDERS

ACID-BASE INTERPRETATION

- Acidemic or alkalemic (normal pH 7.35–7.45)
  - Acidemia represents a pH less than 7.35 and alkalemia is a pH greater than 7.45
- Is the primary problem metabolic or respiratory?
  - Acidosis: $PaCO_2$ greater than 40 is respiratory; HCO_3 less than 24 is metabolic
  - Alkalosis: $PaCO_2$ less than 40 is respiratory; HCO_3 greater than 24 is metabolic

RESPIRATORY DISORDERS

- Acute respiratory acidosis or alkalosis: $\Delta pH = 0.008 \times \Delta PaCO_2$
- Chronic respiratory acidosis: $\Delta pH = 0.003 \times \Delta PaCO_2$
- Chronic respiratory alkalosis: $\Delta pH = 0.002 \times \Delta PaCO_2$
- Also, determine the expected change in HCO_3 as evidence of an acute or chronic process
  - Acute respiratory acidosis: $0.1 \times \Delta PaCO_2 = \Delta HCO_3$
  - Chronic respiratory acidosis: $0.35–0.4 \times \Delta PaCO_2 = \Delta HCO_3$
  - Acute respiratory alkalosis: $0.25 \times \Delta PaCO_2 = \Delta HCO_3$
  - Chronic alkalosis: $0.4 \times \Delta PaCO_2 = \Delta HCO_3$
- Causes of a respiratory acidosis: exacerbations of CHF, COPD, or asthma; PE; pneumonia; oversedation; obesity-hypoventilation syndrome; chronic hypoventilation from restrictive lung disease, neuromuscular disorder, or chest wall disorders; and acute intracranial injury
- Causes of a respiratory alkalosis: early sepsis; salicylate toxicity; pregnancy; cirrhosis; panic attack; severe pain, anxiety, or agitation; and pulmonary embolus

METABOLIC DISORDERS

- For a metabolic acidosis, is there an elevated anion gap or a normal anion gap?
  - Simplified anion gap = $Na – Cl – HCO_3$ (normal anion gap = 12 +/– 2)
    - Conditions that lower the "normal anion gap" include hypoalbuminemia, hypergammaglobu-linemia (e.g., in paraproteinemias), severe hypercalcemia, severe hypermagnesemia, and lithium intoxication
    - In hypoalbuminemia, corrected AG = measured AG + ([4 – albumin] × 2)
  - Expected $PaCO_2 = 8 + (1.5 \times HCO_3) +/– 2$
  - If an anion gap acidosis, is there a mixed acid-base disorder? ("delta delta")
    - Change in anion gap (delta gap) = calculated AG – expected AG (typically 12)
    - Change in HCO_3 (delta HCO_3) = "normal HCO_3" (24) – measured HCO_3
    - Calculated AG-12 + measured HCO_3 = 24 +/– 2 in a **simple** anion gap acidosis
    - Delta delta is greater than 26 = concomitant metabolic alkalosis
    - Delta delta is less than 22 = concomitant nongap metabolic acidosis
  - If an anion gap acidosis, is there an increased osmolal gap? (normal is 10 mosm/kg or less)
    - Osmolal gap = [2 × Na + glucose/18 + BUN/2.8 + EtOH/4.6] – serum osm
    - Increased osmolal gap with alcohol, ketones, lactate, mannitol, ethylene glycol, methanol, or isopropanol (no acidosis with isopropanol)

- Causes of a high anion gap metabolic acidosis (MUDPILERS)
  - **M**: methanol
  - **U**: uremia
  - **D**: diabetic ketoacidosis (or other ketoacidosis: alcoholic, starvation)
  - **P**: paraldehyde
  - **I**: ingestions (isoniazid, iron, or toluene)
  - **L**: lactic acidosis
  - **E**: ethylene glycol, ethanol
  - **R**: rhabdomyolysis (severe)
  - **S**: salicylates or strychnine
- Causes of a nonanion gap metabolic acidosis (HARDUP)
  - **H**: hyperalimentation, and posthypocapneic
  - **A**: acetazolamide use
  - **R**: renal tubular acidosis (RTA)
  - **D**: diarrhea (chronic)
  - **U**: ureterosigmoidostomy
  - **P**: pancreatic fistula
  - Urine anion gap $= U_{Na} + U_k - U_{Cl}$; a negative value = diarrhea, and positive = RTA
- Metabolic alkalosis: calculate expected pCO_2 using $\Delta PaCO_2 = 0.6 \times \Delta HCO_3$
  - Chloride responsive metabolic alkalosis (urine chloride less than 10–20 mmol/L)
    - Vomiting, high nasogastric tube output, diuretics, and rapid correction of chronic hypercapnia (posthypercapneic)
  - Chloride unresponsive metabolic alkalosis (urine chloride greater than 20 mmol/L)
    - Excess mineralocorticoid activity
      - Primary hyperaldosteronism (Conn's syndrome), Cushing disease, black licorice ingestion, ectopic ACTH secretion, or secondary hyperaldosteronism (renovascular disease, malignant hypertension, CHF with diuretic therapy, cirrhosis with diuretic therapy)
    - Significant hypokalemia
    - Significant hypomagnesemia
    - Bartter's syndrome

REFERENCES

N Engl J Med, 1998;338(1):26–34 and *N Engl J Med*, 2002;347(1):43–53.

CHAPTER 76

EVALUATION OF HEMATURIA

EPIDEMIOLOGY

- Prevalence of microscopic hematuria is 0.19–16.1% (more common in females than males)

CLINICAL PRESENTATION

- Microscopic hematuria is often an incidental finding
- Gross hematuria can range from pink-tinged urine to frank blood
- If a urine dipstick is positive for blood, always confirm the presence of RBCs by urine microscopy
- See **Table 76.1**

TABLE 76.1.   Etiologies of Persistent Hematuria in Adults

• Infections: cystitis, pyelonephritis, prostatitis, urethritis, renal tuberculosis, schistosomiasis	• Glomerular causes: IgA nephropathy, hereditary nephritis (Alport syndrome), thin basement membrane disease, glomerulonephritis, Goodpasture's syndrome, granulomatosis with polyangiitis (formerly known as Wegener's granulomatosis), hemolytic uremia syndrome
• Hypercalciuria	
• Hyperuricosuria	
• Cancer: bladder, kidney or urethral	• Sickle cell disease
• Coagulopathy, overanticoagulation	• Medullary sponge kidney
• Thrombocytopenia	• Nephrolithiasis or ureterolithiasis
• Foreign body: urethra or bladder	• Polycystic kidney disease
• Renal vein thrombosis	• Renal arteriovenous malformation
• Drug- or radiation-induced cystitis	• Renal infarction
• Interstitial nephritis	

DIFFERENTIAL DIAGNOSIS

- Glomerulonephritis
- Myoglobinuria
- Hemoglobinuria
- Porphyria

EVALUATION OF HEMATURIA IN ADULTS

- Routine screening urinalyses are not recommended in adults
- If urine dipstick positive for "blood" × 2, check a microscopic exam of urine
- Examine urinary sediment for dysmorphic red blood cells or red blood cell casts, both of which suggest a glomerular source of hematuria
  - Check for renal insufficiency and significant persistent proteinuria (urine protein/creatinine ratio greater than 0.5 or 24-h urine with greater than 500 mg protein)
  - For glomerular bleeding, nephrology consult and renal biopsy are indicated
- Helical CT scan or ultrasound of kidneys to evaluate nonglomerular bleeding
  - CT scan superior for renal masses smaller than 3 cm but more expensive and requires a contrast injection; ultrasound safer screen for children and pregnant women
  - Noncontrast CT urogram superior to ultrasound or IV pyelogram for stones

- First morning urine for cytology with or without acid-fast bacilli culture (if indicated) × 3 days
- Cystoscopy indicated for positive urine cytology, 40 yo or older, or younger if risk factors for bladder or transitional cell cancer (tobacco abuse or history of exposure to benzenes, aromatic amines, aniline dyes, or cyclophosphamide)
- For unexplained hematuria, consider 24-h urine for calcium and uric acid

5. COMPLICATIONS

- Prolonged and significant hematuria, anemia may occur
- Blood clots may cause urinary tract obstruction

REFERENCES

N Engl J Med, 2003;348(23):2330–8; *Urol Clin North Am*, 2004;31(3):559–73; *Med Clin North Am*, 2004;88(2):329–43; *Am Fam Physician*, 2006;73(10):1748–54.

CHAPTER 77

NEPHROTIC SYNDROME

PATHOPHYSIOLOGY

- Glomerular wall normally impermeable to large proteins due to size and charge selection; glomerular damage may allow plasma proteins (albumin, globulin) to leak into urine, causing hypoalbuminemia; hypoalbuminemia then decreases plasma oncotic pressure which leads to edema; decreased effective circulating volume then activates the renin-angiotensin-aldosterone system, increasing Na and H_2O retention and worsening edema (nephrotic syndrome)
- Urinary loss of antithrombin-III leads to hypercoagulability
- Urinary loss of immunoglobulins increases risk of infection
- Compensatory increased hepatic synthesis of lipoprotein results in hyperlipidemia
- Proximal tubule normally resorbs small proteins filtered by glomerulus; but excess production of abnormal protein that may exceed tubular resorption capacity, leading to tubular obstruction and finally renal failure
- Preliminary evidence demonstrates a correlation between the degree of tubulointerstitial damage and the degree of creatinine increase; the theory is that the proteinuria itself causes inflammation that is toxic to the tubulointerstitium
- Plasma cell dyscrasias: multiple myeloma, amyloidosis, lymphomas

CLINICAL PRESENTATION

- Foamy urine
- Edema (peripheral, periorbital)
- Hypercoagulability (DVTs, PE, renal vein thrombosis)
- Hyperlipidemia

DIAGNOSTIC CRITERIA

- Proteinuria greater than or equal to 3–3.5 g/24 h; albumin less than 2.5 g/dL; peripheral edema
- See **Table 77.1**

TABLE 77.1.   Etiologies of Nephrotic Syndrome in Adults

Primary (idiopathic)	Medications	Infections
• Minimal change disease • Membranous nephropathy • Focal segmental glomerulosclerosis	• Antimicrobial agents • Captopril • Gold • Lithium • NSAIDs • Penicillamine • Tamoxifen	• Filariasis • Hepatitis B and C viruses • HIV • Malaria • Mycoplasma • Schistosomiasis • Syphilis • Toxoplasmosis
Systemic diseases • Diabetes mellitus • Amyloidosis • Systemic lupus erythematosus		
Cancer • Multiple myeloma • Lymphoma		

Source: Adapted from *BMJ*, 2008; 336: 1185–9.

4. EVALUATION OF NEPHROTIC SYNDROME

- Urinalysis to check for proteinuria and fatty casts; 24-h urine for protein/CrCl
- Labs: CBC; PT; PTT; chemistry panel; CRP, ESR, ANA, anti-dsDNA, C3, and C4 levels; fasting glucose and lipid panel; with or without glycohemoglobin
- Serologies: HIV, HBV, and HCV
- Serum and urine electrophoresis and quantitative immunoglobulins
- Consider abdominal fat pad aspirate to evaluate for amyloidosis
- Radiology: CXR; renal ultrasound with Doppler study of renal veins to rule out clot
- Renal biopsy if etiology remains unclear

5. TREATMENT

- Treat the underlying cause of nephrotic syndrome
- Diet: 2 g sodium/day; fluid restrict to 1.5 L/day if Na is less than 125 MEq/L or marked edema
  - Normal dietary protein intake
- Edema management: furosemide 40–80 mg PO/IV with or without chlorothiazide 500 mg IV or metolazone 10 mg PO 30 minutes prior to furosemide; administer therapy daily–tid
  - Route is typically PO unless patient is admitted for severe anasarca
  - Anasarca: furosemide 40–80 mg IV bid–tid right after 25% albumin 100 mL IV
- Meds: ACEI with or without ARB; data inconclusive about the safety of combined ACEI/ARB rx
  - Caution with any combination of either ACEI/ARB/renin inhibitor, which may lead to hypotension, hyperkalemia, or progression of renal insufficiency
  - Verapamil or diltiazem can reduce proteinuria if unable to use ACEI/ARBs
  - Statins decrease risk of cardiovascular complications and may slow progression to CKD
  - Aspirin 81 mg PO daily for primary cardiovascular prevention
- Keep blood pressure 125/75 mmHg or less
- Prevention: assure that pneumococcal and influenza vaccinations are up to date
  - Heparin or low-molecular weight heparin for DVT prophylaxis
  - Bone mineral densitometry to screen for osteoporosis

6. COMPLICATIONS OF NEPHROTIC SYNDROME

- Infection is common secondary to hypogammaglobulinemia and decreased complement activity
- Venous thromboembolism and renal vein thrombosis
- Fluid overload: ascites, pleural effusions, and increased risk of CHF
- Hyperlipidemia with eruptive xanthomata and xanthelasmata
- Increased risk of cardiovascular morbidity and mortality
- Possible worsening of renal insufficiency by the proteinuria itself

REFERENCES

Brit Med J, 2008;336:1185–9 and *Nephrology (Carlton)*, 2008;13(1):45–50.

CHAPTER 78

ACUTE KIDNEY INJURY

1. ## EPIDEMIOLOGY
   - Adult inpatient mortality ranges from 30% for drug-induced ARF to 90% for ARF with MODS

2. ## PATHOPHYSIOLOGY
   - Kidneys receive 20% of total cardiac output
   - Prerenal azotemia: hypovolemia, CHF, medications (NSAIDs, ACEIs/ARBs), cirrhosis lead to failure of normal glomerular autoregulation
     - Normally, prostaglandins dilate afferent arteriole and angiotensin II constricts efferent arteriole, maintaining normal GFR
     - Atherosclerosis, HTN, age, CKD, and medications (especially combination of NSAID and ACEI/ARB) reduce autoregulatory response
   - Intrinsic renal disease: most commonly sepsis (hypoperfusion, generalized vasodilation, endothelial damage), ischemia (renal medulla susceptible to hypoxia), or toxins (via direct cytotoxic effects, crystal precipitation, or inflammatory infiltrate)
     - Vascular: glomerulonephritis, vasculitis, TTP/HUS, DIC, atheroemboli, malignant HTN, sepsis, thrombosis, abdominal compartment syndrome
     - Tubular: toxic ATN (rhabdomyolysis, hemolysis, IV contrast, cisplatin, aminoglycosides, acyclovir, ethylene glycol), ischemia, sepsis, precipitation (myeloma, uric acid)
     - Interstitial: allergic (medications), infection, hematologic malignancy, sepsis
   - Postrenal obstruction: retrograde hydrostatic pressure decreases GFR if bilateral obstruction in healthy patients (unilateral obstruction may be sufficient to decrease GFR if underlying CKD)
     - Bladder neck obstruction: prostate disease, neurogenic bladder, anticholinergics
     - Foreign bodies: obstructed catheters, calculi, clots, sloughed renal papillae
     - Strictures
     - Extrinsic compression of ureters

3. ## CLINICAL PRESENTATION
   - Initially asymptomatic
   - Uremia (anorexia, nausea, vomiting, metallic taste, altered mental status, pericardial effusion, pruritus)
   - Volume overload (pulmonary edema and peripheral edema)
   - History to help differentiate between postrenal (BPH, malignancy, nephrolithiasis), prerenal (reasons for volume depletion or poor cardiac output), and intrinsic renal (recent IV contrast, nephrotoxic medications, symptoms of glomerulonephritis or vasculitis)
   - Acidosis (Kussmaul breathing, fatigue, vomiting)

4. ## DEFINITION OF ACUTE KIDNEY INJURY (AKI)
   - AKI should be abrupt (within 1–7 days) and sustained (longer than 24 hours)
   - See **Table 78.1**

TABLE 78.1. RIFLE Classification* of Acute Kidney Injury

Class	GFR Criteria	UO Criteria
Risk	Increased serum creatinine[†] × 1.5	UO less than 0.5 mL/kg/h × 6 h
Injury	Increased serum creatinine[†] × 2	UO less than 0.5 mL/kg/h × 12 h
Failure (acute renal failure)	Increased serum creatinine[†] × 3 or increased to greater than 0.5 mg/dL above 4 mg/dL	UO less than 0.5 mL/kg/h × 24 h[‡]
Loss	Persistent acute renal failure for more than 4 weeks	
End-stage kidney disease	Persistent renal loss for more than 3 months	

* RIFLE class is determined based on the worst of either GFR criteria or urine output criteria
† Represents the **baseline** serum creatinine, GFR = glomerular filtration rate
‡ Or anuria for longer than 12 hours, UO = urine output

Source: Adapted from *Critical Care*, 2006; 10: 73.

5. ETIOLOGIES OF ACUTE KIDNEY INJURY

- Causes of prerenal azotemia (55–60% of cases)
  - Hypovolemia
  - Distributive shock (sepsis, anaphylaxis, or neurogenic)
  - Decreased effective circulating volume (chronic CHF, sepsis, nephrotic syndrome, decompensated cirrhosis, or "third spacing" of fluids)
  - Decreased cardiac output (cardiogenic shock or pericardial tamponade)
  - Chronic hypercalcemia causing renal vasoconstriction
  - Meds: ACEI, ARBs, NSAIDs, COX-2 inhibitors, cyclosporine, amphotericin B, radiocontrast dyes, hydralazine, and minoxidil
- Causes of postrenal or obstructive nephropathy (5–10% of cases)
  - Bilateral ureteral obstruction
  - Bladder outlet obstruction (benign prostatic hyperplasia, bladder stone or cancer of the cervix, bladder or prostate or a urethral stricture)
  - Neurogenic bladder
  - Crystal-forming meds: acetazolamide, acyclovir, indinavir, methotrexate, sulfadiazine, topiramate, and triamterene
- Intrinsic AKI: acute glomerulonephritis, tubular necrosis, or interstitial nephritis
- Causes of acute glomerulonephritis (AGN) (2–3% of cases)
  - Systemic illnesses: systemic lupus erythematosus, granulomatosis with polyangiitis (formerly known as Wegener's granulomatosis), Goodpasture's syndrome, and polyarteritis nodosa
  - Henoch-Schönlein purpura or immunoglobulin A (IgA) nephropathy
  - Infectious: hepatitis B and C viruses, endocarditis, HIV, poststreptococcal
  - Malignancy
  - Mixed cryoglobulinemia (often hepatitis C virus–related)
  - Meds: allopurinol, cytokine therapy, gold, hydralazine, pamidronate, penicillamine
- Causes of acute tubular necrosis (ATN) (35% of cases)
  - Ischemia from renal hypoperfusion
  - Medications/toxins: aminoglycosides, amphotericin B, arsenic, carboplatin, cisplatin, chromium, contrast dyes, cyclosporine, foscarnet, ifosfamide, methotrexate, methoxyflurane, oxaliplatin, pentamidine, plicamycin, rifampin, tetracyclines, and trimetrexate
  - Pigment-related: severe hemolysis or rhabdomyolysis
  - Cast nephropathy from multiple myeloma

- Acute interstitial nephritis (AIN) (2–3% of cases)
  - Medications (90% of AIN): acyclovir, adefovir, allopurinol, azathioprine, carbamazepine, cephalo-sporins, cidofovir, cimetidine, cyclosporine, erythromycin, ethambutol, fluoroquinolones, furosemide, lithium, NSAIDs, omeprazole, penicillins, phenobarbital, phenytoin, ranitidine, rifampin, sulfon-amides, tacrolimus, tetracyclines, thiazides, trimethoprim, vancomycin, and some Chinese herbs (such as aristolochic acid)
  - Miscellaneous causes: infection, lymphomatous or leukemic infiltration
- Other nephrotoxic agents: cytarabine and melphalan (via tumor lysis syndrome), gemcitabine and mitomycin (hemolytic uremic syndrome), interleukin-2 (vascular leak syndrome), gallium nitrate, IV immune globulin, nitrosoureas and streptozocin (unclear etiologies for acute renal failure)
- Causes of pseudo-renal failure (benign elevation of serum creatinine)
  - Cimetidine, glucocorticoids, and trimethoprim
- See **Table 78.2**

ABLE 78.2.   Urinary Studies in Acute Kidney Injury

Subtype	Urinary Sediment	UNa (mmol/L)	Protein (mg/dL)	FENa (%)	FEurea* (%)
Prerenal	Bland	Less than 20	0	Less than 1	Less than 35
Postrenal	Bland	Usually greater than 20	0	Greater than 1	Greater than 35
AGN	RBC casts	Less than 20	100 or higher	Less than 1	Less than 35
ATN	Gran. casts	Greater than 20	30–100	Greater than 1†	Greater than 35
AIN	WBC casts	Greater than 20	30–100	Greater than 1	Greater than 35

= urine, Na = sodium, FENa = fractional excretion of sodium = (UNa x Serum crt)/(Ucrt x Serum Na) x 100,
Eurea = fractional excretion of urea = (Uurea x Serum crt)/(Ucrt x BUN) x 100, crt = creatinine, BUN = blood urea nitrogen,
GN = acute glomerulonephritis, RBC = red blood cell, ATN = acute tubular necrosis, Gran. = granular, AIN = acute interstitial nephritis, WBC = white ood cell
More useful measure when patient receiving diuretics
Contrast nephropathy, sepsis, pigment-induced nephropathy and AKI with underlying cirrhosis all can cause ATN with a FENa less than 1
ource: Information from *AFP*, 2005; 72: 1739 and *AFP*, 2003; 67: 2527.

EVALUATION OF ACUTE KIDNEY INJURY

- Careful effort to find any prior serum creatinine values (if possible)
- Thorough history and physical and careful investigation of medication history
- Calculate FENa or FEurea using previous equations and check urinary sediment
- Place a Foley catheter and measure the postvoid residual after urine studies done
- Renal ultrasound (for size and to check for hydronephrosis/hydroureter)
- Labs to **consider** *depending on* classification of AKI and likely causes: urine eosinophils (present in 30% of AIN), complete blood count, electrolytes, renal panel, calcium, phosphate, hepatitis B and C virus serologies, HIV test, antistreptolysin O titer, antiglomerular basement membrane antibody, antineutrophil cytoplasmic antibody, antinuclear antibody, complement studies, serum cryoglobulins, blood cultures, serum and urine protein electrophoreses
  - Important to be cost conscious and judicious with labs ordered
- When to perform a renal biopsy
  - There is no unanimous consensus about this issue
  - Decision should always be made after consultation with nephrologist
  - Reasonable approach is to biopsy patients with an active urinary sediment or who have an unexplained intrarenal process (AGN, ATN, or AIN)

7. **COMPLICATIONS**
   - Chronic renal failure
   - Hypertension
   - Electrolyte abnormalities (i.e., hyperkalemia, hyperphosphatemia)
   - Uremia/encephalopathy/uremic bleeding
   - Acidosis
   - Fluid overload

8. **PREVENTION OF CONTRAST-INDUCED NEPHROPATHY**
   - Maintain adequate hydration, stop potentially nephrotoxic medications for at least 24–48 hours (e.g., ACEIs, ARBs, diuretics, and NSAIDs)
   - N-acetylcysteine 600 mg PO bid × 4 doses starting a day before the procedure
   - D5W with 3 amps $NaHCO_3$ at 3 mL/kg/h for 1 hour before the procedure and 1 mL/kg/h for 6 hours after the contrast procedure (significant sodium load)
     - Any hydration (normal saline versus sodium bicarbonate) is the most important factor

9. **INDICATION FOR ACUTE DIALYSIS (MNEMONIC AEIOU)**
   - **A:** acidosis: persistent arterial pH less than 7.2 refractory to medical therapy
   - **E:** electrolytes: severe hyperkalemia refractory to medical therapy
   - **I:** intoxications or overdoses
   - **O:** fluid overload
   - **U:** uremia

REFERENCES

J Am Soc Nephrol, 1999;10(8):1833–9; *J Am Soc Nephrol*, 1998;9:506–15, 710–18; *Crit Care*, 2006;10:73; *Am Fam Physician*, 2000;61–88; *Am Fam Physician*, 2005;72(9):1739–46; *Am Fam Physician*, 2003;67:2527–34.

CHAPTER 79

CHRONIC KIDNEY DISEASE*

1. ## EPIDEMIOLOGY
   - 9th leading cause of death in the United States
   - In 2005, incidence was 105,000 cases, mostly due to diabetes (44%) and HTN (27%)
   - Prevalence of Stage 5 CKD was greater than 550,000 in 2009 (greater than 370,000 on dialysis and greater than 180,000 with kidney transplant)
   - Annual mortality for ESRD is 15–20% per year, which is 7 × higher than general Medicare population
   - Annual cost for Medicare ESRD patients in 2009 was $40 billion, which is more than 6% of total Medicare budget

2. ## PATHOPHYSIOLOGY
   - As nephron number decreases, compensatory hypertrophy and hyperfiltration of remaining nephrons fails, leading to increased glomerular flow and pressure, worsening glomerular dysfunction and then progressive nephron loss
   - Uremia: due to accumulation of multiple nitrogenous waste substances (not just urea) and loss of fluid and hormone regulation plus systemic inflammation with atherosclerosis and calcification
   - Secondary hyperparathyroidism: decreased PO_4 excretion increases PTH; decreased calcitriol synthesis decreases Ca, further increasing PTH; increased PTH stimulates bone turnover, leading to renal osteodystrophy
   - Ischemic heart disease: due to traditional risk factors and CKD-related risk factors (anemia, increased PO_4, increased PTH, increased acute phase reactants/proinflammatory state)
     - CKD increases cardiovascular mortality primarily by increasing the prevalence of vascular calcification, LVH, and arrhythmias
   - Hypertension, heart failure: due to hypervolemia/diastolic dysfunction
   - Normocytic anemia: due to decreased erythropoietin production, occult GI losses, and ongoing blood losses with hemodialysis

3. ## CLINICAL PRESENTATION
   - Most are asymptomatic
   - Advanced disease: fatigue, anorexia, nausea, morning vomiting, malnutrition, pruritus, bone pain, impotence, amenorrhea, epistaxis, easy bruising, myopathy, muscle cramps, nail changes, uremic frost, pleurisy, pericarditis, edema, volume overload, lethargy, confusion, asterixis, peripheral neuropathy, seizures, coma
   - Hypertension is common (NaCl retention, high renin levels)
   - Classic signs (rarely seen)
     - Half-and-half (Lindsay) nails: increased melanin production turns the distal nail brown
     - Uremic frost: diffuse, white powdery deposits on the skin (urea accumulates in sweat, crystalizes on skin)

4. ## DIAGNOSIS AND WORKUP
   ### KDIGO Definition of Chronic Kidney Disease (CKD)
   - Structural or functional kidney abnormalities or kidney transplantation for 3 months or longer
     - Hematuria, proteinuria, or abnormal kidneys by imaging or laboratory studies **OR**
     - Glomerular filtration rate (GFR) less than 60 mL/min/1.73 m² for 3 months or longer
   - See **Tables 79.1** and **79.2**

* Adapted from kdoqi guidelines at www.kidney.org/professionals/kdoqi/index.cfm and the kdigo guidelines available at www.kdigo.org

TABLE 79.1. National Kidney Foundation Stages of Chronic Kidney Disease

Stage	Description	GFR* (mL/min/1.73 m²)	Action
1	Kidney damage (NL GFR)	90 or higher	Treat comorbid conditions, slow progression, and CVD risk reduction
2	Mildly decreased GFR	60–89	Estimate/slow disease progression
3	Moderately decreased GFR	30–59	Treat disease complications Refer to nephrologist†
4	Severely decreased GFR	15–29	Prepare for dialysis/transplantation
5	Renal failure	Less than 15	Dialyze if uremic or GFR less than 10

NL = normal, GFR = glomerular filtration rate (expressed in mL/min/1.73 m²), CVD = cardiovascular disease
* GFR calculated with the MDRD equation. Advise people not to eat meat for 12 hours before GFR estimation. Interpret GFR with caution in bodybuilders, amputees, or people with muscle wasting disorders. MDRD equation is available at www.kidney.org/professionals/kdoqi/gfr_calculator.cfm.
† Consider nephrology referral when patients reach advanced Stage 2 CKD
Source: Adapted from the kdoqi guidelines available at www.kidney.org/professionals/kdoqi/pdf/ckd_evaluation_classification_stratification.pdf

TABLE 79.2. Select Etiologies of CKD

• Diabetes mellitus	• Hypertension	• Polycystic kidney disease
• Glomerulonephritis	• Alport syndrome	• Medullary sponge kidney
• Reflux nephropathy	• Myeloma kidney	• Analgesic nephropathy
• Sarcoidosis	• Amyloidosis	• Chronic obstructive uropathy
• Lupus nephritis	• IgA nephropathy	• Hypercalcemic nephropathy
• HIV nephropathy	• Hepatorenal syndrome	• Nephrolithiasis
• Nephrotoxic meds	• Genetic syndromes	

Source: Information from *NEJM*, 2006; 355: 2088–98 and *Ann Intern Med*, 2006; 145(4): 247–54.

Screening for Chronic Kidney Disease in Adults

- Risk factors for CKD: age older than 60 yo, family history of CKD, history of low birth weight, ethnic minorities, HIV, Tb, HBV or HCV infection, diabetes, HTN, cardiovascular disease, autoimmune disease, systemic infections, recurrent UTIs, nephrolithiasis, recovery from acute renal failure, reduction in kidney mass, cancer, exposure to nephrotoxic drugs, or obstructive uropathy
- All patients with risk factors for CKD should be screened annually
- Screen with urine albumin-to-creatinine ratio and estimation of GFR
  - Urine albumin-to-creatinine ratio 30–300 mg/g indicates microalbuminuria
  - Urine albumin-to-creatinine ratio greater than 300 mg/g indicates macroalbuminuria
- MDRD (modification of diet in renal disease) equation for estimating GFR to determine the stage of CKD; not validated for drug dosing in renal insufficiency
  - Calculator available at www.kidney.org/professionals/kdoqi/gfr_calculator.cfm
  - Cockcroft-Gault equation is used to determine CrCl for drug dosing in CKD
  - CKD-EPI equation may be better in early CKD to reduce false-positives
    - Online calculator available at www.qxmd.com/calculate-online/nephrology/ckd-epi-egfr
- Urinalysis and microscopy to assess for hematuria, pyuria, and casts
- Renal ultrasound if obstructive uropathy, severe HTN, recurrent UTIs, active urinary sediment, persistent hematuria, suspected renal artery stenosis, Stage 4 or 5 CKD, or if older than 20 years old and have a family history of polycystic kidney disease

Monitoring Patients with Chronic Kidney Disease

- Follow urine protein-to-creatinine (mg/mg) ratio once overt proteinuria develops
  - First morning urine collection is preferred
- Fasting lipid panel annually (or every 6 months while on therapy)
- Assess for proteinuria annually (urine albumin/creatinine ratio or 24-h urine collection)
- See **Table 79.3**

ABLE 79.3. Laboratory Screening Intervals for Complications by CKD Stage

CKD Stage	Hgb	iPTH	Phos/Calcium	Bicarbonate
3	12 months*	12 months*	12 months*	12 months*
4	6 months	3 months	3 months	3 months
5	3 months	3 months	1 months	3 months
Dialysis	3 months	3 months	1 months	1 months

If GFR is 35 mL/min, these parameters should be checked every 3–6 months

ource: Adapted from *J Amer Board Fam Med*, 2010; 23(4): 542–50.

Screening for Diabetic Kidney Disease

- Patients with diabetes should be screened annually for diabetic nephropathy
- Screening for CKD, as described earlier, 5 years after diagnosis of DM 1 and at diagnosis of DM 2
- Consider other causes of CKD if: absence of DM retinopathy, rapidly decreasing GFR, refractory HTN, active urinary sediment, or signs of another systemic disease

5. TREATMENT

Management of Diabetes with Chronic Kidney Disease Stages 1–4

- Target HgbA1c less than 7%
- ACEI/ARB for HTN or albuminuria; BP goal less than 130/80 mmHg (less than 125/75 if overt proteinuria)
- Indications for treadmill or myocardial perfusion test: chest pain, possible anginal equivalent, older than 35 yo and plans to begin vigorous exercise, carotid artery/peripheral vascular disease

Management of Anemia of Chronic Kidney Disease

- Epoetin α 50–100 U/kg IV three times a week with hemodialysis
  - Give weekly prior to dialysis
  - Target hemoglobin 11 g/dL; avoid hemoglobin levels greater than 12 gm/dL
- PO/IV iron to maintain transferrin saturation greater than 20% and ferritin above 100 ng/mL

Surgical Referrals

- Refer patient to surgeon for dialysis access when CrCl is less than 25 mL/min
  - Protect arm most suitable for access from venipunctures, IVs, or BP checks
- Refer for transplant evaluation once CrCl is less than or equal to 20 mL/min even if *not* on dialysis

Metabolic Acidosis

- Maintain serum bicarbonate at 20 mmol/L with sodium bicarbonate 0.5–1 MEq/kg/day
  - Initiate PO NaHCO$_3$ if HCO$_3$ is less than 18 as chronic metabolic acidosis may hasten reduction of GFR
- May use diuretics to control hypertension, fluid retention, and hyperkalemia (which itself can cause decreased ammoniagenesis and metabolic acidosis)

Nutrition

- 2 g sodium, low potassium, and low phosphate for all patients with CKD
- Protein intake
  - 1.2 g/kg/day protein with chronic hemodialysis
  - 1.2–1.3 g/kg/day for peritoneal dialysis
  - 0.8–1 g/kg/day protein in Stage 4–5 CKD predialysis
  - 0.8 g/kg/day protein and urinary protein losses if pt has nephrotic syndrome predialysis
- Periodic assessment of predialysis albumin and weekly weight checks
- Vitamins: initiate multivitamin 1 tablet PO daily and folic acid 1 mg PO daily

Management of Secondary Hyperparathyroidism in CKD

- Goal phosphorus 2.7–4.6 mg/dL (Stage 3–4); keep 3.5–5.5 mg/dL if Stage 5 or on dialysis
  - Hyperphosphatemia is associated with increased mortality in all stages of CKD
- Maintain serum calcium-phosphorus product less than 55
- Goal iPTH: Stage 3 (35–70 pg/mL), Stage 4 (70–110 pg/mL), Stage 5 (150–300 pg/mL)
  - Oversuppression of iPTH below these ranges may lead to increased incidence of adynamic bone disease, which may cause increased fractures and possibly increased cardiovascular risk
- Annual dual energy X-ray absorptiometry in patients to rule out osteoporosis
- Calcium-containing phosphate binders (use if pt hypocalcemic; avoid if calcium is greater than 10.2 mg/dL)
  - Calcium acetate (Phoslo) 1–3 tabs PO tid with meals; calcium carbonate is alternative (watch for premature development of vascular calcifications)
- Non–calcium-containing phosphate binders
  - Preferred over calcium-containing binders, especially if hyperphosphatemia in setting of higher calcium levels
  - Sevelamer hydrochloride 800–3200 mg PO tid with meals
  - Sevelamer bicarbonate 800–1600 mg PO tid with meals
  - Lanthanum 250–1250 mg PO tid with meals (*alternative if highly increased hyperphosphatemia*)
- Vitamin D analogs (start if increased iPTH and 25-hydroxyvitamin D [25-(OH)D] is 30 ng/mL or less)
  - Calcitriol (Rocaltrol) 0.25–2 mcg PO daily **or** paricalcitol (Zemplar) 1–4 mcg PO every other day **or** doxercalciferol (Hectoral) 2–6 mcg IV/PO 3 ×/week
  - Titrate dose to appropriate iPTH levels based on stage of CKD
  - Use with caution if serum calcium is greater than 9.5 mg/dL and phosphate is greater than 4.6 mg/dL
- Options for refractory secondary hyperparathyroidism on dialysis (iPTH greater than 300 pg/mL); may use with or without Vitamin D
- Cinacalcet 30–180 mg PO daily; use if calcium normal/high; also for calciphylaxis
  - Only approved for dialysis patients with above parameters
  - See www.sensipar.com/optima_approach.html for specifics of usage
- Parathyroidectomy for severe, refractory hyperparathyroidism (iPTH greater than 800 pg/mL)
- Ergocalciferol 50,000 IU PO q week–month for Vitamin D deficiency (25-[OH]D) less than 30 ng/mL

Lifestyle Changes

- Cessation of smoking
- Target LDL-cholesterol less than 100 mg/dL; statins are the recommended agents
  - Consider monitoring CK and ALT every 3 months for moderate–high dose statin use
- Target body mass index is 18.5–24.9 kg/m^2; waist circumference less than 102 cm in men and less than 88 cm in women
- Aspirin 75–162 mg/day
- Aerobic exercise for 30 minutes on most days of the week

Vaccinations

- Hepatitis B, influenza, tetanus, and pneumococcal vaccines

Medications to Avoid

- Meperidine, fleets enemas, milk of magnesia, magnesium citrate, magnesium-aluminum antacids, nitrofurantoin, NSAIDs, COX-2 inhibitors, and caution with digoxin or antiarrhythmics

Indications for Initiation of Dialysis

- Estimated GFR less than 10 mL/min/1.73 m^2; uremia; unexplained weight loss, malnutrition, or decline in functioning; intractable fluid overload; refractory hypertension; and hyperkalemia, hyperphosphatemia, or metabolic acidosis refractory to treatment

6. PROGNOSIS

- The 5-year survival rate for a patient undergoing chronic dialysis in the United States is approximately 35%, 25% in patients with diabetes

REFERENCES

National Institute for Health and Clinical Excellence (NICE) 2008 guidelines available at www.nice.org.uk/nicemedia/live/12069/42116/42116.pdf; *Can Med Assoc J*, 2008;179(11):1154–62; *J Am Board Fam Med*, 2010;23(4):542–50.

CHAPTER 80

NEPHROLITHIASIS

1. **EPIDEMIOLOGY**
   - United States: prevalence is 12% men and 7% women
   - Recurrence rates after the first episode are 14%, 35%, and 52% at 1, 5, and 10 years, respectively
   - Mean age 20–49 yo, peak around 35–45 yo

2. **PATHOPHYSIOLOGY**
   - Balance between solubility and precipitation; supersaturation causes crystallization
   - Pyrophosphate, citrate, and glycoprotein keep cations in solution; reductions can increase substrate concentration above saturation point
   - Dehydration, even transient, can also lead to supersaturation
   - pH changes also determine solubility for some stones (not Ca oxalate)
   - Ca stones (most common) start as apatite (Randall's) plaques on papillae, serving as nucleus for crystal formation

3. **CLINICAL PRESENTATION**
   - Flank pain, severe and unilateral, comes in waves, radiates to lower abdomen and groin
   - Migrates medially and caudally with time; cannot find a comfortable position
   - Dysuria and urinary frequency from ureteral stones
   - May be accompanied by nausea/vomiting, hematuria, malaise, fever/chills
   - See **Table 80.1**

TABLE 80.1. Risk Factors for Nephrolithiasis

• Distal renal tubular acidosis	• Hypertension
• Positive family history of stones	• Hyperthyroidism
• Gout or secondary hyperuricemia	• UTI with urease-positive bacteria*
• Hot climate and dehydration	• Obesity
• Primary hyperparathyroidism	• Vitamin D intoxication
• Inflammatory bowel disease	• Insulin resistance

• Diet: low calcium, high sodium, high animal protein, and low fluid intake

• Meds: acyclovir, ceftriaxone, darunavir, indinavir, saquinavir, sulfadiazine, topiramate, triamterene, varenicline, and zonisamide

* UTI = urinary tract infection; *Proteus*, *Klebsiella*, and *Pseudomonas*

4. **EVALUATION**
   - Helical CT scan without contrast is preferred imaging for suspected stones
   - Stone analysis and examine medication list for any offending medications
   - Labs for calcium stones
     - Serum calcium, phosphate, potassium, magnesium, bicarbonate (screen for renal tubular acidosis), intact parathyroid hormone, and Vitamin D metabolites
     - 24-h urine for calcium, potassium, magnesium, citrate, uric acid, oxalate, sodium, and creatinine
   - Urate stones: serum uric acid, CBC, and 24-h urine for uric acid and creatinine
   - Staghorn calculi: 24-h urine for cystine and creatinine and check urine pH

5. **TREATMENT**
   - Drink 2–3 liters of noncaffeinated beverages daily (preferably water)
   - NSAIDs and often opioids for symptomatic therapy of ureteral colic

- Stones smaller than 5 mm have a 90% chance of spontaneous passage
- Trial of medical expulsion therapy if **distal ureteral** stones are smaller than 1 cm
  - α-blockers (e.g., tamsulosin 0.4 mg PO daily)
  - Calcium channel blockers (nifedipine, verapamil, or diltiazem)

Management of Calcium Stones (70–80%)

- Hypercalciuria (urinary calcium greater than 250–300 mg/day): treat with thiazides
  - Diet: low sodium, low animal protein, **normal** calcium, and avoid grapefruit juice and dark sodas
  - A low-calcium diet increases the risk of calcium oxalate stones by causing more GI oxalate absorption and increased urinary oxalate excretion
- Parathyroid surgery for primary hyperparathyroidism
- Hyperoxaluria: diet with low oxalate/high calcium/low Vitamin C
  - Minimize black tea, chocolate, soy milk, nuts, berries, beans, beets, carrots, celery
  - Pyridoxine 100 mg PO daily
- Hypocitraturia: potassium citrate 10–20 MEq PO tid with meals
  - Increase intake of fruits and vegetables and reduce animal protein intake

Management of Urate Stones (10–15%)

- Allopurinol 300–600 mg PO daily for hyperuricosuria (urinary uric acid greater than 600–700 mg/day)
- Potassium citrate 10–30 MEq PO tid or sodium bicarbonate (titrated to urine pH 6.5 or higher)
- Low purine and animal protein diet

Management of Cystine Stones (less than 1%)

- Potassium citrate 10–30 MEq PO tid or sodium bicarbonate (titrated to urine pH 6.5–7 or higher)
- Tiopronin 300–500 mg PO tid OR penicillamine 125–250 mg PO qid

Management of Struvite or Staghorn Calculi (10–15%)

- Surgical removal of stone and fluid intake should exceed 3 liters/day
- Struvite stones: long-term antibiotic prophylaxis; acetohydroxamic acid (Lithostat) for patients who cannot tolerate surgical intervention
- Staghorn calculi: potassium citrate for urine pH 7.5 or higher and tiopronin 300–500 mg PO tid OR penicillamine 125–250 mg PO qid plus pyridoxine 50 mg PO 2 ×/week

Interventional Techniques for Nephrolithiasis and Ureterolithiasis

- Symptomatic renal stones: larger than 2 cm usually requires percutaneous nephrostolithotomy and smaller than 2 cm can be treated with ESWL
- Proximal ureteral stones: 5–20 mm can be treated with ESWL or flexible ureteroscopy and larger than 2 cm often require percutaneous nephrostolithotomy
- Mid-distal ureteral stones: usually treated by ureteroscopy and stenting

6. **COMPLICATIONS**

- Urinary obstruction
- Hydronephrosis
- Acute renal failure
- Infection

7. **PROGNOSIS**

- 80–85% of stones pass spontaneously; prognosis is worse in the setting of concomitant urinary tract infection, as it can lead to pyelonephritis and urosepsis
- Recurrence rate for nephrolitis is 50% within 5 years and 70% or higher within 10 years
- A stone less than 4 mm in diameter has an 80% chance of spontaneous passage; this falls to 20% for stones larger than 8 mm in diameter

REFERENCES

Am J Kidney Dis, 2005;45(2):422–8; *N Engl J Med*, 2002;346(2):77–84; *Endocrinol Metab Clin North Am*, 2002;31(4):1051–64; *Am Fam Physician*, 2006;74(1):86–94; *South Med J*, 2011;104(2):133–9; *Kidney Int*, 2011;79(4):385–92; *Cleve Clin J Med*, 2009;76(10):583–91; *Ann Emerg Med*, 2007;50(5):552–63.

SECTION 10

RHEUMATOLOGY

CHAPTER 81

EVALUATION OF ACUTE MONOARTICULAR ARTHRITIS

1. **EPIDEMIOLOGY**
   - Top 3: infection, crystalline, trauma
   - Gonococcal is the most common type of nontraumatic infectious arthritis; it is 2–4 × more common in women than men
   - Nongonococcal septic arthritis is mostly Staph species 60% of the time, 80% monoarticular, and 50% of the time it affects the knees

2. **CLINICAL PRESENTATION**
   - History
     - Fracture, ligamentous or meniscal tears: history of trauma, acute onset, mild-to-moderate swelling, worse with movement, improved with rest
     - Infections, bacterial: onset over hours to days
     - Infections, fungal or mycobacterial: indolent and protracted
     - Crystal-induced: onset over hours to days; presence of tophi (firm, subcutaneous depositions of monosodium urate crystals); history of renal stones, alcohol binges, diuretic use
     - Osteoarthritis: gradual onset
     - Tumor: gradual onset
     - Gonococcal arthritis: most common acute nontraumatic monoarthritis in young people; sequential monoarthritis in several joints; predilection for wrist extensor tenosynovitis
     - Inflammatory arthritis: monoarthritis may be initial presentation in psoriatic arthritis; spondyloarthritides such as ankylosing spondylitis; and rarely in rheumatoid
   - Examine for joint effusion or inflammation
     - "Bulge" sign for knee effusions: compress the medial or lateral compartment; sign is positive (effusion is present) if the opposite compartment bulges
     - Ankle effusions are palpable anteriorly
     - Elbow effusions are palpable in the triangular recess (between lateral epicondyle, olecranon process, radial head)
   - See **Figure 81.1**

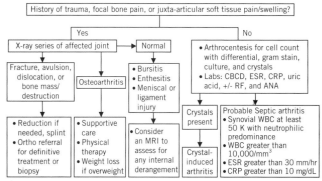

FIGURE 81.1. Approach to Monoarticular Arthritis

Source: Adapted from *AFP*, 2003; 68(1): 83–90, *CMAJ*, 2000; 162: 1577–83, and *JAMA*, 2007; 297(13): 1478–88.

CHAPTER 82

EVALUATION OF ACUTE BACK PAIN

1. **EPIDEMIOLOGY**
   - Prevalence is 70% in industrialized countries, peak at age 35–55 yo
   - 85% pain does not correlate with pathology or neurological encroachment
   - 4% present with compression fracture, 1% with neoplasm, 1–3% with intervertebral disc prolapsed
   - Do not miss these emergent ones: 1–4% older than 50 yo may have aortic aneurysm, MI, ectopic pregnancy with 20% presenting in shock
   - 90% are self-limiting and recover within 6 weeks but 2–7% develop into chronic pain; 75–85% worker absenteeism is attributed to chronic recurrent low back pain

2. **PATHOPHYSIOLOGY**
   - Anatomy and function
     - Anterior spine: vertebral bodies, intervertebral disk serve as shock absorbers
     - Posterior spine: vertebral arches, facet joints are attachments of muscles and ligaments allowing for flexion/extension and lateral bending
   - Types of back pain
     - Local pain: from irritation of sensory nerve from spinal nerve at each spine segment
     - Periosteum, dura, facet joints, annulus fibrosus, epidural vessels, and posterior longitudinal ligaments have pain fibers
     - Nucleus pulposus has no pain fibers but may herniate and compress a nerve root
     - Referred pain: from abdominal or pelvic organs, no variation with posture
     - Spinal pain: upper lumbar spine affects lumbar region, groin, anterior thighs; lower lumbar spine affects buttocks, posterior thighs
     - Radicular pain: radiates to leg in nerve root distribution, may worsen with positions that stretch nerve roots
     - Muscular pain: secondary to spasm

3. **CLINICAL PRESENTATION**
   - "Red flags": TUNA FISH
     - **T:** trauma (significant)
     - **U:** unexplained weight loss
     - **N:** neurological signs (motor or sensory loss, saddle anesthesia, bowel/bladder incontinence, urinary retention)
     - **A:** age older than 50
     - **F:** fever
     - **I:** IV drug use or immunosuppression
     - **S:** steroids
     - **H:** history of cancer
   - Serious etiologies
     - Cancer: history of cancer metastatic to bone, pain increased/unrelieved by rest, vertebral tenderness, limited ROM in spine
     - Cauda equina syndrome: bowel or bladder incontinence, urinary retention, progressive motor/sensory loss, major weakness or sensory deficit on exam, loss of anal tone, saddle anesthesia
     - Fracture: history or significant trauma, prolonged use of steroids, vertebral tenderness, limited ROM, age older than 70, osteoporosis
     - Infection: severe pain, lumbar spine surgery in past year, IVDU, immunosuppression, pain increased/unrelieved by rest, fever, urinary tract infection

- Less serious etiologies
  - Compression fracture: history of trauma or osteoporosis, point tenderness, pain worse with flexion
  - Herniated nucleus pulposus: leg pain is worse than back pain, worse with sitting, radiates to hip/anterior thigh (L1–L3) or below the knee (L4–S1)
  - Lumbar strain/sprain: diffuse back pain, with or without buttock pain, worsens with movement, improves with rest
  - Spinal stenosis, spondylolisthesis: leg pain greater than back pain, worse with standing/walking, improves with rest or flexion of spine
  - Spondylosis (degenerative disk): diffuse back pain, worse with flexion or sitting
  - Inflammatory spondyloarthropathy: intermittent pain at night, morning pain and stiffness
- Referred sources of back pain
  - AAA: abdominal discomfort, pulsatile abdominal mass
  - GI (pancreatitis, PUD, cholecystitis): abdominal pain, nausea/vomiting
  - Herpes zoster: dermatomal pain, allodynia, vesicular rash
  - Pelvic conditions (endometriosis, PID, prostatitis): discomfort in lower abdomen, pelvis, or hip
  - Retroperitoneal (renal colic, pyelonephritis): costovertebral angle pain, abnormal urinalysis

4. DIFFERENTIAL DIAGNOSIS OF BACK PAIN

- Emergent conditions
  - Dissecting aortic aneurysm
  - Ectopic pregnancy
  - Myocardial infarction
  - Pulmonary embolism
  - Epidural abscess
  - Vertebral fracture
- Urgent conditions
  - Acute pancreatitis
  - Duodenal ulcer
  - Pyelonephritis
  - Perforated viscus
  - Pelvic inflammatory disease
  - Nephrolithiasis
  - Vertebral osteomyelitis or diskitis
  - Spondylolisthesis
  - Gynecologic malignancy (uterus, cervix, ovary)
  - Colon cancer
  - Bony mets to the spine
- Other conditions
  - Cholelithiasis
  - Endometriosis
  - Uterine fibroids
  - Pregnancy
  - Prostatitis
  - Paget's disease
  - Ankylosing spondylitis
  - Urinary tract infection
- See **Figure 82.1**

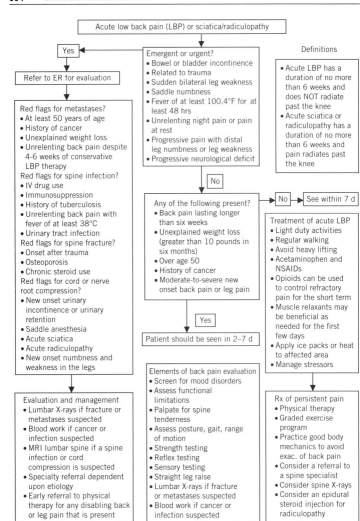

Acute low back pain (LBP) or sciatica/radiculopathy

Yes → Refer to ER for evaluation

Emergent or urgent?
• Bowel or bladder incontinence
• Related to trauma
• Sudden bilateral leg weakness
• Saddle numbness
• Fever of at least 100.4°F for at least 48 hrs
• Unrelenting night pain or pain at rest
• Progressive pain with distal leg numbness or leg weakness
• Progressive neurological deficit

Definitions
• Acute LBP has a duration of no more than 6 weeks and does NOT radiate past the knee
• Acute sciatica or radiculopathy has a duration of no more than 6 weeks and pain radiates past the knee

Red flags for metastases?
• At least 50 years of age
• History of cancer
• Unexplained weight loss
• Unrelenting back pain despite 4-6 weeks of conservative LBP therapy
Red flags for spine infection?
• IV drug use
• Immunosuppression
• History of tuberculosis
• Unrelenting back pain with fever of at least 38°C
• Urinary tract infection
Red flags for spine fracture?
• Onset after trauma
• Osteoporosis
• Chronic steroid use
Red flags for cord or nerve root compression?
• New onset urinary incontinence or urinary retention
• Saddle anesthesia
• Acute sciatica
• Acute radiculopathy
• New onset numbness and weakness in the legs

No

Any of the following present?
• Back pain lasting longer than six weeks
• Unexplained weight loss (greater than 10 pounds in six months)
• Over age 50
• History of cancer
• Moderate-to-severe new onset back pain or leg pain

No → See within 7 d

Treatment of acute LBP
• Light duty activities
• Regular walking
• Avoid heavy lifting
• Acetaminophen and NSAIDs
• Opioids can be used to control refractory pain for the short term
• Muscle relaxants may be beneficial as needed for the first few days
• Apply ice packs or heat to affected area
• Manage stressors

Yes

Patient should be seen in 2–7 d

Evaluation and management
• Lumbar X-rays if fracture or metastases suspected
• Blood work if cancer or infection suspected
• MRI lumbar spine if a spine infection or cord compression is suspected
• Specialty referral dependent upon etiology
• Early referral to physical therapy for any disabling back or leg pain that is present

Elements of back pain evaluation
• Screen for mood disorders
• Assess functional limitations
• Palpate for spine tenderness
• Assess posture, gait, range of motion
• Strength testing
• Reflex testing
• Sensory testing
• Straight leg raise
• Lumbar X-rays if fracture or metastases suspected
• Blood work if cancer or infection suspected

Rx of persistent pain
• Physical therapy
• Graded exercise program
• Practice good body mechanics to avoid exac. of back pain
• Consider a referral to a spine specialist
• Consider spine X-rays
• Consider an epidural steroid injection for radiculopathy

FIGURE 82.1.   Evaluation and Management of Acute Low Back Pain. ICSI, November 2010

Source: Adapted from ICSI, November 2010. Available at www.icsi.org/low_back_pain/adult_low_back_pain_8.html

REFERENCES

Cleve Clin J Med, 2007;74(12):905–13; *Current Med Res and Opin*, 2010;26:170; *Am Fam Physician*, 2012;85(4):343–50.

CHAPTER 83

EVALUATION OF POLYARTICULAR ARTHRITIS

1. **CLINICAL PRESENTATION**
   - Evaluate for: acuity, inflammation (erythema, warmth, pain, swelling, morning stiffness), distribution, symmetry, extraarticular manifestations
   - Features of various etiologies
     - Parvovirus B19: acute, inflammatory, symmetric, small joints; associated lacy, malar "slapped-cheeks" rash
     - Rheumatoid arthritis: chronic, inflammatory, symmetric, small and large joints; associated subcutaneous nodules, carpal tunnel syndrome
     - Systemic lupus erythematosus: chronic, inflammatory, symmetric, small joints; associated malar rash, oral ulcers, serositis
     - Osteoarthritis: chronic, noninflammatory, lower extremity, PIP, DIP, 1st carpometacarpal joints, usually asymmetric; no associated systemic symptoms
     - Fibromyalgia: chronic, noninflammatory, symmetric, diffuse; associated myalgias/poorly localized, tender points, irritable bowel symptoms
     - Ankylosing spondylitis: chronic, inflammatory, symmetric, large joints; associated iritis, tendonitis, aortic insufficiency
     - Psoriatic arthritis: chronic, inflammatory, usually asymmetric, large and small joints; associated psoriasis, dactylitis (sausage digits), tendonitis, onychodystrophy (pitted nails)
   - See **Tables 83.1** and **83.2**

TABLE 83.1.   Different Causes of Polyarthritis

Arthritis	Patient Profile	History and Onset	Pattern of Arthritis and Joints Involved	X-ray Findings	Supporting Tests
RA	Female more often than Male Age: 35–50 yo	Insidious, additive-increased morning stiffness	Symmetric, inflammatory PIP, MCP, wrist, MTP, knees, and ankles	Joint space narrowing, bony erosions	Positive RF Positive anti-CCP Elevated CRP/ESR
UPA	Females more than males	Insidious polyarthritis	Inflammatory arthritis, same joint involvement as for RA	Joint space narrowing, bony erosions	↑ CRP/ESR
Psoriatic arthritis	History of psoriasis	Insidious additive	Inflammatory, asymmetric, DIP, PIP, knee, feet, and spine	Erosions, periostitis, osteolysis	Increased CRP/ESR, negative RF, increased uric acid
Gout	Males: 2–40 yo Females: older than 60 yo	Intermittent; Oligo: earlyl Poly: later	Sudden, severe attacks; joints involved are the first MTP, toes, ankle, knees, and hands (late)	"Punched out" bony erosions or tophi	Synovial fluid: + monosodium urate crystals
Pseudogout	Elderly, same in men and women	Intermittent; oligo or poly	Intermittent or chronic arthritis; Knee, wrist, finger, and MTP	Chondrocalcinosis	Synovial fluid: CPPD crystals
Osteoarthritis	Females more than males, older pts, obesity	Insidious, additive, oligo or poly	Asymmetric; noninflammatory; joints involved are the DIP, PIP, knee, hip, MTP, and spine	Osteophytes, joint space narrowing, subchondral sclerosis	Normal lab tests
PMR	Same in men and women, older Caucasians	Increased morning stiffness, weight loss	Chronic and inflammatory, hip and shoulder girdles	Normal X-rays	Increased CRP/ESR, anemia, increased LFTs
Reactive arthritis	1–4 weeks after GI/GU infection	Fever; malaise; intermittent; & extra-articular	Inflammatory; oligoarthritis; spine; knees; digits; and enthesitis	Possible sacroiliitis; periostitis; erosions; joint space narrowing	Increased CRP/ESR 40% HLA-B27-positive
SLE	Females more than males, young	Rash, serositis, additive	Inflammatory, joints involved are the PIP and knees	Normal X-rays of affected joints	Positive ANA, increased CRP and ESR, positive dsDNA
Gonococcal arthritis	Females more than males, sexually active	Migratory polyarthritis	Inflammatory; wrist, knee, and tenosynovitis	Normal X-rays of affected joints	Increased CRP/ESR and WBC

RA = rheumatoid arthritis, PIP = proximal interphalangeal, MCP = metacarpophalangeal, MTP = metatarsophalangeal, RF = rheumatoid factor, CCP = cyclic citrullinated peptide antibody, Ab = antibody, CRP = c-reactive protein, ESR = erythrocyte sedimentation rate, UPA = undifferentiated polyarthritis, DIP = distal interphalangeal, CPPD = calcium pyrophosphate dehydrate, PMR = polymyalgia rheumatica, LFT = liver function test, GI = gastrointestinal, GU = genitourinary, HLA-B27 = Human Leukocyte Antigen-B27, SLE = systemic lupus erythematosus, ANA = antinuclear antibody, dsDNA = double-stranded DNA, WBC = white blood cell

Source: Adapted from Best Practice & Research Clinical Rheumatology, 2006; 20(4): 653–72.

TABLE 83.2.   Rheumatology Serologic Tests

Disease	Test	Disease Activity	Tests for End-Organ Damage and Comments	Specificity	Sensitivity	Positive Predictive Value	Diagnosis
Systemic lupus erythematosus (SLE)	Antinuclear antibodies (ANA), anti–double stranded DNA	No	Positive anti-SSA (Sjögren's syndrome A) in cutaneous lupus erythematosus; follow serial renal panel, urinalysis with micro and complete blood count with differential	57%	93%	Moderate	Yes
		Yes		97%	57%	95%	Yes
	Anticardiolipin/lupus anticoagulant	No		Yes	No	Low	No
	Anti-Smith antibodies	No		High	25–30%	97%	Yes
Drug-induced LE	Antihistone antibodies*	No	Causes: carbamazepine, chlorpromazine, clindamycin, **hydralazine**, **isoniazid**, methyldopa, oxcarbazepine, phenytoin, and **procainamide**	High	95%	High	Yes
Rheumatoid arthritis	Rheumatoid factor anticitrulline antibodies	No	X-rays of affected joints, baseline PPD and pulmonary function tests; follow complete blood count with differential and liver panel with most therapies	No	50–85%	Moderate	Yes
		No		90–95%	50–85%	High	No

Disease	Test		Description				
Scleroderma (CREST)	ANA Anticentromere† Anti-Scl70‡	No No No	Anticentromere specific for CREST syndrome; chest X-ray, screening pulmonary function tests, blood pressure checks, renal panel, urinalysis with micro, baseline barium swallow and EGD for any dysphagia, echo to screen for pulmonary HTN	54% 99.9% 100%	85% 65% 20%	High High High	Yes Yes Yes
Mixed connective tissue disease	ANA Ant–U1-RNP (ribonucleoprotein)*	No No	Renal panel, complete blood count, creative phosphokinase (CK), blood pressure checks and screen for pulmonary hypertension and interstitial lung disease	No High	93% Moderate	High High	Yes Yes
Polymyositis dermatomyositis	CK Anti-o-1 antibodies Muscle biopsy	Yes No No	Note: electromyogram can help to diagnose myositis; consider search for malignancy in adult dermatomyositis; follow CK in response to therapy	No Yes Yes	High 30–50% Moderate	Low High High	No Yes Yes

(Continued)

TABLE 83.2 (Continued)

Disease	Test	Disease Activity	Tests for End-Organ Damage and Comments	Specificity	Sensitivity	Positive Predictive Value	Diagnosis
Sjögren's syndrome	ANA	No	Schirmer test for decreased tear production; Saxon test for decreased saliva production; needs dental care and eye exams	52%	48%	Moderate	Yes
	Anti-SSA/Ro (Sjögren's syndrome A)§	No		87%	8–70%	~40%	Yes
	Anti-SSB/La (Sjögren's syndrome B)	No		94%	16–40%	~40%	Yes
Granulomatosis with polyangiitis	Antiproteinase 3 antibody	Possible	Diagnosis secured with biopsy of nasopharyngeal lesion; ear/nose/throat exam, chest X-ray, renal panel and urinalysis with or without pulmonary function tests	High	Moderate	High	Yes
	c-antineutrophil cytoplasmic antibodies	Possible		50%	95%	High	Yes

CREST = calcinosis, Raynaud's phenomenon, esophageal dysmotility, sclerodactyly and telangiectasias, SSA = Sjögrens syndrome antibody A, DNA = deoxynucleic acid, PPD = purified protein derivative, anti-SCL70 = anti-topoisomerase 1 antibody, EGC = Esophagoduodenoscopy, HTN = hypertension, RNP = ribonucleoprotein, SSB = Sjögrens syndrome antibody B
* False positives from SLE
† Anticentromere antibodies are associated more with limited systemic sclerosis (CREST syndrome)
‡ Anti-Scl70 is associated more with systemic scleross
§ False positive in cutaneous lupus erythematosus; Dis. = disease

Source: Adapted from *S. Medical J,* 2005; 98(2): 185–91.

CHAPTER 84

RHEUMATOID ARTHRITIS

1. **EPIDEMIOLOGY**
   - Prevalence is 1% in general population, 2% in older than 60 yo; it affects about 2.1 million people
   - Age of onset is 30–50 yo; female-to-male ratio is 2–3:1
   - Standardized mortality ratio 1.28–2.98 times higher than general population with more than 50% of premature deaths, attributable to cardiovascular disease
   - After 10–20 years of having disease, 80% show compromise in ADL; with treatment, this improves to around 60%
   - Within 2–3 years of diagnosis, 20–30% become permanently disabled

2. **PATHOPHYSIOLOGY**
   - Genetic factors associated with major histocompatibility complex (HLA-DRB1, the shared epitope) and environmental factors (smoking, infection)
   - Failure of self-tolerance results in autoreactive T-cells, which drive dysregulated inflammation
   - Stress (smoking) induces peptidylarginine deaminase, which results in citrullination of proteins leading to autoreactive antibodies (anti-CCP)
   - Rheumatoid factor IgM directed against Fc portion of IgG forms immune complexes in joints
   - Chronic inflammation causes synovial hyperplasia and invasive pannus
   - Osteoclast activation causes bony erosions
   - Loss of proteoglycan results in thinning of cartilage

3. **CLINICAL PRESENTATION**
   - Pain and stiffness in multiple joints
   - Most common locations: wrists, PIP, MCP joints
   - Morning stiffness lasts more than 1 hour
   - Synovitis (boggy swelling) or synovial thickening on exam
   - Associated subcutaneous nodules (firm, rubbery, on pressure areas)
   - Fatigue, weight loss, low-grade fever with active disease
   - Extraarticular manifestations: atherosclerosis, pericarditis, episcleritis/scleritis, amyloidosis, Felty syndrome (splenomegaly, neutropenia, thrombocytopenia), C1–C2 cervical subluxation, neuropathy, interstitial lung disease, pleural effusion, pulmonary nodules, rheumatoid nodules, vasculitis)
   - See **Table 84.1** and **Figure 84.1**

TABLE 84.1.   The 2010 American College of Rheumatology/European League Against Rheumatism Classification Criteria for Rheumatoid Arthritis

Classification Criteria for RA*	Score
Category 1: joint involvement†	
1 large joint	0
2–10 large joints	1
1–3 small joints (with or without involvement of large joints)	2
4–10 small joints (with or without involvement of large joints)	3
More than 10 joints (with at least 1 small joint)	5
Category 2: serology (at least 1 test result is needed for classification)‡	
Negative RF and negative ACPA	0
Low-positive RF or low-positive ACPA	2
High-positive RF or high-positive ACPA	3
Category 3: acute-phase reactants (at least 1 test result is needed for classification)	
Normal CRP *and* normal ESR	0
Elevated CRP *or* elevated ESR	1
Category 4: duration of symptoms (patient's self report of arthritic symptoms)	
Less than 6 weeks	0
At least 6 weeks	1

RA = rheumatoid arthritis, RF = rheumatoid factor, ACPA = anticitrulinated protein antibody, CRP = c-reactive protein, ESR = erythrocyte sedimentation rate

* Patients presenting with at least 1 joint with **definite synovitis** not better explained by another disease

• Patients with erosive or longstanding disease typical of RA who fit the prior criteria for RA should be classified as having RA

• 2010 score-based algorithm for RA: **add score of categories 1–4**; a score of at least 6/10 is needed for **definite** RA)

• A score of less than 6/10 is not definite RA, but the criteria can be fulfilled over time

† Joint involvement refers to any *swollen* or *tender* joint on examination or imaging evidence of synovitis. Excluded joints: distal interphalangeal joints, first carpometacarpal joints, and first metatarsophalangeal joints

• "Large joints" refers to shoulders, elbows, hips, knees, and ankles

• "Small joints" refers to the metacarpophalangeal joints, proximal interphalangeal joints, second through fifth metatarsophalangeal joints, thumb interphalangeal joints, and wrists

‡ Negative refers to values not exceeding the upper limit of normal (ULN)

Low-positive refers to values that are higher than the upper limit of normal but not exceeding 3 times the ULN

High-positive refers to values that exceed 3 times the ULN

Where rheumatoid factor (RF) information is only scored as positive or negative, a positive result should be scored as low-positive result

Source: Adapted from 2010 ACR RA Classification Criteria in Arthritis and Rheumatism. 2010; 62(9): 2569–81.

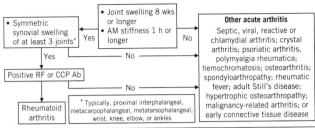

FIGURE 84.1. Early Arthritis Diagnostic Algorithm

Source: Adapted from *J Rheumatology,* 2005; 32(2): 203–7.

4. DIAGNOSIS OF RA

Other Clinical Features of Rheumatoid Arthritis (RA)

- Labs: anemia of chronic disease (33–60%), leukocytosis, and/or thrombocytosis
  - Anticyclic citrullinated peptide antibody (CCP Ab) has a 98% specificity and a superior positive likelihood ratio to rheumatoid factor (RF) for RA
- Symptoms: fatigue, tactile fevers, weight loss, and depression are common
- Late exam findings: ulnar deviation, "swan neck" finger deformities, volar subluxation, and radial drift of the carpal bones; olecranon or retrocalcaneal bursitis
- Subluxation of C1 on C2 can lead to spinal cord compression or radicular pain
- Cricoarytenoid joint arthritis (seen in up to 30%) causes hoarseness or stridor
- Erythrocyte sedimentation rate or C-reactive protein can assess disease activity

Disease Activity in RA

- Disease activity scale-28 (DAS-28) score estimates the RA disease activity
  - Incorporates assessment at 28 joints, global assessment of wellbeing, and ESR
  - DAS-28 calculator available at www.4s-dawn.com/DAS28/DAS28.html
  - Disease remission less than 2.6; low activity is 2.6–3.1; moderate is 3.2–5.1; severe greater than 5.1
- See **Figures 84.2** and **84.3** and **Tables 84.2** through **84.4**

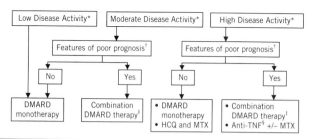

FIGURE 84.2.   Management of Early RA (More Than 6 months Duration)

Source: Adapted from 2012 ACR guidelines in *Arthritis Care and Res*, 2012; 64(5): 625–39.

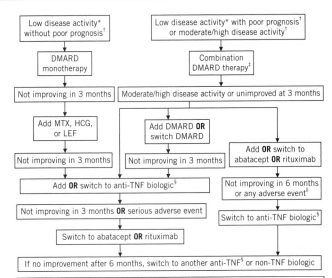

FIGURE 84.3. Management of Established RA

Source: Adapted from 2012 ACR guidelines in *Arthritis Care and Res*, 2012; 64(5): 625–39.

TABLE 84.2.   Disease-Modifying Antirheumatic Drugs (DMARDS) and Biologic Agents for RA

Medication	Dosing	Side Effects	Things to Follow
Methotrexate*	7.5–20 mg PO q week	Nausea, hepatitis, bone marrow reduced, diarrhea	LFTs and CBC
Hydroxychloroquine	200–400 mg PO daily	Retinopathy, headache, nausea, and myopathy	Retinal/visual acuity checks q 6–12 months
Leflunomide*	20 mg PO daily	Increased LFTs, cytopenias, HTN	LFTs, CBC, and BP
Sulfasalazine	1–1.5 g PO bid	Diarrhea, hepatitis, leukopenia, HA, nausea	CBC and LFTs
Azathioprine	1–2.5 mg/kg/day PO	Nausea and vomiting, bone marrow reduced, lymphoma	CBC and baseline LFTs plus renal panel
Infliximab	3–10 mg/kg IV at 0, 2, and 6 wks, then q 8 wks	Reactivation TB, HA, nausea and infections	PPD or any active infection
Etanercept	50 mg SQ q week	Reactivation TB, injection site reaction	PPD or any active infection
Adalimumab	40 mg SQ q 2 weeks	Reactivation TB, infection and injection reaction	PPD or any active infection
Abatacept	500–1000 mg IV q 2 wks × 3, then q 4 wks	Infections, HA, nausea, transient hyperglycemia	CBC or infection
Certolizumab	400 mg SQ q month	Reactivation TB, infection, and injection reaction	PPD or any active infection
Golimumab	50 mg SQ q month	Reactivation TB, infection, and injection reaction	PPD or any active infection
Tocilizumab	4–8 mg/kg IV q 4 wks	Reactivation TB, infection, and injection reaction	PPD or any active infection
Anakinra	100 mg SQ daily	Reactivation TB, infection, and neutropenia	CBC or infection
Minocycline	100 mg PO bid	Hyperpigmentation, dizzy	Skin exam
Cyclosporine	2.5 mg/kg PO daily	Nausea, HA, HTN, and renal insufficiency	CBC, renal panel, and blood pressure
Rituximab	1 g IV q 2 wks × 2 q 6 months	Serious infections	CBC and infections

LFTs = liver function tests, CBC = complete blood count, HTN = hypertension, BP = blood pressure, TB = tuberculosis, PPD = purified protein derivative, HA = headache
* Teratogenic; therefore good contraception essential during use by either woman or partner

TABLE 84.3.   2012 ACR Recommendations for the Use of Biologic Agents in Patients Otherwise Qualifying for RA Treatment Who Have a History of Hepatitis, Malignancy, or CHF

Comorbidity/Clinical Circumstance	Recommended	Not Recommended	Level of Evidence
Hepatitis			
Hepatitis C	Etanercept		C
Untreated chronic hepatitis B or treated chronic hepatitis B with Child-Pugh class B and higher*		Any biologic agent	C
Malignancy			
Treated solid malignancy at least 5 years ago or treated nonmelanoma skin cancer at least 5 years ago	Any biologic agent		C
Treated solid malignancy within the last 5 years or treated nonmelanoma skin cancer within the last 5 years[†]	Rituximab		C
Treated skin melanoma[†]	Rituximab		C
Treated lymphoproliferative malignancy	Rituximab		C
Congestive heart failure			
NYHA class III/IV and with an ejection fraction of no more than 50%[‡]		Anti-TNF biologic	C

NYHA = New York Heart Association, anti-TNF = antitumor necrosis factor.

*Therapy defined as an antiviral regimen deemed appropriate by an expert in liver diseases. The Child-Pugh classification liver disease scoring system is based on the presence of albumin, ascites, total bilirubin, prothrombin time, and encephalopathy. Patients with a score of 10 or more (in the class C category) have a prognosis with 1-year survival being ~50%. Patients with class A or B have a better prognosis of 5 years, with a survival rate of 70–80%.

† Little is known about the effects of biologic therapy on solid cancers treated within the past 5 years, due to exclusion of these patients from most randomized controlled trials.

‡ NYHA class III = patients with cardiac disease resulting in marked limitation of physical activity; they are comfortable at rest; less than ordinary physical activity causes fatigue, palpitation, dyspnea, or anginal pain; NYHA class IV = patients with cardiac disease resulting in inability to carry out any physical activity without discomfort; symptoms of cardiac insufficiency or of anginal syndrome may be present even at rest; if any physical activity is undertaken, discomfort is increased.

Source: Singh, Daniel. 2012 Update of the 2008 American College of Rheumatology recommendations. Arthritis Care and Research. 2012; 64(5): 625–39. Printed with permission from John Wiley and Sons.

TABLE 84.4.   2012 ACR Recommendations for the Use or Vaccines in Patients with RA Starting or Currently Receiving DMARDs or Biologic Agents*

	Killed Vaccines			Recombinant Vaccine	Live Attenuated Vaccine
	Pneumococcal[†]	Influenza (intramuscular)	Hepatitis B[‡]	Human Papillomavirus	Herpes Zoster
Before initiating therapy					
DMARD monotherapy	✓	✓	✓	✓	✓
Combination DMARDs[§]	✓	✓	✓	✓	✓
Anti-TNF biologics[‖]	✓	✓	✓	✓	✓
Non-TNF biologics[¶]	✓	✓	✓	✓	✓
While already taking therapy					
DMARD monotherapy	✓	✓	✓	✓	✓
Combination DMARDs	✓	✓	✓	✓	✓
Anti-TNF biologics[‖]	✓	✓	✓	✓	Not recommended[#]
Non-TNF biologics[¶]	✓	✓	✓	✓	Not recommended[#]

* Evidence level was C for all of the vaccination recommendations. ACR = American College of Rheumatology, RA = rheumatoid arthritis, DMARD = disease-modifying antirheumatic drugs, anti-TNF = antitumor necrosis factor, ✓ = recommended vaccination when indicated (based on age and risk)

† The Centers for Disease Control and Prevention also recommends a one-time pneumococcal revaccination after 5 years for persons with chronic conditions such as RA. For persons at least 65 years of age, one-time revaccination is recommended if they were vaccinated at least 5 years previously and were older than 65 years at the time of the primary vaccination.

‡ If hepatitis risk factors are present (e.g., intravenous drug abuse, multiple sex partners in the previous 6 months, healthcare personnel).

§ DMARDs include hydroxychloroquine, leflunomide, methotrexate, minocycline, and sulfasalazine (listed alphabetically) and combination DMARD therapy included double (most methotrexate-based, with few exceptions) or triple therapy (hydroxychloroquine + methotrexate + sulfasalazine).

‖ Anti-TNF biologics include adalimumab, certolizumab pegol, etanercept, golimumab, and infliximab (listed alphabetically).

¶ Non-TNF biologics include abatacept, rituximab, and tocilizumab (listed alphabetically).

According to the RAND/UCLA Appropriateness Method, panel members judged it as "not appropriate" and therefore it qualifies as "not recommended" (median score on appropriateness scale was 1).

Source: Singh, Daniel. 2012 Update of the 2008 American College of Rheumatology recommendations. Arthritis Care and Research. 2012; 64(5): 625–39. Printed with permission from John Wiley and Sons.

5. COMPLICATIONS

- Increased risk of cardiovascular disease (i.e., MI, pericardial effusion more common than coronary vasculitis, valvular dysfunction, myo-/pericarditis)
- Joint disability/deformity
- Chronic pain
- Peripheral neuropathy
- Anemia
- Scleritis
- Infection
- Osteoporosis
- Sjögren's syndrome
- Felty syndrome
- Malignancies such as lymphoma
- Macrophage activation syndrome (MAS)

6. PROGNOSIS

- 40% of patients become disabled after 10 years, but there is a huge variability of the disease presentation.
- The overall mortality rate in patients with RA is reportedly 2.5 times that of the general population

REFERENCES

Am Fam Physician, 2011;84(11):1245–52; *Arthritis Rheum*, 2002;46:328–46; *N Engl J Med*, 2004;350(21):2167–79; *N Engl J Med*, 2004;350(25):2572–81; *N Engl J Med*, 2004;350(25):2591–602; *Ann Intern Med*, 2007;146(6):406–15; *Ann Intern Med*, 2007;146(11):797–808; *Am Fam Physician*, 2005;72:1037–47; *N Engl J Med*, 2006;355:704–12; *J Rheumatol*, 2005;32(2):203–7; *Prim Care Clin Office Pract*, 2010;37(4):779–92; *J Manag Care Pharm*, 2011;17(9 Suppl B):S14–8; *Arthritis Care Res (Hoboken)*, 2012;64(5):625–39.

CHAPTER 85

SYSTEMIC LUPUS ERYTHEMATOSUS

1. **EPIDEMIOLOGY**
   - Adult onset is around 36 yo; child onset is around 14 yo
   - Prevalence is 56.3/100,000 for adults older than 18 yo
   - Female to male ratio is 10:1

2. **PATHOPHYSIOLOGY**
   - Genetic susceptibility (multiple loci) and environmental factors (UV light, female sex, EBV) interact to yield dysregulated immune response, which produces autoantibodies, immune complexes, and maladaptive inflammation, leading to end-organ damage
   - Autoantibodies against self-antigens: nucleosomal DNA/protein (anti-dsDNA, antihistone), RNA/protein (anti-Sm, anti-Ro, anti-La), phospholipids (anticardiolipin)
   - Increased proinflammatory cytokines, decreased anti-inflammatory cytokines
   - Decreased threshold for activation of innate and adaptive immune responses
   - Decreased suppressor T-cell function
   - Decreased clearance of immune complexes

3. **DIAGNOSIS**
   ### ACR Criteria for Systemic Lupus Erythematosus Classification
   4 or More of the following 11 criteria serially or simultaneously for diagnosis
   - Malar rash: fixed erythematous rash over malar eminences
   - Discoid rash: erythematous plaques with adherent scale and follicular plugging; atrophy and scarring can occur in older lesions
   - Photosensitivity
   - Oral ulcers: usually painless and may involve the nasopharyngeal area
   - Arthritis: nonerosive, oligoarticular with swelling and tenderness of joints
   - Serositis
     - Pleuritis: pleuritic pain, pleural rub, or unexplained pleural effusion
     - Pericarditis: documented by rub, electrocardiogram of pericardial effusion
   - Nephritis
     - Overt proteinuria more than 500 mg/day or 3 or more proteins on dipstick **OR**
     - Active urinary sediment (cellular casts)
   - Neuropsychiatric disorder
     - Seizures in the absence of offending drugs or metabolic derangements
     - Psychosis in the absence of offending drugs or metabolic derangements
   - Hematologic
     - Hemolytic anemia with reticulocytosis
     - Leukopenia (white blood cells less than 4000/mm^3) on 2 or more occasions
     - Lymphopenia (lymphocytes less than 1,500/mm^3) on 2 or more occasions
     - Thrombocytopenia (platelets less than 100,000/mm^3) in the absence of offending drugs
   - Immunologic
     - Anti–double-stranded DNA antibodies
     - Anti-Sm (Smith) antibodies
     - Antiphospholipid antibodies (positive lupus anticoagulant or anticardiolipin antibodies or false-positive venereal disease research laboratory test)
   - Antinuclear antibody (ANA)–positive (titer of 1:40 or higher)

4. <u>TREATMENT GUIDELINES FOR SYSTEMIC LUPUS ERYTHEMATOSUS</u>

- Options for cutaneous lupus erythematosus
  - Hydroxychloroquine 200–400 mg PO daily **OR** chloroquine 100 mg PO tid
  - Pimecrolimus 1% cream under hydrocolloid dressing bid × 3 weeks
  - Tacrolimus
  - Sunscreen against UVA and UVB recommended for all patients
  - Topical corticosteroids: fluorinated steroids for thick facial plaques of discoid lupus × 2 weeks; 1% hydrocortisone cream bid for facial patches or thin plaques
    - Lotions are more appropriate for scalp lesions
- Options for lupus nephritis
  - Prednisone 0.5–1 mg/kg PO daily indicated for all types of lupus nephritis except for mesangial WHO class 1–2 nephritis that usually requires no specific therapy
  - Cyclophosphamide 750 mg/m² BSA IV q month × 6 months added for WHO classes 3–5 glomerulone-phritis (500 mg/m² dosing for elderly, obese, or CrCl less than 40 mL/min)
  - Mycophenolate 500 mg PO bid, then 3 g/day is an alternative agent for WHO classes 3–5
  - Maintenance therapy: prednisone and mycophenolate **or** azathioprine **or** cyclosporine
- Lupus vasculitis, cerebritis, hemolytic anemia, or thrombocytopenia rx
  - Prednisone 0.5–1 mg/kg PO daily with or without pulse cyclophosphamide as above
- Options for lupus oral ulcers
  - 0.1% triamcinolone in Orabase paste applied daily as needed
- Options for lupus arthritis or serositis
  - Mild arthritis/serositis rx: NSAIDs, acetaminophen, or hydroxychloroquine
  - Moderate–severe disease treated with prednisone 0.5–1 mg/kg PO daily
- See **Table 85.1**

TABLE 85.1. Monitoring for Medications Used in SLE

Drug	Baseline Tests	Interval Monitoring
NSAIDs/salicylates	CBC, crt	Annual CBC, crt, and BP
Glucocorticoids	Fasting glc, lipid panel	Fasting glc, lipid panel, and BP annually
Hydroxychloroquine	Fundoscopic exam if greater than 40, CBC, LFTs, crt	Fundoscopic exam and visual fields annually; DEXA-bone mineral densitometry after 12 months
Azathioprine	CBC, crt, LFTs	CBC and LFTs within 4 weeks, then q 2 months once on stable dose
Cyclophosphamide	CBC, crt, UA	CBC and UA q 1–3 months, urine cytology yearly if hematuria present, PAP smear yearly
Methotrexate	CBC, crt, LFTs, CXR, with or without HBV/HCV serologies	CBC, crt, and LFTs q 2 months
Mycophenolate	CBC, chemistry panel, and CXR	CBC q 1–3 months

NSAID = nonsteroidal anti-inflammatory drug, CBC = complete blood count, crt = creatinine, BP = blood pressure, glc = glucose, LFT = liver function test, UA = urinalysis, CXR = chest X-ray, HBV = hepatitis B virus, HCV = hepatitis C virus

Source: Adapted from *Semin Arthritis Rheum*, 2011; 40(6): 559–75.

5. COMPLICATIONS

- Lupus cerebritis, psychosis, seizures
- Lupus glomerulonephritis
- Vasculitis

- Increased risk of infections
- Pericarditis, pericardial effusions, CAD
- Pleurisy, diffuse alveolar hemorrhage, pulmonary hypertension
- Increased risk of malignancy
- Increased risk of miscarriage, preeclampsia, preterm labor
- Thromboembolic events (i.e., stroke/pulmonary embolism)
- Anemia, leucopenia, thrombocytopenia
- Visual disturbances: uveitis, retinal vasculitis

6. PROGNOSIS

- Worse prognosis with renal and CNS disease, milder course with isolated skin and musculoskeletal disease
- Mortality in the first few years of illness is typically from severe SLE disease (e.g., CNS, renal, or cardiovascular involvement) or infection related to immunosuppressive treatment
- Infections account for 29% of all deaths in these patients
- Women aged 35–44 years with SLE were 50 times more likely to develop myocardial ischemia than healthy women

REFERENCES

Arthritis Rheum, 1982;25(11):1271–7; *J Am Acad Dermatol*, 2004;51(3):427–39; *Clin Nephrol*, 2002; 57(2): 120-6; *Am Fam Physician*, 2003;68(11):2179–86; *Clin Fam Practice*, 2005;7:209; *Clin J Am Soc Nephrol*, 2006;1(4):863–8; *Semin Arthritis Rheum*, 2011;40(6):559–75; *Dermatol Clin*, 2010;28(3):489–99.
J Amer Soc Nephrol, 2010; 21(12): 2028–35.

CHAPTER 86

SYSTEMIC VASCULITIS

1. ### EPIDEMIOLOGY
   - Giant cell arteritis and polymyalgia rheumatic is most common type, highest in Scandinavian descent affecting 15–35 per 100,000 over age 50 yo
   - Takayasu's arteritis has global incidence of 1–2 per million
   - ANCA-associated vasculitides have total incidence of 20 million, with peak age of onset around 65–74 yo
   - Wegener's granulomatosis is more common in northern Europe
   - Microscopic polyangiitis is more common in southern Europe and Japan
   - Henoch-Schönlein purpura is most common form in children in the West with incidence 20/100,000 for 17 yo or younger
   - Kawasaki is mostly in Southeast Asia 500/million children under 5 yo, more than 50% are younger than 2 yo
   - Behcet's occur along the Silk Road and Mediterranean, prevalence in Turkey is around 380/100,000
   - Temporal arteritis exclusively affect older than 50 yo, mean age of onset is 70 yo; it causes permanent blindness in 25–50% of those affected

2. ### PATHOPHYSIOLOGY
   - Antigen (e.g., HBV in polyarteritis nodosa, but more often than not unknown) and antibody form immune complexes, which deposit in blood vessel walls and activate complement, leading to inflammatory damage to vessel walls
   - Acute: neutrophils release toxic enzymes
   - Chronic: lymphocytes infiltrate vessel walls
   - ANCA represents autoantibodies against components of neutrophil granules
   - Granulomatosis with polyangiitis (formerly known as Wegener's granulomatosis): cytoplasmic ANCA (cANCA) represents autoantibody against proteinase-3
   - Microscopic polyangiitis, Churg-Strauss syndrome: perinuclear ANCA (pANCA) represents autoantibody against myeloperoxidase
   - Deranged cell-mediated immunity against unknown antigen results in mononuclear granuloma, as in giant cell arteritis, granulomatosis with polyangiitis (formerly known as Wegener's granulomatosis)
   - End organs affected depend on diameter of vessels involved
   - Small: hypersensitivity vasculitis, Henoch-Schönlein purpura, cryoglobulinemia
   - Medium: polyarteritis nodosa and Kawasaki
   - Large: giant cell (temporal), Takayasu's arteritis

3. ### CLINICAL PRESENTATION
   - Small vessel
     - Churg-Strauss: allergic rhinitis, asthma, peripheral eosinophilia (age 50–60)
     - Cryoglobulinemic vasculitis: recurrent palpable purpura, polyarthralgia, glomerulonephritis (age 40–50)
     - Cutaneous leukocytoclastic angiitis: palpable purpura, cutaneous infarcts, necrotic papules, urticarial (any age)
     - Microscopic polyangiitis: palpable purpura, pulmonary hemorrhage, glomerulonephritis (age 50–60)
     - Wegener's granulomatosis: pneumonitis (bilateral nodular and cavitary infiltrates), nasopharyngeal ulcerations, chronic sinusitis, glomerulonephritis (age 40–50)
   - Medium vessel
     - Polyarteritis nodosa: fever, weight loss, hypertension, abdominal pain, melena, peripheral neuritis, renal ischemia (age 30–40)

- Large vessel
  - Giant cell/temporal arteritis (age 50–60)
    - Jaw claudication [LR+ 4.2, LR– 0.7]
    - Diplopia [LR+ 3.4, LR– 0.9]
    - Headache (severe, throbbing, temporal) [LR+ 1.5, LR– 0.8]
    - Fever [LR+ 1.2, LR– 0.9]
    - Fatigue [LR+ 1.2, LR– 0.9]
    - Beaded temporal artery [LR+ 4.6, LR– 0.9]
    - Prominent or enlarged temporal artery [LR+ 4.3, LR– 0.7]
    - Tender temporal artery [LR+ 2.6, LR– 0.8]
  - Takayasu's arteritis (aorta and major branches): low blood pressure, weak upper extremity pulses, cold/numb fingers, visual disturbances, hypertension, neuro defects (age 30–40, Asian women)
- See **Tables 86.1** and **86.2**

TABLE 86.1.   Small Vessel Vasculitis

Condition	Renal	Lung	Heart	Skin	Granulomas	ANCA Type*	ANCA +
Granulomatosis with polyangiitis (formerly known as Wegener's granulomatosis)[†]	Yes	Yes	+/–	No	Yes	c-ANCA (anti-PR3)	90%
Microscopic polyangiitis[‡]	Yes	Yes	+/–	Yes	No	p-ANCA (anti-MPO)	70%
Churg-Strauss syndrome[§]	Yes	Yes	Yes	No	Yes	p-ANCA (anti-MPO)	50%
Cryoglobulinemic vasculitis[‖]	Yes	No	No	Yes	No	–	–
Leukocytoclastic vasculitis[¶]	No	No	No	Yes	No	–	–
Henoch-Schonlein purpura[#]	Yes	No	No	Yes	No	–	–

* Primary ANCA type seen although either c-ANCA or p-ANCA can be found in granulomatosis with polyangiitis (formerly known as Wegener's granulomatosis), microscopic polyangiitis, or Churg-Strauss syndrome
[†] Presents with chronic sinusitis, saddle-nose deformity, pulmonary nodular and cavitary infiltrates, nasopharyngeal ulcerations, hematuria, neuropathy, or pauci-immune RPGN
[‡] Presents with cough, hemoptysis, hematuria, pauci-immune RPGN, mononeuritis multiplex, and palpable purpura
[§] Presents with eosinophilia, "asthma," neuropathy, transient lung infiltrates, coronary arteritis, and myocarditis
[‖] Presents with recurrent palpable purpura, polyarthralgia, and glomerulonephritis
[¶] Presents with palpable purpura, cutaneous infarcts, necrotic papules, and urticaria
[#] Presents younger than 20 yo with purpura, arthritis, abdominal pain, GI bleeding, and glomerulonephritis

Source: Adapted from *NEJM*, 1997; 337(21): 1512–23 and *AFP*, 2011; 83(5): 556–65.

TABLE 86.2. Medium-Large Vessel Primary Vasculitis in Adults

Condition	Vessels Affected	Clinical Features	Diagnostic Testing
Large Vessel Vasculitis			
Takayasu's arteritis	Aorta and its branches	"Pulseless disease," younger than 40 yo, Asians, young women, fever, weight loss, limb claudication, unequal arm BP, renovascular hypertension	• Aortogram with stenosis or occlusion of branches off aorta • Elevated ESR/CRP
Giant cell arteritis	Temporal artery and its branches	HA, jaw claudication, monocular visual loss, temporal artery tenderness, older than 50 yo	• Elevated ESR • Positive temporal artery biopsy
Medium Vessel Vasculitis			
Polyarteritis nodosa	Medium-sized arteries	30% HBV+, fever, weight loss, myalgias, hypertension, renal failure, mononeuritis multiplex, abdominal pain	• "Beaded vessels" on mesenteric angiogram • Positive sural nerve biopsy • Increased ESR and WBC
Primary CNS vasculitis	Small–medium arteries	HA, confusion, disorientation, bulbar palsies, weakness, or seizures	• Cerebral angiogram with "beaded vessels" • Brain biopsy with vasculitis

HA = headache, BP = blood pressure, ESR = erythrocyte sedimentation rate, CRP = C-reactive protein, HBV = Hepatitis B virus, WBC = white blood cells

Source: Information from *Curr Opin Rheum,* 2006; 18: 1, *NEJM,* 2003; 349: 160–9, *JAMA,* 2002; 288(13): 1632–9 and *Arth Rheum,* 1990; 33: 1065 and 1129

4. TREATMENT OF SYSTEMIC VASCULITIS

- Leukocytoclastic vasculitis
  - Antihistamines and NSAIDs in localized disease
  - Prednisone 1 mg/kg PO daily in severe disease
- Cryoglobulinemic vasculitis
  - Interferon α and ribavirin (HCV-related)
  - Non–HCV-related disease treated as ANCA-associated vasculitides
- Henoch-Schönlein purpura
  - Prednisone 1 mg/kg PO daily and cyclophosphamide
- ANCA-associated localized or early disease
  - Prednisone 1 mg/kg PO daily and methotrexate
- ANCA-associated generalized or organ-threatening disease
  - Steroids and cyclophosphamide
  - Plasmapheresis for glomerulonephritis
  - Refractory disease options: IVIG, azathioprine, rituximab, or infliximab
- Polyarteritis nodosa
  - Prednisone 1 mg/kg PO daily plus cyclophosphamide
  - Methylprednisolone 1 g IV daily × 3 days for fulminant disease
  - Interferon α plus lamivudine and plasmapheresis (HBV-related PAN)
- Takayasu's arteritis
  - Prednisone 1 mg/kg PO daily × 3 months with gradual taper
  - Refractory cases may require cyclophosphamide or methotrexate
- Temporal arteritis
  - Prednisone 40–60 mg PO daily × 1 month, then taper by 50% each month for a very slow taper over 12–24 months
  - Methylprednisolone 1 g IV daily × 3 days for patients with acute visual loss

- Life-threatening vasculitis
  - Solu-Medrol 1 g IV daily × 3 days, then prednisone 1 mg/kg PO daily
  - Cyclophosphamide

5. COMPLICATIONS

- Renal failure (due to activation of RAS from ischemia to kidneys)
- Cardiovascular disease: hypertension
- Claudication
- Seizure, stroke
- Optic neuritis, orbital inflammation
- Mesenteric ischemia, which leads to bowel necrosis

6. PROGNOSIS

- Isolated hypersensitivity vasculitis usually resolves spontaneously
- ANCA-associated vasculitis is associated with a poorer prognosis, as is polyarteritis nodosa, which has a 60% 5-year survival rate
- Henoch-Schönlein purpura resolves in almost all patients
- Patients with granulomatosis with polyangiitis (formerly known as Wegener's granulomatosis) who are appropriately treated will have a 5-year survival of approximately 70%

REFERENCES

Curr Opin Rheumatol, 2006;18(1):3–9; *N Engl J Med*, 2003;349:160–9; *JAMA*, 2002;288(13):1632–9; *Arthritis Rheum*, 1990;33(8):1065–7, 1129–34; *N Engl J Med*, 1997;337(21):1512–23; *Am Fam Physician*, 2011;83(5):556–65; *Neurol Clin*, 2010;28(1):171–84; *J Allergy Clin Immunol*, 2009;123(6):1226–36.

SECTION 11

SUBSTANCE ABUSE ABSTINENCE DISORDERS

CHAPTER 87

ALCOHOL WITHDRAWAL SYNDROMES

TABLE 87.1. Alcohol Abstinence Syndromes

Syndrome	Time from Last Drink	Clinical Presentation
Withdrawal tremulousness	6–36 h (typically 6–12 h)	Tremulousness, anxiety, insomnia, headache, palpitations, nausea, anorexia, and palpitations
Withdrawal hallucinosis	12–48 h (typically 12–24 h)	Visual more so than auditory or tactile hallucinations, orientation and sensorium usually maintained
Withdrawal seizures	6–48 h (typically 24–48 h)	Generalized, tonic-clonic, and typically self-limited
Delirium tremens	48–96 h (peaks at 120 h)	Hallucinations, disorientation, sensorium clouded, and marked autonomic instability

Source: Adapted from Signae Vitae 2008; 3: 24 and AFP 2004; 69: 1443.

TABLE 87.2. Clinical Institute Withdrawal Assessment for Alcohol (CIWA-Ar) Scale

Nausea/Emesis	Tremor	Diaphoresis	Anxiety	Agitation
0—None	0—None	0—None	0—None/calm	0—None
1—Mild nausea	1—Can be felt	1—Palms moist	1—Mild anxiety	1—Slight
4—Occasional nausea/dry heaves	4—Moderate tremor	4—Beads of sweat on forehead	4—Moderate anxiety	4—Moderate, fidgety, restless
7—Constant nausea/ vomiting	7—Severe tremor	7—Drenching sweats	7—Severe, or panic state	7—Severe, pacing, thrashing about

Tactile Disturbance	Auditory Disturbance	Visual Disturbance	Headache or Head Fullness	Level of Orientation
0—None	0—None	0—None	0—None	0—Oriented and can do serial additions
1—Mild itching or paresthesias	1—Very mild sounds	1—Mild sensitivity to light	1—Very mild headache	1—Unsure of date or unable to add
4—Moderate occasional hallucinosis	4—Moderate occasional hallucinosis	4—Moderate occasional hallucinosis	4—Moderate headache	2—Date disorientation within 2 days
7—Continuous hallucinosis	7—Continuous hallucinosis	7—Continuous hallucinosis	7—Extremely severe	4—Disoriented to place or person

Score 0–7 for each category except level of orientation where range is 0–4. Minimal withdrawal if score is less than 8; mild withdrawal if score 8–15; and moderate symptoms for score 16–29; severe symptoms for score 30–39 and extremely severe for score 40 or higher.
Source: Adapted from CIWA-Ar scale in Brit J Addiction 1989; 84(11): 1353–7.

TABLE 87.3. Suggested Treatment Regimen for Alcohol Abstinence Syndrome

CIWA-Ar Score*	Intervention†
6–9	Lorazepam 1 mg IV
10–19	Lorazepam 2 mg IV; chlordiazepoxide 25 mg or diazepam 5 mg PO
20–29	Lorazepam 4 mg IV; chlordiazepoxide 50 mg or diazepam 10 mg PO
30–39	Lorazepam 6 mg IV; chlordiazepoxide 100 mg or diazepam 20 mg PO
Greater than 40	Lorazepam 8 mg IV q 1 h until score is less than 30; may need continuous infusion

* Assess CIWA-Ar score q 1 h × 8 h if initial score is 8 or higher; then if stable assess q 2 h × 8 h, then assess q 4 h; assess CIWA-Ar score q 4 h if initial score is less than 8

† Consider adjunctive baclofen 10 mg PO tid × 10 days for mild–moderate abstinence syndrome. Consider adjunctive haloperidol 2.5–5 mg IV/IM q 2 h prn severe hallucinations, agitation, or combative behavior refractory to benzodiazepines (assure that at least 8 mg lorazepam given in preceding 2 h). All patients require thiamine 100 mg, folate 1 mg, pyridoxine 100 mg daily, and a multivitamin.

Note: Recommend ICU care for any of the following: CIWA-Ar score 35 or higher, respiratory distress, hemodynamic instability, unresponsiveness, if pt requires more than 4 mg/h lorazepam for 3 h, or if pt requires hourly assessment for longer than 8 h

Source: Adapted from *J Addictive Diseases* 2006; 25(2): 17–24, *Pharmacotherapy*, 2007; 27(4): 510–8, and *Crit Care Clin*, 2008; 24(4): 767–88.

CHAPTER 88

OPIATE WITHDRAWAL SYNDROME

- Clinical presentation: flulike symptoms, mydriasis, lacrimation, rhinorrhea, piloerection, yawning, sneezing, anorexia, nausea, vomiting, and diarrhea
- Onset (peak/duration): heroin (36–72 h/7–10 days), methadone (72–96 h/14 days)
- Treatment options
  - Opioid agonist: PO methadone 20–35 mg/day or morphine SR 45–120 mg/day; taper over wks
  - Nonopioid agents: clonidine 0.1–0.2 mg PO q 4 h × 3 days, then 0.2 mg PO tid and hydroxyzine 25–50 mg PO tid; or lofexidine 0.2 mg PO qid × 6–8 days then taper; treatment duration is 10–14 days
    - Caution with lofexidine for history of cardiovascular disease, cerebrovascular disease, or renal insufficiency
  - Alternative medications: naltrexone and Suboxone should be administered by addiction specialists

CHAPTER 89

SYMPATHOMIMETIC (COCAINE AND AMPHETAMINES) WITHDRAWAL SYNDROME

- Clinical presentation: insomnia, dysphoria, anorexia, nausea, vomiting, fatigue, malaise, restlessness, depression, and craving
- Onset: peak symptoms at 48–96 hours and lasts for 7 days
- Medications for acute withdrawal syndrome
  - Insufficient evidence to support bromocriptine or amantadine for cocaine withdrawal/craving
  - Consider use of desipramine or bupropion for severe depression
  - Minimize use of benzodiazepines, but can use if severe restlessness/agitation

REFERENCES

N Engl J Med, 2003;348(18):1786–95.

SECTION 12

APPENDIX

ACLS ALGORITHMS

TABLE A1.1. Basic Life Support for Healthcare Providers

Maneuver	Adolescent and Older	One Year to Adolescent	Infant Under 1 yo
Airway	If no suspected neck trauma: head-tilt, chin-lift If suspected neck trauma: jaw thrust		
Rescue breathing without chest compressions	1 breath q 5–6 seconds	1 breath q 3 seconds	
Rescue breathing for CPR with advanced airway	1 breath q 6–8 seconds; 1 second per breath Desire visible chest rise Asynchronous with chest compressions		
Airway obstructed by foreign body	Abdominal thrusts	Up to 5 repetitions of back slaps and chest thrusts	
Circulation	Check carotid pulse for up to 10 seconds	Check brachial or femoral pulses for up to 10 seconds	
Compression site	Lower sternum between nipples	Sternum just below nipple line	
Compression method: push hard and fast and allow complete recoil; if 2 providers, no pauses for ventilation	Heel of one hand with other hand on top	Heel of one hand	2 fingers (lone provider) or 2 thumbs and encircling hands (2 providers)
Compression depth	At least 2 inches	At least $\frac{1}{3}$ the depth of the chest	
Compression rate	100 beats/min; allow full chest recoil after each compression		
Compression to ventilation ratio	30:2 (1 or 2 providers)	30:2 (lone provider) 15:2 (2 providers)	
Defibrillation AED	Use adult pads	Witnessed collapse or hospital arrest: use AED immediately with pediatric pads (if available)	No recommendation

Source: Adapted from 2010 American Heart Association Guidelines for Cardiopulmonary Resuscitation and Emergency Cardiovascular Care. *Circulation.* 2010; 122(18 Suppl 3): S729–67.

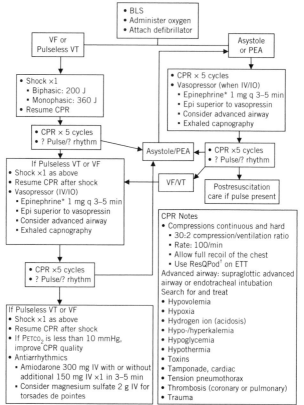

* Meds may be given via endotracheal tube if vascular access unavailable at 2–2.5× standard IV doses.
† ResQPOD is an impedance threshold device that increases blood flow to the heart and brain during CPR.

FIGURE A1.1. Pulseless Arrest Algorithm

Source: Adapted from 2010 American Heart Association Guidelines for Cardiopulmonary Resuscitation and Emergency Cardiovascular Care. *Circulation.* 2010; 122(18 Suppl 3): S729–67 and *NEJM,* 2008;359(1): 21–30.

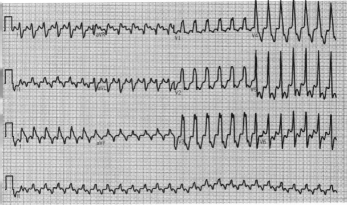

IGURE A1.2.   ECG Demonstrating Sustained Ventricular Tachycardia

ource: Courtesy of Daniel Clark, M.D., Director of Medicine and Cardiology, Ventura County Medical Center, Ventura, California.

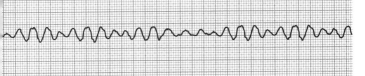

IGURE A1.3.   Rhythm Strip Demonstrating Coarse Ventricular Fibrillation

ource: Courtesy of Daniel Clark, M.D., Director of Medicine and Cardiology, Ventura County Medical Center, Ventura, California.

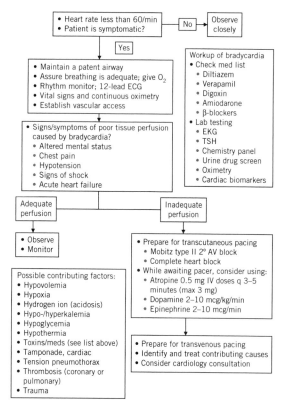

FIGURE A1.4. Bradycardia Algorithm

Source: Adapted from 2010 American Heart Association Guidelines for Cardiopulmonary Resuscitation and Emergency Cardiovascular Care. *Circulation.* 2010; 122(18 Suppl 3): S729–67.

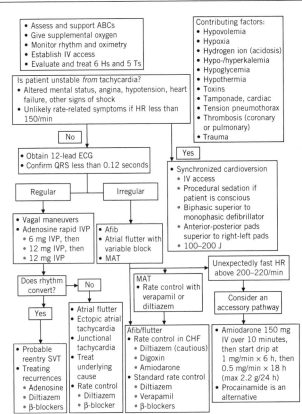

FIGURE A1.5. Narrow-Complex Tachycardia with a Pulse

Source: Adapted from 2010 American Heart Association Guidelines for Cardiopulmonary Resuscitation and Emergency Cardiovascular Care. Circulation. 2010; 122(18 Suppl 3): S729–67.

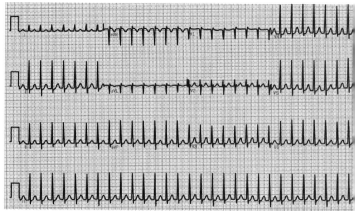

FIGURE A1.6.   ECG Demonstrating Supraventricular Tachycardia (SVT)

Source: Courtesy of Daniel Clark, M.D., Director of Medicine and Cardiology, Ventura County Medical Center, Ventura, California.

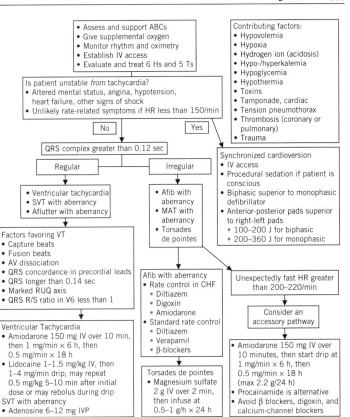

- Assess and support ABCs
- Give supplemental oxygen
- Monitor rhythm and oximetry
- Establish IV access
- Evaluate and treat 6 Hs and 5 Ts

Contributing factors:
- Hypovolemia
- Hypoxia
- Hydrogen ion (acidosis)
- Hypo-/hyperkalemia
- Hypoglycemia
- Hypothermia
- Toxins
- Tamponade, cardiac
- Tension pneumothorax
- Thrombosis (coronary or pulmonary)
- Trauma

Is patient unstable *from* tachycardia?
- Altered mental status, angina, hypotension, heart failure, other signs of shock
- Unlikely rate-related symptoms if HR less than 150/min

No   Yes

QRS complex greater than 0.12 sec

Regular   Irregular

- Ventricular tachycardia
- SVT with aberrancy
- Aflutter with aberrancy

- Afib with aberrancy
- MAT with aberrancy
- Torsades de pointes

Synchronized cardioversion
- IV access
- Procedural sedation if patient is conscious
- Biphasic superior to monophasic defibrillator
- Anterior-posterior pads superior to right-left pads
  - 100–200 J for biphasic
  - 200–360 J for monophasic

Factors favoring VT
- Capture beats
- Fusion beats
- AV dissociation
- QRS concordance in precordial leads
- QRS longer than 0.14 sec
- Marked RUQ axis
- QRS R/S ratio in V6 less than 1

Afib with aberrancy
- Rate control in CHF
  - Diltiazem
  - Digoxin
  - Amiodarone
- Standard rate control
  - Diltiazem
  - Verapamil
  - β-blockers

Unexpectedly fast HR greater than 200–220/min

Consider an accessory pathway

Ventricular Tachycardia
- Amiodarone 150 mg IV over 10 min, then 1 mg/min × 6 h, then 0.5 mg/min × 18 h
- Lidocaine 1–1.5 mg/kg IV, then 1–4 mg/min drip; may repeat 0.5 mg/kg 5–10 min after initial dose or may rebolus during drip
SVT with aberrancy
- Adenosine 6–12 mg IVP

Torsades de pointes
- Magnesium sulfate 2 g IV over 2 min, then infuse at 0.5–1 g/h × 24 h

- Amiodarone 150 mg IV over 10 minutes, then start drip at 1 mg/min × 6 h, then 0.5 mg/min × 18 h (max 2.2 g/24 h)
- Procainamide is alternative
- Avoid β blockers, digoxin, and calcium-channel blockers

FIGURE A1.7. Wide-Complex Tachycardia with a Pulse

Source: Adapted from 2010 American Heart Association Guidelines for Cardiopulmonary Resuscitation and Emergency Cardiovascular Care. Circulation. 2010; 122(18 Suppl 3): S729–67.

APPENDIX A2

FORMAT FOR ADMISSION ORDERS

- Admit: to where? ICU, other monitored unit, floor status
- Diagnosis (just one needed for order set)
- Condition: good, fair, serious, guarded, or critical (stable implies not getting worse but does not adequate describe current condition)
- Code status: DNR/DNI, comfort measures, or full code
- Allergies/intolerances: including reaction type
- Vitals: how often?
- Activity: bed rest, bathroom privileges, ad lib; weight-bearing status, fall, or seizure precautions
- Nursing: parameters that you want to be called about (e.g., vital sign abnormalities); care for wound dressings, tubes, and lines; fluid restrictions; daily weights; ins and outs; calorie counts; and other nursing care go here
- Diet: NPO, clears, diabetic, renal, cardiac, low sodium, low fat, calorie restricted, nutritional supplement (e.g., Ensure)
- IV: IV fluid type and rate
- In-hospital services: PT, social services, chaplain, some other consults
- Medication: all medicines—review home medication list for reconciliation, all medications for the acute condition, and prn orders such as pain, fever, nausea. Remember all medications need the route, timing, and dose. All as-needed meds need an indication. Two routes may be written (PO and IV for example) but need the preferred route (e.g., "may give PO if no IV access" or "give IV if patient unable to take PO"). Some hold orders are standard, but be sure you know if you need to write, "hold f somnolence," if scheduled narcotics, benzodiazepines, or H1 blockers; hold parameters for meds that lower heart rate and blood pressure, especially on scheduled medications
- Labs: kook over your diagnoses, interventions, and decide what labs add to your clinical information; you want information reflecting pretreatment values, such as ESR, reticulocyte counts, iron studies, o BNP, be sure to add these to the initial blood draw while it is still possible
- Special studies: radiology, stress testing, nuclear medicine, etc.

FORMAT FOR HISTORY AND PHYSICAL EXAM

- CC/ID: age, main complaint
- HPI: describe patient's baseline level of function in reference to the acute condition
- Medications and allergies
- Past medical problems: should be comprehensive; top of the list should include most relevant problems (often also the most recent or most active)
- Past surgical history
- OB/GYN history
- Immunizations
- Substance abuse history (current and remote history)
- Social history
- Family history
- Review of systems; relevant should be in HPI
- Physical exam: do not forget your vital signs
- Labs and studies
- ER course if significant changes, including procedures
- Assessment and plan—by problems (by systems if in ICU): If a final diagnosis has not been reached, keep the problems generalized by complaints and discuss your differential and the workup as well as the plan and treatment goals. Examples: fever, chest pain, or altered mental status. Altered mental status and other problems can also be multifactorial. If this is the case, then list separately the known causes and if needed, include a separate altered mental status problem. Example: 1) hypothyroidism, 2) alcohol intoxication, and 3) head trauma. Include a timeframe and parameters for further workup if mental status does not return to baseline as expected. In your HPI should be the patient's baseline as best you can determine, and include reference to that here. Additional categories should include disposition and criteria for disposition and prophylaxis.

APPENDIX A4

FORMAT FOR SOAP PROGRESS NOTE

S—Subjective: interval history, overnight events, current status from patient and nursing reports

O—Objective: vital signs, including ins and outs, ACCU-CHEK for diabetics, drains or tubes present and for how long, number of bowel movements (if relevant); physical exam for the day—again relevance is key; labs and studies, including any from the day before, and updated cultures

A/P—Assessment/Plan: brief summary statement followed by (relevant) problem list, how the patient is doing in this regard, what you are doing, and what you plan to do about it. Your problem list evolve throughout the hospitalization. A separate medication list can be helpful in medically complex patients and should be reviewed daily as part of the assessment and plan.

FORMAT FOR TRANSFER SUMMARY

- Date of admission
- Date of transfer
- Attending physician
- Resident physician/medical student
- Admission diagnoses
- Diagnoses at time of transfer
- Consultants and their specialty
- Procedures (include transfusions), date, and by whom
- Brief summary of HPI—approximately 2–3 sentences
- Hospital course by diagnoses: brief assessment and plan for each diagnosis, including current and recommended future plan especially if discussed with patient, continuity-care doctors, or consultants' recommendations

APPENDIX A6

FORMAT FOR DISCHARGE SUMMARY

Same as for transfer summary, except additionally at the end, include:

- Discharge condition: clinically, the next time a patient sees a physician who reads your note, what relevant info may help—ambulatory status, mental status, extent of cellulitis, how short of breath are they? Some of this may be in the hospital course, but quick reference of most clinically relevant info can be here.
- Discharge to? home, SNF, home nursing
- Discharge medications: may want to highlight changes, new meds, discontinued meds, changed doses, and specify how many days in a course (e.g., levofloxacin 750 mg PO daily × 3 days to complete a 5-day course)
- Follow-up appointments
- Follow-up needs/instructions for primary MD: summarize important follow-up. Include if labs or imaging have been ordered for the interim. Imagine yourself in a clinic seeing this patient after their hospitalization—what would you want to know in a time-crunch without reading your entire, fascinating hospital story?

APPENDIX A7

PROCEDURE NOTE TEMPLATES

LL procedure notes should include:
- Procedure (include which side)
- Preprocedure diagnosis
- Postprocedure diagnosis (usually the same)
- Operator(s)
- Anesthesia (lidocaine 1% with or without epinephrine 5 mL)
- Findings
- Specimens
- Details of procedure
- EBL
- Complications

Radial Arterial Line Insertion Procedure Note

INDICATION: _____

PROCEDURE OPERATOR: _____

ATTENDING PHYSICIAN: _____ IN ATTENDANCE (Y/N): _____

CONSENT:

    Consent was obtained from _____ prior to the procedure.
    Indications, risks, and benefits were explained at length.

    The procedure was performed emergently and the permission was implied because of the emergent
    nature.

PROCEDURE SUMMARY:

A timeout was performed. My hands were washed immediately prior to the procedure. I wore a surgical cap, mask with protective eyewear, sterile gown, and sterile gloves throughout the procedure. After an Allen test was performed to ensure adequate perfusion, the LEFT/RIGHT wrist was prepped using chlorhexidine scrub and draped in sterile fashion using a 3/4-sheet drape and sterile towels. The radial pulse was identified and the wrist was positioned in the usual fashion. Anesthesia was achieved using 1% lidocaine. Using the Arrow Radial Arterial Line Kit, a needle was inserted into the radial artery. Arterial blood was seen to pulsate in the flash chamber. The internal guidewire was advanced easily into the radial artery. The catheter was then advanced over the wire and the needle and wire were withdrawn. The catheter was sutured in place. A sterile OpSite was placed over the catheter at the insertion site. The patient tolerated the procedure without any hemodynamic compromise. At the time of procedure completion, the catheter was connected to the cardiac monitor and calibrated. Appropriate waveform and blood pressure tracing was observed.

COMMENT:

ESTIMATED BLOOD LOSS: _____ mL

FIGURE A7.1.   Radial Arterial Line Insertion Procedure Note

Subclavian Central Venous Catheter Insertion Procedure Note

INDICATION: _____

PROCEDURE OPERATOR: _____

ATTENDING PHYSICIAN: _____ **IN ATTENDANCE (Y/N):** _____

CONSENT:

Consent was obtained from _____ prior to the procedure.
Indications, risks, and benefits were explained at length.

The procedure was performed emergently and the permission was implied because of the emergent nature.

PROCEDURE SUMMARY:
The CDC Central Line Insertion Practices form was completed by the nurse prior to starting the procedure. A timeout was performed. My hands were washed immediately prior to the procedure. I wore a surgical cap, mask with protective eyewear, sterile gown, and sterile gloves throughout the procedure. The patient was placed in Trendelenburg position. LEFT/RIGHT chest region was prepped using chlorhexidine scrub and draped in sterile fashion using a three-quarter sheet drape and sterile towels. Anesthesia was achieved with 1% lidocaine. The introducer needle was inserted approximately 2 cm lateral to and 1 cm inferior to the normal curvature of the patient's clavicle. Venous blood was withdrawn. The syringe was removed and a guidewire was advanced into the introducer needle. A small incision was made at the skin surface with a scalpel and the introducer needle was exchanged for a dilator over the guidewire. After appropriate dilation was obtained, the dilator was exchanged over the wire for a _____ central venous catheter. The wire was removed and the catheter was sutured in place at _____ cm. A sterile SorbaView shield was placed over the catheter at the insertion site. The patient tolerated the procedure without any hemodynamic compromise. At time of procedure completion, all ports aspirated and flushed properly. Post-procedure chest X-ray is pending at this time.

COMMENT:

ESTIMATED BLOOD LOSS: _____ mL

FIGURE A7.2. Subclavian Central Venous Catheter Insertion Procedure Note

Internal Jugular Central Venous Catheter Insertion Procedure Note: Ultrasound-Guided

INDICATION: _____

PROCEDURE OPERATOR: _____

ATTENDING PHYSICIAN: _____ IN ATTENDANCE (Y/N): _____

CONSENT:

Consent was obtained from _____ prior to the procedure. Indications, risks, and benefits were explained at length.

The procedure was performed emergently and the permission was implied because of the emergent nature.

PROCEDURE SUMMARY:

The CDC Central Line Insertion Practices form was completed by the nurse prior to starting the procedure. A timeout was performed. My hands were washed immediately prior to the procedure. I wore a surgical cap, mask with protective eyewear, full gown, and sterile gloves throughout the procedure. The patient was placed in the Trendelenburg position. LEFT/RIGHT chest region was prepped using chlorhexidine scrub and draped in sterile fashion using a 3/4-sheet drape and sterile towels. The medial and lateral heads of the sternocleidomastoid muscle were identified, as was the carotid pulse. The internal jugular vein was identified using the ultrasound. Anesthesia was achieved over the vein using 1% lidocaine. Using real-time out of plane guidance, the introducer needle was inserted into the internal jugular vein under direct ultrasound visualization. Venous blood was withdrawn. The syringe was removed and a guidewire was advanced into the introducer needle. The guidewire was visualized in the internal jugular vein by ultrasound. A small incision was made at the skin surface with a scalpel and the introducer needle was exchanged for a dilator over the guidewire. After appropriate dilation was obtained, the dilator was exchanged over the wire for a _____ central venous catheter. The wire was removed and the catheter was sutured in place at _____ cm. A sterile SorbaView shield was placed over the catheter at the insertion site. The patient tolerated the procedure without any hemodynamic compromise. At time of procedure completion, all ports were aspirated and flushed properly. Postprocedure chest X-ray is pending at this time.

COMMENT:

ESTIMATED BLOOD LOSS: _____ mL

FIGURE A7.3.   Internal Jugular Central Venous Catheter Insertion Procedure Note: Ultrasound-Guided

Femoral Venous Catheter Insertion Procedure Note

INDICATION: _____

PROCEDURE OPERATOR: _____

ATTENDING PHYSICIAN: _____ IN ATTENDANCE (Y/N): _____

CONSENT:

Consent was obtained from _____ prior to the procedure. Indications, risks, and benefits were explained at length.

The procedure was performed emergently and the permission was implied because of the emergent nature.

PROCEDURE SUMMARY:

The CDC Central Line Insertion Practices form was completed by the nurse prior to starting the procedure. A timeout was performed. My hands were washed immediately prior to the procedure. I wore a surgical cap, mask with protective eyewear, sterile gown, and sterile gloves throughout the procedure. The LEFT/RIGHT inguinal region was prepped using chlorhexidine scrub and draped in sterile fashion using a 3/4-sheet drape and sterile towels. The femoral pulse was identified. Anesthesia was achieved using 1% lidocaine. Palpating the femoral pulse throughout the procedure, the introducer needle was inserted medial to the femoral artery, inferior to the inguinal crease and into the femoral vein. Venous blood was withdrawn. The syringe was removed and a guidewire was advanced into the introducer needle. A small incision was made at the skin surface with a scalpel and the introducer needle was exchanged for a dilator over the guidewire. After appropriate dilation was obtained, the dilator was exchanged over the wire for a _____ central venous catheter. The wire was removed and the catheter was sutured in place at _____ cm. A sterile SorbaView shield was placed over the catheter at the insertion site. The patient tolerated the procedure without any hemodynamic compromise. At time of procedure completion, all ports were aspirated and flushed properly.

COMMENT:

ESTIMATED BLOOD LOSS: _____ ml

FIGURE A7.4. Femoral Venous Catheter Insertion Procedure Note

Thoracentesis Procedure Note

INDICATION: ____________________

PROCEDURE OPERATOR: ____________________

ATTENDING PHYSICIAN: ____________________ **IN ATTENDANCE (Y/N):** __________

CONSENT:

Consent was obtained from ____________________ prior to the procedure. Indications, risks, and benefits were explained at length.

The procedure was performed emergently and the permission was implied because of the emergent nature.

PROCEDURE SUMMARY:

A timeout was performed and the chest X-ray was reviewed, the appropriate side was confirmed and marked. My hands were washed immediately prior to the procedure. I wore a surgical cap, mask with protective eyewear, sterile gown, and sterile gloves throughout the procedure. The patient was prepped and draped in a sterile manner using chlorhexidine scrub after the appropriate level was determined by percussion and confirmed by ultrasound. 1% lidocaine was used to anesthesize the skin, subcutaneous tissue, superior aspect of the rib periosteum, and parietal pleura. A finder needle was then introduced over the superior aspect of the rib to locate the pleural fluid; ____________________-colored fluid was aspirated at a depth of approximately __________ cm. A 10-blade scalpel was used to nick the skin at the insertion site. The Safe-T-Centesis needle was then introduced through the skin incision into the pleural space using negative aspiration pressure and the red colometric indicator to confirm appropriate positioning of the needle. The thoracentesis catheter was then threaded without difficulty. __________ mL of ____________________-colored fluid was removed without difficulty. The catheter was then removed. No immediate complications were noted during the procedure. A postprocedure chest X-ray is pending at the time of this note. The fluid will be sent for studies.

COMMENT:

ESTIMATED BLOOD LOSS: __________ mL

FIGURE A7.5. Thoracentesis Procedure Note

Paracentesis Procedure Note

INDICATION: _____

PROCEDURE OPERATOR: _____

ATTENDING PHYSICIAN: _____ IN ATTENDANCE (Y/N): _____

CONSENT:

Consent was obtained from _____ prior to the procedure. Indications, risks, and benefits were explained at length.

The procedure was performed emergently and the permission was implied because of the emergent nature.

PROCEDURE SUMMARY:

A timeout was performed. My hands were washed immediately prior to the procedure. I wore a surgical cap, mask with protective eyewear, sterile gown, and sterile gloves throughout the procedure. The area was cleansed and draped in usual sterile fashion using chlorhexidine scrub. Anesthesia was achieved with 1% lidocaine. The _____ of the abdomen was prepped and draped in a sterile fashion using chlorhexidine scrub. 1% lidocaine was used to numb the skin, soft tissue, and peritoneum. The paracentesis catheter was inserted and advanced with negative pressure until _____ -colored fluid was aspirated. Approximately 60 mL of ascitic fluid was collected and sent for laboratory analysis. The catheter was then connected to the Vacutainer and _____ liters of additional ascitic fluid were drained. The catheter was removed and no leaking was noted. A Band-Aid was placed over the puncture wound. The patient tolerated the procedure well without any immediate complications.

COMMENT:

ESTIMATED BLOOD LOSS: _____ mL

FIGURE A7.6. Paracentesis Procedure Note

Lumbar Puncture Procedure Note

INDICATION: _____

PROCEDURE OPERATOR: _____

ATTENDING PHYSICIAN: _____ IN ATTENDANCE (Y/N): _____

CONSENT:

Consent was obtained from _____ prior to the procedure. Indications, risks, and benefits were explained at length.

The procedure was performed emergently and the permission was implied because of the emergent nature.

PROCEDURE SUMMARY:

A timeout was performed. My hands were washed immediately prior to the procedure. I wore a surgical cap, mask with protective eyewear, sterile gown, and sterile gloves throughout the procedure. The patient was placed in the _____ position with help from the nursing staff. The area was cleansed and draped in usual sterile fashion using betadine scrub. Anesthesia was achieved with 1% lidocaine. A 20-gauge 3.5-inch spinal needle was placed in the _____ lumbar interspace. On the _____ attempt, _____ -colored cerebral spinal fluid was obtained. The opening pressure was _____ cm H_2O. CSF was collected into 4 tubes. These were sent for the usual tests, including 1 tube to be held for further analysis if needed. A sterile Band-Aid was placed over the puncture site. The patient had no immediate complications and tolerated the procedure well.

COMMENT:

ESTIMATED BLOOD LOSS: _____ mL

FIGURE A7.7.   Lumbar Puncture Procedure Note

Tube Thoracostomy Procedure Note

INDICATION: _____

PROCEDURE OPERATOR: _____

ATTENDING PHYSICIAN: _____ IN ATTENDANCE (Y/N): _____

CONSENT:

    Consent was obtained from _____ prior to the procedure. Indications, risks, and benefits were explained at length.

    The procedure was performed emergently and the permission was implied because of the emergent nature.

PROCEDURE SUMMARY:

A timeout was performed and after the chest X-ray was reviewed, the appropriate side was confirmed and marked. My hands were washed immediately prior to the procedure. I wore a surgical cap, mask with protective eyewear, sterile gown, and sterile gloves throughout the procedure. The patient was prepped and draped in a sterile manner using chlorhexidine scrub after the patient was positioned in the usual fashion. A total of _____ mL of 1% lidocaine was used to anesthetize the skin, subcutaneous tissue, superior aspect of the rib periosteum, and parietal pleura. A 2-cm incision was then made parallel to the rib in the midaxillary line at the level of the _____ rib. The subcutaneous tissue superficial and superior to the rib was dissected bluntly to the level of the pleura. The pleura was then entered bluntly. _____ was noted from the pleural space. The disruption in the parietal pleura was expanded bluntly and a finger was inserted and swept carefully in all directions. A _____ French chest tube was then inserted using my finger as a guide. The chest tube was directed _____ and inserted easily. The chest tube was sutured to the skin at the insertion site, and connected securely with tape to a Pleurovac. A sterile occlusive dressing was placed over the insertion site. No immediate complications were noted. A postprocedure chest X-ray is pending at the time of this note.

COMMENT:

ESTIMATED BLOOD LOSS: _____ mL

FIGURE A7.8.   Tube Thoracostomy Procedure Note

Endotracheal Intubation Procedure Note

INDICATION: _____

PROCEDURE OPERATOR: _____

ATTENDING PHYSICIAN: _____ IN ATTENDANCE (Y/N): _____

CONSENT:

Consent was obtained from _____ prior to the procedure. Indications, risks, and benefits were explained at length.

The procedure was performed emergently and the permission was implied because of the emergent nature.

PROCEDURE SUMMARY:

A timeout was performed. My hands were washed immediately prior to the procedure. I wore a surgical cap, mask with protective eyewear, sterile gown, and sterile gloves throughout the procedure. The patient was placed on a cardiac monitor including continuous pulse oximetry. Rapid sequence intubation was conducted. The patient received _____ mg of _____ for induction and _____ mg of _____ for adequate paralysis. Cricoid pressure was maintained from time induction agent was given to time of cuff balloon inflation. Using a _____ laryngoscope and a size _____ endotracheal tube with stylet, the patient was intubated on the _____ attempt. The stylet was removed and cuff balloon was inflated. Appropriate endotracheal tube position was confirmed by direct visualization of vocal cord passage, fogging of the tube, CO_2 colorimetric indicator, and symmetric breath sounds. The tube was secured at _____ cm at the lips. Postintubation chest X-ray is pending at this time.

COMMENT:

ESTIMATED BLOOD LOSS: _____ mL

FIGURE A7.9.   Endotracheal Intubation Procedure Note

Swan-Ganz Catheter Insertion

INDICATION: _____

PROCEDURE OPERATOR: _____

ATTENDING PHYSICIAN: _____ **IN ATTENDANCE (Y/N):** _____

CONSENT:

Consent was obtained from _____ prior to the procedure. Indications, risks, and benefits were explained at length.

The procedure was performed emergently and the permission was implied because of the emergent nature.

PROCEDURE SUMMARY:

A timeout was performed. My hands were washed immediately prior to the procedure. I wore a surgical cap, mask with protective eyewear, sterile gown, and sterile gloves throughout the procedure. The patient was placed in the Trendelenburg position. LEFT/RIGHT chest region was prepped using chlorhexidine scrub and draped in sterile fashion using a 3/4-sheet drape and sterile towels. The Swan-Ganz catheter was removed in sterile fashion from its package and the sheath was applied. All ports were flushed by the nurse, and the catheter was calibrated and connected to the monitor. The pressure transducer was moved and an appropriate artifact was noted on the monitor. The catheter was then inserted through the diaphragm of the introducer catheter in a sterile fashion. At 15 cm, the balloon was inflated and the catheter was floated through the right atrium and right ventricle into the pulmonary artery. Appropriate waveforms were seen on the monitor at each step. The catheter was advanced in the pulmonary artery until a wedge position pressure tracing was obtained. The balloon was then deflated and return of the pulmonary artery pressure tracing was confirmed. During the floating procedure the position of the catheter tip was confirmed by continuous pressure monitoring through the distal tip of the catheter. The catheter was locked to the introducer catheter at the insertion site with the tip of the catheter at a distance of _____ cm from the lock. A sterile dressing was applied. Postprocedure chest X-ray and hemodynamic values are pending at this time.

COMMENT:

ESTIMATED BLOOD LOSS: _____ mL

FIGURE A7.10.   Swan-Ganz Catheter Insertion

APPENDIX A8

ECG INTERPRETATION

- Rate, rhythm, axis, intervals (PR, QT), waves (P wave, QRS, ST segment, T waves)
- First: is the amplitude correct? The scale at the beginning of the ECG should be 10 boxes high.
- Normal width: small box = 0.04 seconds; large box = 0.20 seconds. Height: 1 small box = 1 mm.
- Low voltage: QRS is less than 5 mm in I, II, III, aVR, aVL, aVF, and less than 10mm in V1–V6
- See **Figure A8.1**

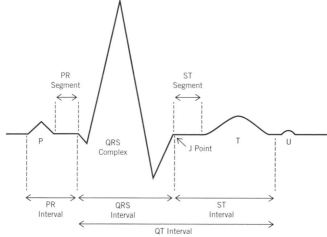

FIGURE A8.1.   ECG Interpretation Graph

1. <u>RATE</u>
   - Regular or irregular? How fast? Normal is 60 to 100. 1500 divided by the number of small boxes between each QRS. You can memorize the number of beats corresponding to each large box. See **Table A8.1**.

TABLE A8.1.   ECG Interpretation Table

Large boxes between QRS complexes	1	2	3	4	5	6
Rate (beats per minute)	300	150	100	75	60	50

   - For irregular rhythm, count the number of QRS complexes in 6 seconds of a rhythm strip and multiply by 10
   - Tachycardia is rate greater than 100, bradycardia is rate less than 60

2. **RHYTHM**

- Sinus: yes or no? Sinus rhythm has a P wave preceding every QRS, QRS for every P, P upright in I and II

3. **AXIS**

- Normal, left, or right? Look at the direction of the QRS complex in I, II, avF. Up in all 3 means normal
- Down in I, up in aVF: right axis deviation
- Up in I, down in aVF: leftward axis; look at lead II: upward in lead II makes it a normal left axis, downward in lead II makes it an abnormal left-axis deviation

4. **PR INTERVAL**

- Normal is 0.12–0.20 seconds (3–5 small boxes)
- Long PR interval is first-degree AV block
- Short PR interval is junctional (P wave inverted in II) or preexcitation (P wave upright in II: think of Wolff-Parkinson-White syndrome)

5. **QT INTERVAL (QT CORRECTED)**

- From beginning of the QRS to the end of the T wave; correct for heart rate; should be less than ½ of the R-R interval or less than 0.46 seconds

6. **P WAVE**

- Normal is up in leads I and II, sine wave configuration in lead V1
- Peaked in lead II or marked upward deflection in V1 indicates right atrial abnormality
- Notched or wide in lead II marked downward deflection in V1 indicates left atrial abnormality

7. **Q WAVES**

- Initial downward deflection in the QRS complex
- *ALWAYS* abnormal in V1 and V2
- Pathologic Q waves in any other leads are larger than 1 small box wide or more than ⅓ the height of the R wave in that lead

8. **QRS COMPLEX**

- Narrow or wide? Narrow is less than 3 small boxes
- R wave progression: QRS should be more upright than down by lead V4.
- See **Figures A8.2 and A8.3**

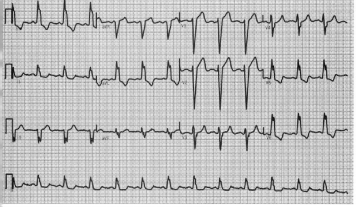

FIGURE A8.2.   ECG Demonstrating a Left Bundle Branch Block Pattern

Source: Courtesy of Daniel Clark, M.D., Director of Medicine and Cardiology, Ventura County Medical Center, Ventura, California.

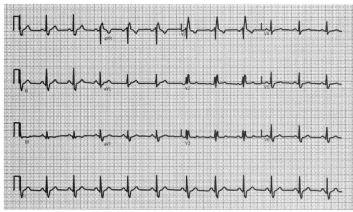

FIGURE A8.3.   ECG Demonstrating a Right Bundle Branch Block Pattern

Source: Courtesy of Daniel Clark, M.D., Director of Medicine and Cardiology, Ventura County Medical Center, Ventura, California.

9. ST SEGMENT

- Elevation (suggests myocardial injury) or depression (suggests ischemia) and is defined as at least 1 box above or below the PR segment isoelectric line

10. T WAVES

- Same direction as QRS (except V1, V2)
- Opposite direction is abnormal, which is consistent with ischemia, drug effect, or electrolyte disorder
- Tall and peaked suggests hyperkalemia or ischemia

11. ANATOMIC CORRELATION

- ST segment elevation, depression, and T wave changes in groups of leads indicate ischemia in certain coronary vessels.
- II, III, aVF: inferior wall (right coronary artery, or RCA)
- V1, V2: septum (left anterior descending, or LAD)
- V3, V4: anterior (left anterior descending, or LAD)
- I, aVL, V5, V6: lateral wall (circumflex)

REFERENCES

Dr. Daniel Clark's *Family Practice Cardiology: Core Curriculum Study Guide,* 19th ed.

Dr. Gary Martin and Eric Feigl's University of Washington School of Medicine HuBio 540 ECG Syllabus

APPENDIX A9

HOW TO READ A CHEST X-RAY

1. SYSTEM OF READING: TECHNIQUE, QUALITY, ANATOMY

Technique

- PA: standard chest X-ray view; the beam is directed from behind the person onto the cassette in front of them
- AP: commonly performed on patients not able to stand up for an X-ray; portable chest X-rays and trauma X-rays are usually A; the mediastinum appears wider on this view
- Lateral upright: looks at the lung tissue behind the heart, as well as the spine and hemidiaphragms
- Lateral decubitus: used to image pleural effusions and see if they move (layering) or are stuck (loculated)

Quality

- Should be at full inspiration; the diaphragm should be visible between the 8th and 10th ribs
- Penetration should be such that the bronchovascular structures can be seen through the heart and the thoracic spine disc spaces should be barely visible on an AP view (in the chest but disc spaces should not be visible in the abdomen on a well penetrated CXR)
- Look at the clavicles and make sure they are equidistant from the spinous processes of the thoracic vertebral bodies to ensure there is no rotation
- On a lateral view, the spine should appear darker at lower spinal levels

Anatomy

ABCDE Technique

- **A** Airway: trachea, bronchi, and lung fields; trachea midline or deviated, caliber, masses; lung fields: look for pneumothorax, consolidations, effusions, infiltrates
- **B** Bones and soft tissue: fractures, dislocations, lytic lesions, subcutaneous air, soft tissue swelling
- **C** Cardiac contours and mediastinum: the cardiac silhouette should be less than 1/2 the width of the entire chest (on AP film)
- **D** Diaphragms and costophrenic angles: symmetric elevation of the diaphragm, free air under the diaphragm, pleural effusion blunting the costophrenic angles
- **E** Examine technique
- **F** Foreign bodies, tubes, wires: look for placement of endotracheal tubes (should be above the carina), nasogastric tubes (should go past the diaphragm), external leads

Outside to Inside Technique

- External leads and wires
- Soft tissue
- Bones
- Lungs and diaphragms
- Trachea
- Mediastinum

2. NOT TO BE MISSED

- Free air below the diaphragm suggests bowel perforation or recent abdominal surgery
- Widened mediastinum suggests aortic aneurysm or dissection
- Mediastinal air suggests esophageal rupture
- Mediastinal shift supports tension pneumothorax (contralateral shift) or mucous plugging (ipsilateral shift)
- Air in the pleural space suggests pneumothorax

3. SIGNS AND WHAT THEY MEAN

- Silhouette sign: loss of the difference in light and dark at borders indicating a change in the composition of tissue adjacent to each other; that is, a right middle lobe pneumonia will obscure the right heart border because it rests against it, and a pneumonia changes the normally dark lung to lighter white like the heart
- Kerley B lines: thin horizontal linear densities of the periphery of the lung fields caused by edema, indicating volume overload (often from congestive heart failure)
- Air bronchogram: a tubular outline of an airway made visible by filling the surrounding alveoli by fluid or inflammatory exudate
- Double-bubble sign: air in the stomach and the duodenum with constriction in between; looks like 2 bubbles or a lopsided bowtie in the left upper quadrant; indicates duodenal atresia
- See **Figure A9.1**

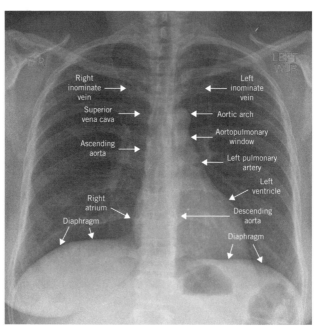

FIGURE A9.1. X-ray of chest

APPENDIX A10

HOW TO READ AN ABDOMINAL X-RAY

1. **INDICATIONS FOR AN ABDOMINAL X-RAY**
   - Abdominal distension, suspected bowel perforation, suspected bowel obstruction, suspected ingestion of foreign body, confirming placement of a feeding tube, ileus, constipation

2. **WHAT COMPRISES AN "ACUTE ABDOMEN X-RAY SERIES"**
   - Supine abdomen, upright abdomen, AP chest

3. **THINGS TO LOOK FOR**
   - Upright abdomen: look for an air-fluid level in the stomach (right side of the image, under the diaphragm) to confirm you are looking at an upright film
   - AP chest: best for seeing free air under the diaphragm indicating viscous rupture

4. **READING THE X-RAYS: *HAVE A SYSTEM***
   - One approach is to look at
     - Bones: integrity of the bones (ribs, spinal column, pelvis)
     - Stones: look for calcifications (kidney stones, aortic plaque, chronic pancreatitis deposits) or foreign bodies
     - Gas
       - Extraluminal: subdiaphragmatic (free air) between bowel loops, in the bowel wall (pneumatosis)
       - Intraluminal: dilation of bowel, thickness of wall, air-fluid levels, displacement of bowel loops
     - Normal caliber of intestines: small bowel is 3 cm, transverse colon is 6 cm, cecum is 9 cm
     - Small bowel: located in the center, circumferential lines across the entire bowel
     - Large bowel: located around the edges, haustra create a scalloped border
       - Mass: look at the normal organs (liver, spleen, bladder), and look for any abnormal masses

5. **ABDOMINAL X-RAY FINDINGS**
   - Free air under the diaphragm (generally the left side of the image; do not be confused by the gastric bubble on the right): indicates either recent surgery (laparoscopic), or perforated viscous
   - Dilated loops of bowel with air-fluid levels: often indicates ileus or small bowel obstruction

REFERENCES

Department of Radiology and Medical Imaging, University of Virginia Health System. Introduction to Radiology: An Online Interactive Tutorial. Available at: www.med-ed.virginia.edu/courses/rad.

Paauw DS, Burkholder LR, Migeon MB. *Internal Medicine Clerkship Guide*. 3rd ed. New York, NY: Mosby; 2007.

EMPIRIC ANTIBIOTICS FOR COMMON INFECTIONS IN IMMUNOCOMPETENT ADULTS

TABLE A11.1. Empiric Antibiotics for Common Infections in Immunocompetent Adults

Infection	First Choices	Alternatives	Duration
Bite, dog	• Amoxicillin-clavulanate • Ampicillin-sulbactam	• Ciprofloxacin plus clindamycin	10 days
Bite, cat	• Amoxicillin-clavulanate • Ampicillin-sulbactam	• Ciprofloxacin plus doxycycline	10 days
Bite, human	• Amoxicillin-clavulanate • Ampicillin-sulbactam	• Piperacillin-tazobactam • Ciprofloxacin plus clindamycin	10 days
Cellulitis, extremity (no MRSA risk factors*)	• Cefazolin	• Nafcillin	10–14 days
Cellulitis, extremity (if MRSA risk factors*)	• Vancomycin	• Linezolid	10–14 days
Cellulitis, facial	• Vancomycin	• Linezolid	10 days
Cellulitis, orbital	• Nafcillin (or Vanco if MRSA RFs*) plus Ceftriaxone plus Metronidazole	• Vancomycin plus levofloxacin plus metronidazole	10–14 days
Erysipelas	• Nafcillin	• Cefazolin	10 days
Chancroid	• Ceftriaxone	• Azithromycin	1 day
Cholecystitis, acute	• Piperacillin-tazobactam • Carbapenem	• Ciprofloxacin plus metronidazole	Until 24 h postop
Cholangitis, acute	• Piperacillin-tazobactam • Carbapenem	• Ciprofloxacin plus metronidazole	7–10 days
Colitis, *Clostridiumdifficile*	• PO metronidazole	• PO vancomycin	10 days
Diabetic foot infection, mild	• Nafcillin	• Cefazolin	10–14 days
Diabetic foot infection, limb-threatening	• Vancomycin plus piperacillin-tazobactam • Vancomycin plus carbapenem	• Linezolid plus carbapenem • Vancomycin plus gentamicin plus metronidazole	10–14 days
Diabetic foot infection, life-threatening	• Vancomycin plus piperacillin-tazobactam • Vancomycin plus ciprofloxacin plus clindamycin	• Linezolid pluscarbapenem • Vancomycin plus gentamicin plus metronidazole	10–14 days
Diverticulitis, acute	• Ampicillin-sulbactam • Piperacillin-tazobactam	• Ciprofloxacin plus metronidazole	7–10 days
Endocarditis, native valve	• Nafcillin plus gentamicin†	• Nafcillin plus gentamicin† • Vancomycin plus gentamicin†	4–6 weeks

(Continued

TABLE A11.1. *(Continued)*

Infection	First Choices	Alternatives	Duration
Epididymo-orchitis	• Ceftriaxone plus doxycycline (less than 35) • Fluoroquinolone (more than 35)	• Ampicillin-sulbactam (more than 35)	10–14 days
Gastroenteritis, bacterial	• Ciprofloxacin	• Azithromycin	3–5 days
Gonorrhea urethritis	• Ceftriaxone	• Azithromycin	1 day
Gonorrhea, disseminated	• Ceftriaxone • Cefotaxime	• Spectinomycin	7 days
Herpes, genital	• Acyclovir	• Valacyclovir • Famciclovir	7–10 days
Leptospirosis	• Penicillin G	• Ceftriaxone	7 days
Liver abscess, pyogenic	• Ampicillin plus gentamicin plus metronidazole	• Metronidazole plus ceftriaxone or ampicillin-sulbactam or fluoroquinolone	7–10 days
Liver abscess, amebic	• Metronidazole	• Tinidazole plus paromomycin	10 days
Lyme disease	• Doxycycline	• Amoxicillin	14–21 days
Lyme disease involving heart/CNS	• Ceftriaxone	• Penicillin G	14–28 days
Lymphogranulomavenereum	• Doxycycline	• Erythromycin	21 days
Mastitis	• Nafcillin	• Vancomycin	10 days
Meningitis less than 1 month old	• Ampicillin plus cefotaxime	• Ampicillin plus gentamicin	7–21 days‡
Meningitis 1 month–50 years	• Ceftriaxone plus vancomycin plus dexamethasone	• Meropenem plus vancomycin plus dexamethasone	7–21 days‡
Meningitis more than 50 years or immunocompromised or alcoholism	• Ampicillin plus ceftriaxone plus vancomycin plus dexamethasone	• Meropenem plus vancomycin plus dexamethasone	7–21 days‡
Necrotizing fasciitis	• Penicillin G plus clindamycin plus piperacillin-tazobactam or carbapenem	• Vancomycin plus gentamicin plus clindamycin	10–14 days
Odontogenic infection	• Amoxicillin-clavulanate	• Penicillin G • Clindamycin	10 days
Osteomyelitis, vertebral	• Nafcillin	• Vancomycin	4–6 weeks
Otitis media	• Amoxicillin	• Fluoroquinolone	7 days
Pelvic inflammatory disease	• Clindamycin plus gentamicin then doxycycline	• Cefotetan or cefoxitin plus doxycycline	14 days
Pneumonia, community-acquired	• Ceftriaxone plus azithromycin	• Respiratory fluoroquinolone	5–8 days
Pneumonia, healthcare-associated or nosocomial	• Vancomycin plus respiratory fluoroquinolone plus antipseudomonal β-lactam	• Linezolid plus antipseudomonal β-lactam plus aminoglycoside	8 days

(Continued)

TABLE A11.1. *(Continued)*

Infection	First Choices	Alternatives	Duration
Pneumonia, aspiration	• Ampicillin-sulbactam	• Ceftriaxone plus clindamycin	7–10 days
Prostatitis, acute	• Ceftriaxone plus doxycycline (less than 35) • Fluoroquinolone (greater than 35)	• Ampicillin-sulbactam (older than 35 yo)	10–14 days
Pyelonephritis	• Ceftriaxone • Ampicillin plus Gentamicin	• Fluoroquinolone	14 days
Septic arthritis	• Cefazolin (no MRSA RFs*) • Vancomycin (MRSA RFs*)	• Nafcillin (no MRSA RFs*)	14–28 days
Sinusitis, acute	• Amoxicillin	• Fluoroquinolone	5–10 days
Spontaneous bacterial peritonitis	• Cefotaxime	• Ceftriaxone	7 days
Syphilis, latent	• Benzathine penicillin G weekly × 3	• Ceftriaxone × 10 days • Doxycycline × 28 days	10–28 days
Syphilis, primary or secondary	• Benzathine penicillin G × 1	• Doxycycline × 14 days	1–14 days
Neurosyphilis	• Penicillin G	• Ceftriaxone	10–14 days

* MRSA risk factors: IVDU, history of MRSA colonization, sickle cell anemia, residence in a long-term care facility
† Gentamicin at 1.5 mg/kg IV q 12 h × 2 weeks (maintain gentamicin peak 3–4 mcg/mL)
‡ 7 days for *N. meningitidis* and *H. influenzae*; 10 days for *S. pneumonia*; 21 days for *L. monocytogenes*

Source: Information from *The Sanford Guide to Antimicrobial Therapy*, 2nd Edition. NJ: 2012 Ed. Gilbert DN et al. Royalty Press. Sperryville; 2012, *CID*, 2007; 44: S27, *Amer J Resp Crit Care Med*, 2005; 171: 388, *CID*, 2011; 52: e103, *Clin Infect Dis CID*, 2005; 41: 1373, *CID*, 2011; 52: e18, *NEJM*, 2006; 354: 44, *Circulation*, 2005; 111: e394, *Lancet*, 2004; 364: 369, *Infect Dis Clin N Amer*, 2005; 19: 799, *NEJM*, 2008; 358: 2804, and *MMWR*, 2010; 59(RR-12): 1.

ANTIBIOTIC COVERAGE BY CLASS

TABLE A12.1.   Antimicrobial Coverage by Class

Penicillins (penicillin VK or penicillin G)	**Typical coverage**: *Streptococcus pneumoniae*; Groups A, B, C, G *Streptococcus*; *Streptococcus milleri*; *Enterococcus faecalis*; *Haemophilus ducreyi*; *Pasteurella multocida*; *Actinomyces*; non-*difficile Clostridia*; oral anaerobes; *Treponema pallidum* (syphilis) **+/– coverage**: *Listeria monocytogenes*; *Neisseria meningitidis*; *Streptococcus viridians*; *Enterococcus faecium*
Antistaphylococcal Penicillins (dicloxacillin, nafcillin, oxacillin, methicillin)	**Typical coverage**: *Streptococcus pneumoniae*; Groups A, B, C, G *Streptococcus*; *Streptococcus milleri*; methicillin-susceptible *Staphylococcus aureus*; *Staphylococcus epidermidis*; oral anaerobes **+/– coverage**: *Streptococcus viridians*
Aminopenicillins (ampicillin and amoxicillin)	**Typical coverage**: *Streptococcus pneumoniae*; Groups A, B, C, G *Streptococcus*; *Streptococcus milleri*; *Enterococcus faecalis*; *Enterococcus faecium*; *Listeria monocytogenes*; *Neisseria meningitidis*; *Pasteurella multocida*; *Proteus mirabilis*; *Actinomyces*; non-*difficile Clostridia*; oral anaerobes **+/– coverage**: *Streptococcus viridians*; *Haemophilus influenza*; *E. coli*; *Salmonella*; *Shigella*
Aminopenicillins + β-Lactamase Inhibitor (amoxicillin-clavulanate and ampicillin-sulbactam)	**Typical coverage**: *Streptococcus pneumoniae*; Groups A, B, C, G *Streptococcus*; *Streptococcus milleri*; *Enterococcus faecalis*; *Enterococcus faecium*; methicillin-susceptible *Staphylococcus aureus*; *Listeria monocytogenes*; *Neisseria meningitidis*; *Neisseria gonorrhea*; *Moraxella catarrhalis*; *Haemophilus influenza*; *Haemophilus ducreyi*; *Pasteurella multocida*; *E. coli*; *Klebsiella*; *Proteus*; *Providentia*; *Aeromonas*; *Salmonella*; *Shigella Actinomyces*; non-*difficile Clostridia*; oral anaerobes; *Bacteroides fragilis* **+/– coverage**: *Streptococcus viridians*; *Morganella*; *Acinetobacter*; *Yersinia*
Antipseudomonal Penicillins (ticarcillin-clavulanate and piperacillin-tazobactam)	**Typical coverage**: *Streptococcus pneumoniae*; Groups A, B, C, G *Streptococcus*; *Streptococcus milleri*; methicillin-susceptible *Staphylococcus aureus*; *Listeria monocytogenes*; *Neisseria meningitidis*; *Neisseria gonorrhea*; *Moraxella catarrhalis*; *Haemophilus influenza*; *Haemophilus ducreyi*; *Pasteurella multocida*; *E. coli*; *Klebsiella*; *Enterobacter*; *Morganella*; *Serratia*; *Citrobacter*; *Proteus*; *Providentia*; *Pseudomonas aeruginosa*; *Aeromonas*; *Salmonella*; *Shigella*; *Yersinia*; *Actinomyces*; non-*difficile Clostridia*; oral anaerobes; *Bacteroides fragilis* **+/– coverage**: *Streptococcus viridians*; *Staphylococcus epidermidis*; *Enterococcus faecalis*; *Enterococcus faecium*; *Acinetobacter*; *Xanthomonas maltophilia*
1st-Generation Cephalosporins (cefazolin)	**Typical coverage**: *Streptococcus pneumoniae*; Groups A, B, C, G *Streptococcus*; *Streptococcus viridians* methicillin-susceptible *Staphylococcus aureus*; *Neisseria gonorrhea*; *Moraxella catarrhalis*; *Haemophilus influenza*; *E. coli*; *Klebsiella*; *Proteus* **+/– coverage**: *Staphylococcus epidermidis*
2nd-Generation Cephalosporins (cefuroxime, cefoxitin, cefotetan)	**Typical coverage**: *Streptococcus pneumoniae*; Groups A, B, C, G *Streptococcus*; *Streptococcus viridians* methicillin-susceptible *Staphylococcus aureus*; *Haemophilus influenza*; *E. coli*; *Klebsiella*; *Proteus*; *Enterobacter*; *Morganella*; *Serratia*; *Citrobacter*; *Providentia*; *Aeromonas*; *Yersinia*; *Hemophilus ducreyi*; *Pasteurella multocida*; non-*difficile Clostridia*; oral anaerobes; *Bacteroides fragilis* (only cefoxitin and cefotetan cover *B. fragilis*) **+/– coverage**: *Staphylococcus epidermidis*; *Neisseria gonorrhea*; *Neisseria meningitidis*

(Continued)

TABLE A12.1. *(Continued)*

3Rd-Generation Cephalosporins Without Pseudomonal Coverage (ceftriaxone, cefotaxime, ceftizoxime)	**Typical coverage**: *Streptococcus pneumoniae*; Groups A, B, C, G *Streptococcus; Streptococcus viridans*; methicillin-susceptible *Staphylococcus aureus; Moraxella catarrhalis; Haemophilus influenza; Neisseria gonorrhea; Neisseria meningitidis; Haemophilus ducreyi; Pasteurella multocida; E. coli; Klebsiella; Enterobacter; Morganella; Serratia; Citrobacter; Proteus; Providentia; Aeromonas; Salmonella; Shigella; Yersinia; Actinomyces*; non-*difficile Clostridia*; oral anaerobes **+/– coverage**: *Staphylococcus epidermidis; Pseudomonas aeruginosa; Burkholderia cepacia*
3Rd-Generation Cephalosporins with Pseudomonal Coverage (ceftazidime)	**Typical coverage**: *Streptococcus pneumoniae*; Groups A, B, C, G *Streptococcus; Moraxella catarrhalis; Haemophilus influenza; Haemophilus ducreyi; Pasteurella multocida; E. coli; Klebsiella; Enterobacter; Morganella; Serratia; Citrobacter; Proteus; Providentia; Pseudomonas aeruginosa; Burkholderia cepacia; Aeromonas; Salmonella; Shigella*; non-*difficile Clostridia*; oral anaerobes **+/–coverage**: *Streptococcus viridians*; methicillin-susceptible *Staphylococcus aureus; Staphylococcus epidermidis; Neisseria gonorrhea; Neisseria meningitidis; Acinetobacter; Xanthomonas maltophilia; Yersinia*
4th-Generation Cephalosporins (cefepime)	**Typical coverage**: *Streptococcus pneumoniae*; Groups A, B, C, G *Streptococcus; Streptococcus viridians*; methicillin-susceptible *Staphylococcus aureus; Moraxella catarrhalis; Haemophilus influenza; Pasteurella multocida; Neisseria gonorrhea; Neisseria meningitidis; E. coli; Klebsiella; Enterobacter; Morganella; Serratia; Citrobacter; Proteus; Providentia; Pseudomonas aeruginosa; Aeromonas; Salmonella; Shigella; Yersinia*; oral anaerobes **+/– coverage**: *Staphylococcus epidermidis; Acinetobacter; Burkholderia cepacia*
5th-Generation Cephalosporins (ceftobiprole and ceftaroline)	**Typical coverage**: *Streptococcus pneumoniae*; Groups A, B, C, G *Streptococcus; Streptococcus viridians*; methicillin-susceptible *Staphylococcus aureus*; methicillin-resistant *Staphylococcus aureus; Staphylococcus epidermidis; Enterococcus faecalis; Moraxella catarrhalis; Haemophilus influenza; Neisseria gonorrhea; Neisseria meningitidis; E. coli; Klebsiella; Enterobacter; Morganella; Serratia; Citrobacter; Proteus; Providentia; Aeromonas; Salmonella; Shigella* **+/– coverage**: *Acinetobacter; Pseudomonas aeruginosa*
Carbapenems (imipenem, meropenem, doripenem)	**Typical coverage**: *Streptococcus pneumoniae*; Groups A, B, C, G *Streptococcus; Streptococcus viridians*; methicillin-susceptible *Staphylococcus aureus; Staphylococcus epidermidis; Listeria monocytogenes; Moraxella catarrhalis; Haemophilus influenza; Neisseria gonorrhea; Neisseria meningitidis; Pasteurella multocida; E. coli; Klebsiella; Enterobacter; Morganella; Serratia; Citrobacter; Proteus; Providentia; Pseudomonas aeruginosa; Aeromonas; Salmonella; Shigella; Yersinia; Actinomyces*; non-*difficile Clostridia*; oral anaerobes; *Bacteroides fragilis* **+/– coverage**: *Acinetobacter; Enterococcus faecalis; Burkholderia cepacia*
Aztreonam	**Typical coverage:** *Moraxella catarrhalis; Haemophilus influenza; Neisseria gonorrhea; Neisseria meningitidis; Pasteurella multocida; E. coli; Klebsiella; Enterobacter; Morganella; Serratia; Citrobacter; Proteus; Providentia; Pseudomonas aeruginosa; Aeromonas; Salmonella; Shigella; Yersinia*
Respiratory Fluoroquinolones (levofloxacin, gatifloxacin, gemifloxacin, moxifloxacin)	**Typical coverage**: *Streptococcus pneumoniae*; Groups A, B, C, G *Streptococcus; Streptococcus milleri; Streptococcus viridians; Staphylococcus epidermidis*; methicillin-susceptible *Staphylococcus aureus; Enterococcus faecalis; Listeria monocytogenes; Neisseria meningitidis; Neisseria gonorrhea; Moraxella catarrhalis; Haemophilus influenza; Legionella pneumophila; Chlamydia pneumonia; Mycoplasma; Pasteurella multocida; E. coli; Klebsiella; Enterobacter; Morganella; Serratia; Citrobacter; Proteus; Providentia; Aeromonas; Salmonella; Shigella; Yersinia*; non-*difficile Clostridia*; oral anaerobes **+/– coverage**: *Enterococcus faecium; Acinetobacter; Pseudomonas aeruginosa; Xanthomonas maltophilia; Actinomyces*

(Continued)

TABLE A12.1. *(Continued)*

Nonrespiratory Fluoroquinolones (ciprofloxacin, ofloxacin)	**Typical coverage**: *Staphylococcus epidermidis*; methicillin-susceptible *Staphylococcus aureus*; *Listeria monocytogenes*; *Neisseria meningitidis*; *Neisseria gonorrhea*; *Moraxella catarrhalis*; *Haemophilus influenza*; *Legionella pneumophila*; *Chlamydia pneumonia*; *Mycoplasma*; *Pasteurella multocida*; *E. coli*; *Klebsiella*; *Enterobacter*; *Morganella*; *Serratia*; *Citrobacter*; *Proteus*; *Providentia*; *Salmonella*; *Shigella*; *Aeromonas*; *Yersinia* **+/– coverage**: *Streptococcus pneumoniae*; Groups A, B, C, G *Streptococcus*; *Acinetobacter*; *Pseudomonas aeruginosa*; *Actinomyces*; non-*difficile Clostridia*; oral anaerobes
Aminoglycosides (gentamicin, tobramycin, amikacin)	**Typical coverage**: methicillin-susceptible *Staphylococcus aureus*; *Moraxella catarrhalis*; *Haemophilus influenza*; *Pasteurella multocida*; *E. coli*; *Klebsiella*; *Enterobacter*; *Serratia*; *Citrobacter*; *Proteus*; *Providentia*; *Pseudomonas aeruginosa*; *Salmonella*; *Shigella*; *Yersinia* **+/– coverage**: *Staphylococcus epidermidis*; *Vibrio*
Clindamycin	**Typical coverage**: *Streptococcus pneumoniae*; Groups A, B, C, G *Streptococcus*; methicillin-susceptible *Staphylococcus aureus*; methicillin-resistant *Staphylococcus aureus*; *Haemophilus ducreyi*; *Actinomyces*; oral anaerobes
Macrolides (erythromycin, azithromycin, clarithromycin)	**Typical coverage**: *Streptococcus pneumoniae*; *Listeria monocytogenes*; *Neisseria meningitidis*; *Moraxella catarrhalis*; *Haemophilus influenza*; *Legionella pneumophila*; *Chlamydia pneumonia*; *Mycoplasma*; *Haemophilus ducreyi*; mycobacterium avium complex; *Actinomyces*; *Treponema pallidum* (syphilis) **+/– coverage**: methicillin-susceptible *Staphylococcus aureus*; Groups A, B, C, G *Streptococcus*; *Neisseria gonorrhea*; non-*difficile Clostridia*; oral anaerobes
Tetracyclines (doxycycline, minocycline)	**Typical coverage**: *Streptococcus pneumoniae*; methicillin-resistant *Staphylococcus aureus*; *Listeria monocytogenes*; *Neisseria meningitidis*; *Moraxella catarrhalis*; *Haemophilus influenza*; *Legionella pneumophila*; *Chlamydia pneumonia*; *Mycoplasma*; *Haemophilus ducreyi*; *Aeromonas*; *Borrelia burgdorferi*; *Brucella*; *Vibrio*; *Rickettsia*; *Actinomyces*; non-*difficile Clostridia*; oral anaerobes **+/– coverage**: methicillin-susceptible *Staphylococcus aureus*; Groups A, B, C, G *Streptococcus*; *Neisseria gonorrhea*; *E. coli*; *Klebsiella*; *Salmonella*; *Shigella*; *Bacteroides fragilis*
Tigecycline	**Typical coverage**: *Streptococcus pneumoniae*; Groups A, B, C, G *Streptococcus*; *Streptococcus milleri*; *Streptococcus viridians*; *Staphylococcus epidermidis*; methicillin-susceptible *Staphylococcus aureus*; methicillin-resistant *Staphylococcus aureus*; *Enterococcus faecalis*; *Enterococcus faecium*; *Listeria monocytogenes*; *Neisseria gonorrhea*; *Moraxella catarrhalis*; *Haemophilus influenza*; *Legionella pneumophila*; *Chlamydia pneumonia*; *Mycoplasma*; *E. coli*; *Klebsiella*; *Enterobacter*; *Morganella*; *Serratia*; *Citrobacter*; *Providentia*; *Aeromonas*; *Salmonella*; *Shigella*; *Yersinia*; non-*difficile Clostridia*; oral anaerobes; *Bacteroides fragilis* **+/– coverage**: *Acinetobacter*; *Xanthomonas maltophilia*; *Proteus*
Vancomycin	**Typical coverage**: *Streptococcus pneumoniae*; Groups A, B, C, G *Streptococcus*; *Streptococcus viridians*; *Staphylococcus epidermidis*; methicillin-susceptible *Staphylococcus aureus*; methicillin-resistant *Staphylococcus aureus*; *Enterococcus faecalis*; *Listeria monocytogenes*; *Actinomyces*; *Clostridium difficile* (PO vancomycin) **+/– coverage**: *Enterococcus faecium*
Trimethoprim-Sulfamethoxazole	**Typical coverage**: *Streptococcus pneumoniae*; methicillin-susceptible *Staphylococcus aureus*; methicillin-resistant *Staphylococcus aureus*; *Listeria monocytogenes*; *Neisseria meningitidis*; *Moraxella catarrhalis*; *Legionella pneumophila*; *Aeromonas*; *Burkholderia cepacia*; *Xanthomonas maltophilia*; *Yersinia*; *Francisella tularensis*; *Brucella* **+/– coverage**: *Staphylococcus epidermidis*; *Neisseria gonorrhea*; *Haemophilus influenza*; *E. coli*; *Klebsiella*; *Salmonella*; *Shigella*; *Serratia*; *Acinetobacter*; *Haemophilus ducreyi*

(Continued)

TABLE A12.1. *(Continued)*

Nitrofurantoin	**Typical coverage**: *Streptococcus pneumoniae; methicillin-susceptible Staphylococcus aureus*; methicillin-resistant *Staphylococcus aureus; Enterococcus faecalis; Enterococcus faecium; Neisseria meningitidis; E. coli; Salmonella; Shigella* **+/− coverage:** *Enterobacter; Klebsiella*
Metronidazole	**Typical coverage:** non-*difficile Clostridia*; oral anaerobes; *Bacteroides fragilis; Clostridium difficile; Entamoeba histolytica*
Rifampin	**Typical coverage**: *Streptococcus pneumoniae*; Groups A, B, C, G *Streptococcus*; methicillin-susceptible *Staphylococcus aureus*; methicillin-resistant *Staphylococcus aureus; Staphylococcus epidermidis; Neisseria gonorrhea; Neisseria meningitidis; Moraxella catarrhalis; Haemophilus influenza; Listeria monocytogenes; Francisella tularensis; Brucella; Mycobacterium leprae; Mycobacterium tuberculosis* **+/− coverage:** *Enterococcus faecalis*
Linezolid	**Typical coverage**: *Streptococcus pneumoniae*; Groups A, B, C, G *Streptococcus*; methicillin-susceptible *Staphylococcus aureus*; methicillin-resistant *Staphylococcus aureus; Staphylococcus epidermidis; Enterococcus faecalis; Enterococcus faecium; Listeria monocytogenes*; non-*difficile Clostridia* **+/−coverage:** *Moraxella catarrhalis; Haemophilus influenza*
Daptomycin	**Typical coverage**: *Streptococcus pneumoniae*; Groups A, B, C, G *Streptococcus*; methicillin-susceptible *Staphylococcus aureus*; methicillin-resistant *Staphylococcus aureus; Staphylococcus epidermidis; Enterococcus faecalis; Enterococcus faecium* **+/− coverage:** *Listeria monocytogenes*

Typical coverage = more than 60% susceptibility; with or without coverage = 30–60% susceptibility

Note: This coverage is based on national statistics. Always refer to your institutional antibiogram for specifics about your institutional sensitivities for different pathogens.

Source: Adapted from the individual product inserts of each medication.

APPENDIX A13

GRAM-STAIN INTERPRETATION

TABLE A13.1. Gram Stain Interpretation

Gram-Positive Aerobic Cocci	*Staphylococcus, Streptococcus, Enterococcus*
Gram-Negative Aerobic Diplococci	*Moraxella catarrhalis, Neisseria gonorrhea, Neisseria meningitidis*
Gram-Negative Aerobic Coccobacilli	*Haemophilus ducreyi, Haemophilus influenzae*
Gram-Positive Bacilli	*Bacillus, Corynebacterium, Listeria, Nocardia, Erysipelothrix*
Gram-Negative Aerobic Bacilli	*Acinetobacter, Bartonella, Bordetella pertussis, Brucella, Burkholderia cepacia, Campylobacter, Francisella tularensis, Helicobacter pylori, Legionella pneumophila, Pseudomonas aeruginosa, Stenotrophomonas maltophilia, Vibrio, Yersinia*
Gram-Negative Facultatively Anaerobic Bacilli	*Aeromonas hydrophila, Eikenella corrodens, Pasteurella multocida, E. coli, Citrobacter, Shigella, Salmonella, Klebsiella, Enterobacter, Hafnia, Serratia, Proteus, Providencia*
Anaerobes	*Actinomyces, Bacteroides fragilis, Clostridium, Fusobacterium, Lactobacillus, Peptostreptococcus*

APPENDIX A14

COMMON TOXIDROMES AND OVERDOSES

1. <u>TOXIDROMES</u>

- Anticholinergic toxidrome: "red as a beet (flushed), dry as a bone (dry skin), hot as a hare (hyperthermia), blind as a bat (mydriasis), mad as a hatter (delirium), and full as a flask (urinary retention and ileus)"; and hypertension, tachycardia, myoclonus, or seizures
  - Causes: amantadine, tricyclics, antihistamines, antiparkinsonian meds, low-potency antipsychotics, antispasmodics, atropine, and jimson weed
  - Treatment: activated charcoal, supportive care, and physostigmine 1–2 mg slow IVP
- Benzodiazepine overdose: coma, respiratory depression, nystagmus, hypotonia, and decreased BP
  - Treatment: supportive care of cardiopulmonary system
- Cholinergic toxidrome: SLUDGE (salivation, lacrimation, urination, diarrhea, GI cramps, and emesis), bradycardia, bronchoconstriction, miosis, and rhinorrhea
  - Causes: carbamate and organophosphate insecticides and cholinesterase inhibitors
  - Treatment: atropine 2 mg IV; or pralidoxime 2 g IV over 30 min, then 1 g/h infusion
- Opioid overdose: coma, respiratory depression, miosis, pulmonary edema, decreased HR/BP
  - Treatment: naloxone 0.1 mg IV q 30 seconds cautiously titrated to effect; may need a naloxone infusion of approximately 0.4 mg/h for overdoses of long-acting opioids
- Sympathomimetic toxidrome: tachycardia, hypertension, fever, diaphoresis, mydriasis, hyperreflexia, psychosis, and potentially dysrhythmias or seizures
  - Causes: amphetamines, cocaine, ephedrine, pseudoephedrine, and theophylline
  - Treatment: supportive care, hydration, and benzodiazepines
- See **Table A14.1**

TABLE A14.1.   Antidotes for Specific Ingestions

Ingestion or Bite	Antidote
Acetaminophen	N-acetylcysteine
Anticholinergics	Physostigmine
Benzodiazepine	Flumazenil (avoid if chronic benzodiazepine use)
β-blockers	Atropine, glucagon, and calcium
Wound botulism	Botulism antitoxin
Calcium channel blockers	Atropine, glucagon, and calcium
Carbon monoxide	Supplemental O_2 (hyperbaric in severe cases)
Cholinesterase inhibitors	Atropine or pralidoxime
Cyanide	Amyl nitrite, sodium nitrite, sodium thiosulfatec, and/or hydroxocobalamin; plus 100% oxygen
Digitalis	Digoxin immune Fab (Digibind)
Ethylene glycol	Ethanol or fomepizole; pyridoxine, thiamine
Heavy metals (arsenic, lead, mercury)	Dimercaprol, EDTA, or penicillamine (copper, lead, and mercury)
Heparin (or LMWH)	Protamine sulfate
Iron	Deferoxamine
Isoniazid	Pyridoxine
Methanol	Ethanol or fomepizole; folinic acid, folate
Methotrexate	Folinic acid
Methemoglobinemia	Methylene blue
Opioids	Naloxone
Organophosphates (and other insecticides)	Atropine or pralidoxime
Snakebites (crotalids)	Crotalidae polyvalent immune fab
Sulfonylureas	Octreotide, glucagons, and dextrose
Sympathomimetics	Benzodiazepines with or without phentolamine
Thallium	Prussian blue
Warfarin	Vitamin K with or without fresh frozen plasma (if bleeding)

Source: Adapted from *Chest* 2003; 123(2): 577–92.

2. <u>MANAGEMENT OF ACETAMINOPHEN TOXICITY FROM ACUTE INGESTIONS</u>

- Clinical presentation: Stage 1: asymptomatic; Stage 2: nausea, vomiting, anorexia, RUQ pain, jaundice; Stage 3: renal failure, bleeding, ARDS, encephalopathy, then coma
- Treatment: N-acetylcysteine (NAC) 140 mg/kg PO × 1, then 70 mg/kg PO q 4 h × 17 doses **OR** 150 mg/kg IV over 60 min, then 50 mg/kg IV over 4 h, then 100 mg/kg over 16 h if acetaminophen level within possible or probable hepatotoxicity range in nomogram
  - Abbreviated NAC course with 5 doses is acceptable when AST, ALT, and PTT are normal after the fifth dose
- See **Figure A14.1**

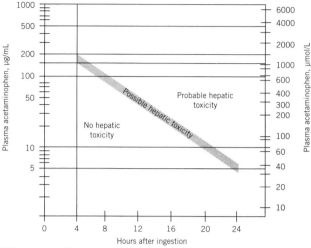

FIGURE A14.1.   Rumack-Matthew Nomogram for Acetaminophen Toxicity from Acute Ingestions

3. MANAGEMENT OF ALCOHOL INTOXICATIONS (ETHYLENE GLYCOL, METHANOL)

- Clinical presentation of alcohols: nausea, confusion, ataxia, slurred speech, sedation, and seizures; severe cases may develop ARDS or cardiac failure
- Ethylene glycol (EG) may cause renal failure, and methanol toxicity causes blindness
- Lab findings: anion-gap acidosis, osmolar gap; ethylene glycol also causes hypocalcemia and urinary calcium oxalate crystals
- Indications for fomepizole or ethanol: serum EG level greater than 20 mg/dL; ingested greater than 100 mL and osmolal gap greater than 10 mOsm/kg; or suspected ingestion and greater than or equal to 2 of following: pH less than 7.3, serum bicarbonate less than 20 MEq/L, osmolal gap greater than 10 mOsm/kg, or urinary oxalate crystals
- Hemodialysis if: worsening vitals, pH less than 7.25, refractory renal failure/electrolyte abnormal

4. MANAGEMENT OF CALCIUM CHANNEL BLOCKER TOXICITY

- Clinical presentation: altered mental status, fatigue, syncope, hypotension, and bradycardia
- Treatment: fluids and dopamine for hypotension with bradycardia; glucagon 10 mg IVP, then 10 mg/h for persistent hypotension; calcium chloride 1 g IVP over 10 min, may repeat × 3

5. MANAGEMENT OF SALICYLATE (ASA) TOXICITY

- Clinical presentation: nausea, vomiting leading to tinnitus, sweating, hyperpnea, delirium leading to lethargy, respiratory failure, and seizures leading to cardiac failure and cerebral edema
- Labs: anion-gap acidosis, respiratory alkalosis, hypokalemia, ASA greater than 20 mg/dL
- Treatment: urinary alkalinization and potassium repletion
- Hemodialysis if: refractory acidosis or hypotension, seizures, pulmonary edema, rhabdomyolysis, renal failure, ASA level greater than 100 mg/dL or if intubation is needed
- Avoid intubation and mechanical ventilation if possible: increases risk of death

6. MANAGEMENT OF TRICYCLIC ANTIDEPRESSANT TOXICITY

- Clinical presentation: anticholinergic toxidrome, sinus tachycardia, drowsiness leading to delirium, rigidity, prolonged PR/QRS/QT resulting in seizures, hypotension leading to VF/VT, coma, and respiratory depression
- Best predictor of seizures or ventricular arrhythmias is a QRS duration greater than 0.16 seconds
  - Drug levels do not correlate with the degree of cardiac or neurologic toxicity
- Treatment: sodium bicarbonate infusion to alkalinize serum to pH 7.45–7.5 for cardiovascular toxicity (indicated if wide QRS), isotonic fluids and norepinephrine for hypotension, lorazepam for seizures, intubation for respiratory failure, and treat arrhythmias with either lidocaine or pacing

REFERENCES

Clin Med, 2008;8(1):89–91; *Am Fam Physician,* 2002;66(5):807–12; *Med Letter,* 2006;4:61; *Emerg Med J,* 2001;18(4):236–41; *Emerg Med Clin North Am,* 2007;25(2):333–46; *Chest,* 2007;123(2):577–92; *Ann Emerg Med,* 2007;50(3):272–9.

APPENDIX A15

ELECTROLYTE REPLETION

1. **POTASSIUM REPLETION**
   - Goal K greater than or equal to 4 MEq/L in critically ill patients or those with cardiac disorders or weakness
   - Total body potassium deficit is approximately 200 mEq for every decrease of 1 mEq/L
   - Conditions/meds that cause potassium to move intracellularly
     - Alkalosis, insulin, β-agonists, and hypothermia
   - Conditions/meds that cause potassium to move extracellularly
     - Acidosis, crush injury, tumor lysis syndrome, and starvation

2. **CALCIUM REPLETION**
   - IV calcium indicated only for symptomatic hypocalcemia (seizures, tetany, ventricular arrhythmias, or hypotension)
   - Oral repletion can be with 2–4 g/day calcium carbonate or calcium gluconate tablets
   - Check for Vitamin D deficiency and treat accordingly if present

3. **MAGNESIUM REPLETION**
   - Causes of hypomagnesemia: loop diuretics, aminoglycosides, amphotericin, digitalis, cisplatin, cyclosporine, alcoholism, chronic diarrhea, uncontrolled diabetes mellitus
   - Goal Mag greater than or equal to 2 MEq/L in critically ill patients or those with cardiac disorders or weakness
   - Indications for treatment: severe hypomagnesemia or symptomatic hypomagnesemia
   - Treatment of mild hypomagnesemia
     - Give 1 mEq/kg magnesium PO on day 1 and then 0.5 mEq/kg magnesium PO on days 2–5
   - Treatment of moderate hypomagnesemia (Mag less than 1 mg/dL)
     - $MagSO_4$ 6 g IV over 3 hours and then 4 g IV daily over 4 hours until normal levels achieved
   - Treatment of life-threatening hypomagnesemia (associated seizures or arrhythmias)
   - $MagSO_4$ 2 g IV over 2 minutes and then 5 g IV q 12 h over 4 hours until level is normal

4. **PHOSPHORUS REPLETION**
   - Causes of hypophosphatemia: glucose loading and refeeding syndrome, alcoholism, sucralfate, Amphojel, uncontrolled diabetes mellitus, sepsis, and respiratory alkalosis
   - Treatment
     - IV replacement with 40 mEq KPhos or NaPhos if Phos less than 1 mg/dL or if cardiac dysfunction, respiratory failure, generalized weakness, or shock
     - Oral replacement with Neutra-Phos 1200–1500 mg daily for mild–moderate hypophosphatemia

APPENDIX A16

CORTICOSTEROID EQUIVALENCY CHART

TABLE A16.1. Coticosteroid Equivalency Chart

Steroid	Approximate equivalent dose (mg)	Relative anti-inflammatory effect	Relative mineralocorticoid effect	Half-life (h)
Betamethasone	0.6–0.75	20–30	0	36–54
Cortisone	25	0.8	2	8–12
Dexamethasone	0.75	20–30	0	36–54
Hydrocortisone	20	1	2	8–12
Methylprednisolone	4	5	0	18–36
Prednisolone	5	4	1	18–36
Prednisone	5	4	1	18–36
Triamcinolone	4	5	0	12–36

Source: Reproduced from Hamilton RJ, ed. *Tarascon Pocket Pharmacopoiea. Burlington, MA:* Jones & Bartlett Publishing; 2012.

ACUTE PAIN CONTROL

1. STEPWISE APPROACH TO MEDICATION MANAGEMENT OF ACUTE PAIN

- Mild pain: acetaminophen, NSAIDs, or salicylates (see **Table A17.1**)
- Moderate pain: add low-dose opioids often as combination pills (acetaminophen with hydrocodone or codeine), or tramadol (if no history of seizures); refer to **Table A17.2**
  - For mild–moderate pain, meds should be titrated to effect, then given on a scheduled basis
- Severe pain: parenteral opioids (see Table A17.2 and **Table A17.3**)
- For moderate–severe pain: give scheduled analgesics with as-needed meds for breakthrough pain
  - Use standardized pain scales and reassess pain with each vital sign check
  - Rescue dose is 10–15% of 24 hour daily dose q 2–4 h as needed
- Neuropathic pain is best managed by adjuvant medications listed in **Table A17.4**

TABLE A17.1. Nonopioid Analgesics

Medication	Usual Oral Adult Dose	Max Daily Adult Dose	Usual Oral Pediatric Dose
Acetaminophen	650 mg q 4–6 h	4000 mg*	10–15 mg/kg q 4–6 h
Salicylates[†]			
Aspirin	325–650 mg q 4–6 h	4000 mg	N/R for younger than 19 yo[‡]
Diflunisal	500 mg q 12 h	1500 mg	N/R
Salsalate	500 mg q 4 h	3000 mg	N/R
Trilisate	1000–1500 mg q 12 h	3000 mg	N/R
Nonsteroidal Anti-inflammatory Drugs (NSAIDs)[§]			
Diclofenac	50 mg q 8 h	150 mg	N/R
Flurbiprofen	50–100 mg bid–tid	300 mg	N/R
Ibuprofen	400–800 mg q 6–8 h	3200 mg	10 mg/kg q 6–8 h
Indomethacin	25–50 mg q 8 h	200 mg	0.3–1 mg/kg q 6–8 h
Ketoprofen	25–75 mg q 6–8 h	300 mg	N/R
Ketorolac[∥¶]	10 mg PO q 6–8 h 30 mg IV/IM q 6 h (younger than 65 yo) 15 mg IV/IM q 6 h (older than 65 yo)	120 mg (younger than 65 yo) 60 mg (older than 65 yo)	0.5 mg/kg PO/IV/IM q 6 h (max 100 mg/day)
Meclofenamate	50–100 mg q 4–6 h	400 mg	N/R
Mefenamic acid	250 mg q 6 h[∥]	1250 mg × 1, then 1 g/day; N/R for peds	
Nabumetone	500–1000 mg bid	2000 mg	N/R
Naproxen	250–500 mg bid	1000 mg	5–10 mg/kg q 12 h
Naproxen sodium	275–550 mg bid	1100 mg	5–10 mg/kg q 12 h
Oxaprozin	1200 mg daily	1800 mg	10–20 mg/kg daily

(Continued)

TABLE A17.1. (Continued)

Medication	Usual Oral Adult Dose	Max Daily Adult Dose	Usual Oral Pediatric Dose
Piroxicam	20 mg daily	20 mg	N/R
Sulindac	150–200 mg q 12 h	400 mg	N/R
Tolmetin	200–600 mg tid	1800 mg	N/R
Medications with Significant Cyclooxenase-2-Selective (COX-2) Inhibition#			
Celecoxib¶	100–200 mg bid	400 mg	N/R
Etodolac	200–400 mg q 6–8 h	1200 mg	N/R
Meloxicam	7.5 mg daily	15 mg	N/R

* Maximum dose of acetaminophen is 2 g/day if the patient is an alcoholic or is severely malnourished

† Salicylates as a class are associated with increased risk of gastritis or peptic ulcer disease, reversible inhibition of platelet aggregation (except aspirin is irreversible) and potential papillary necrosis of kidneys, and can exacerbate asthma

‡ Salicylate use during a viral illness in patient 18 yo or younger may cause Reye's syndrome

§ NSAIDs as a class are associated with increased risk of gastritis or peptic ulcer disease, reversible inhibition of platelet aggregation, and potential papillary necrosis of kidneys, and can cause fluid retention and elevated blood pressure, and ibuprofen can offset the antiplatelet action of aspirin

‖ Duration of use limited to 5 days; Ketorolac is the only NSAID available in a parenteral formulation

¶ Brand name medications only (not available as low-cost generics as is true of the others in this table)

These agents have the same GI toxicity as nonselective NSAIDs, have little effect on platelet aggregation, and can cause papillary necrosis of the kidneys; rofecoxib (Vioxx) and valdecoxib (Bextra) were withdrawn from the market for their association with an increased risk of MI and stroke

Source: Adapted from the Principles of Analgesic Use in the Treatment of Acute Pain and Cancer Pain, 5th Edition. American Pain Society, Glenview, IL: 2003 and *AFP*, 2005; 71:913–18.

TABLE A17.2. Fentanyl Transdermal Dose (Based on Ongoing Morphine Requirement)*†

Morphine (IV/IM)	Morphine (PO)	Transdermal Fentanyl
10–22 mg/day	60–134 mg/day	25 mcg/h
23–37 mg/day	135–224 mg/day	50 mcg/h
38–52 mg/day	225–314 mg/day	75 mcg/h
53–67 mg/day	315–404 mg/day	100 mcg/h

* For higher morphine doses see product insert for transdermal fentanyl equivalencies

† Anticipate a delay in 12–18 hours for full analgesic effect of transdermal fentanyl

Not for use in acute pain management, for opiate-naïve pts, or for pain that is not constant

Source: Adapted from Ortho-McNeil package insert at www.duragesic.com.

TABLE A17.3. Opioid Equivalency*

Opioid	PO	IV/SC/IM	Opioid	PO	IV/SC/IM
Buprenorphine	n/a	0.3–0.4 mg	Meperidine[†]	300 mg	75 mg
Butorphanol	n/a	2 mg	Methadone	5–15 mg	2.5–10 mg
Codeine	130 mg	75 mg	Morphine	30 mg	10 mg
Fentanyl	n/a	0.1 mg	Nalbuphine	n/a	10 mg
Hydrocodone	20 mg	n/a	Oxycodone	20 mg	n/a
Hydromorphone	7.5 mg	1.5 mg	Oxymorphone	10 mg	1 mg
Levorphanol	4 mg	2 mg	Pentazocine	50 mg	30 mg

* Approximate equianalgesic doses as adapted from the 2003 and 2005 American Pain Society (www.ampainsoc.org) guidelines and the 1992 AHCPR guidelines.

† Doses should be limited to less than 600 mg/24 h and total duration of use less than 48 h; meperidine should **not** be used for chronic pain management. Not available = "n/a". See drug entries themselves for starting doses. Recommend using 25% lower than equivalent doses when switching between opioids. IV doses should be titrated slowly with appropriate monitoring. All PO dosing is with **immediate-release** preparations. Individualize all dosing, especially in the elderly, children, and those who are opioid naïve, have chronic pain, or have hepatic/renal insufficiency.

Source: Adapted from Hamilton RJ, ed. *Tarascon Pocket Pharmacopoeia.* Burlington, MA: Jones & Bartlett Learning; 2012.

TABLE A17.4. Adjuvant Medications for Neuropathic Pain

Medication	Starting Oral Adult Dose	Titration/Usual Oral Daily Dose Range in mg	Numbers Needed to Treat (NNT₅₀)*
Antiepileptics			
Carbamazepine	100 mg bid	100 mg q 7 days/ 1000–1600[†]	2.6–3.3
Clonazepam[‡]	0.5 mg daily	0.5 mg q 3–5 days/5–20	–
Gabapentin[§]	100–300 mg at bedtime	300 mg q 7 days/ 1800–3600	3.2–4.1
Lamotrigine	25–50 mg daily	25 mg q 7 days/200–600	2.1
Phenytoin	100 mg at bedtime	100 mg q 7 days/300	–
Pregabalin[‖]	50 mg tid	150 mg q 7 days/300–600	–
Topiramate	25 mg daily	25 mg q 7 days/400–800	–
Tricyclic Antidepressants			
Amitriptyline	10 mg at bedtime	10 mg q 7 days/50–150[†]	1.3–3.0
Desipramine	25 mg at bedtime	25 mg q 7 days/75–200[†]	1.3–3.0
Doxepin	10 mg at bedtime	10 mg q 7 days/75–150	1.3–3.0
Nortriptyline	10 mg at bedtime	10 mg q 7 days/25–75[†]	1.3–3.0
Selective Serotonin Reuptake Inhibitors (SSRIs)[‡]			
Paroxetine	10 mg daily	10 mg q 7 days/20–60	6.7
Citalopram	10 mg daily	10 mg q 7 days/20–60	6.7

(Continued)

TABLE A17.4. *(Continued)*

Medication	Starting Oral Adult Dose	Titration/Usual Oral Daily Dose Range in mg	Numbers Needed to Treat (NNT$_{50}$)*
Other Antidepressants			
Duloxetine^ǁ	30 mg daily	30 mg q 14 days/30–120	–
Milnacipran^ǁ	12.5 mg daily	12.5–25 mg q 7 days/ 100–200	–
Venlafaxine	37.5 mg daily	37.5 mg q 7 days/150–300	–
Topical Anesthetic Creams			
Capsaicin	0.25% tid	Use up to 0.75% 5 times/day	5.3–5.9
5% Lidoderm^ǁ	1 patch bid	Use up to 3 patches bid	4.4
Miscellaneous analgesics			
Dextromethorphan	30 mg bid	30 mg q 7 days/60 mg q6 h	1.9‡
Tramadol	50 mg bid	50 mg q 7 days/200–400	3.1–3.4
Opioid analgesics (as extended-release or controlled-release formulations)			
Morphine SR	15 mg bid	15 mg q 7 days/60–360	–
Oxycodone SR^ǁ	10 mg bid	10 mg q 7 days/20–160	2.5
Methadone	2.5 mg bid	2.5 mg q 7 days until qid/10–80	–

* NNT$_{50}$ is the number needed to treat to decrease the neuropathic pain severity 50% or greater in 1 patient

† Titrate drug dosage to therapeutic effect; serum drug levels useful to guide dosing

‡ Data supporting the efficacy of SSRIs, benzodiazepines, and dextromethorphan for neuropathic or functional pain syndromes is sparse

§ Gabapentin plus sustained-release morphine is more effective than either agent alone (*NEJM*, 2005; 352(13): 1324–34)

ǁ Brand name medication only (not available as a low-cost generi c as is true of the other meds in this table)

Source: References: *NEJM*, 2003; 348: 1243. *NEJM*, 2003; 349: 1943. *Mayo Clin. Proc.*, 2004; 79: 1533, *Pain*, 2003; 106: 151. *Curr Opin Anaesth*, 2006; 19: 573. *Mayo Clin Proc*, 2006; 81: S3. *J Fam Prac*, 2007; 56: 3 and the pain management guidelines of the Institute for Clinical Systems Improvement at www.iscsi.org/pain_acute/pain_acute_assessment_and_management_of_3.html.

2. PATIENT-CONTROLLED ANALGESIA (PCA)

- Neither family nor staff may administer opioid doses to patient
- Administered doses: morphine 1–2 mg, hydromorphone 0.1–0.3 mg, fentanyl 10–20 mcg
  - If pain inadequately controlled after 1 h, increase dose 25–50% until pain controlled
- Lockout interval: typically 10 minutes
- Basal rate: none for opioid-naïve pts, use equianalgesic infusion for pts on chronic opiates
  - May increase basal rate up to 50% q 8 h if needed to optimize pain control

3. MANAGEMENT OF OPIOID SIDE EFFECTS

- Constipation: scheduled docusate and a stimulant agent (e.g., senna 2 tabs PO daily–bid)
- Sedation: tolerance develops in 48–72 h, may reduce dose and hold other sedatives
- Nausea/vomiting: dose reduction, change opioid, or trial of antiemetic (e.g., metoclopramide)
- Pruritus: dose reduction, change opioid, or antihistamine (e.g., diphenhydramine)
- Hallucinations/confusion: dose reduction, change opioid, or trial of haloperidol or risperidone
- Respiratory depression: hold opioid, naloxone 0.1 mg IV q 30–60 seconds titrated to effect

4. ADJUVANT TREATMENTS FOR INFLAMMATORY PAIN SYNDROMES

- Epidural steroid injections for cervical or lumbar radiculopathy
- Pain from bone metastases: radiation therapy with or without dexamethasone 4–8 mg PO q 8–12 h
- Acute vertebral compression fractures: calcitonin and use of a TLSO brace
- Muscle spasticity: start baclofen 5–10 mg PO tid–qid (titrate to max of 120 mg/day)

5. EPIDURAL ANALGESIA

- Consider for postoperative analgesia after major abdominal, thoracic, orthopedic, or gynecologic operations
- Avoid all antithrombotics for 24 hours **prior to discontinuation** of epidural catheter
- Wait times before restarting antithrombotics **after discontinuation** of epidural catheter
  - 2 hours for unfractionated heparin
  - 6 hours for LMWH, antiplatelets, direct thrombin inhibitors, or warfarin
  - 6–12 hours for fondaparinux
  - 24–48 hours for GP IIb/IIIa inhibitors
  - 10 days for thrombolytics

REFERENCES

Mayo Clin Proc, 2004;79(12):1533–45; *N Engl J Med*, 2003;348(13):1243–55; *N Engl J Med*, 2003;349(20):1943–53; *Ann Intern Med*, 2004;140(6):441–51; *Cancer J*, 2006;12(5):330–40; *J Palliat Med*, 2006;9(6):1414–34; *J Am Coll Surg*, 2006;202(1):169–75; *Reg Anesth Pain Med*, 2010;35(1):64–101; *Eur J Anaesthesiol*, 2010;27(12):999–1015.
Institute for Clinical Systems Improvement 2004 guidelines at www.iscsi.org/pain_acute/pain_acute_assessment_and_management_of_3.html.

HOW TO WRITE AN ORDER AND A PRESCRIPTION

- Verify that all order forms have the patient's name and birth date or medical record number
- The basics elements of a prescription include the drug, route of administration, dosing interval, and duration of therapy
- Sign, date, and time all orders
- Avoid **trailing** zeros (e.g., use 1 instead of 1.0)
- Use **leading** zeros (e.g., use 0.1 instead of .1)
- Avoid banned abbreviations: cc, D/C, Mg, MgSO$_4$, MSO$_4$, OD, TIW, QD, QOD, qhs, subq, SC, U, IU, MTX, HCTZ, ZnSO$_4$, TAC
- Medications prescribed "as needed" should have clear indications for usage (e.g., prn mild pain, prn anxiety, prn insomnia, prn nausea)
- If more than one medication is prescribed "as needed" for the same indication, it must be very clear in what order the medications should be used (avoid therapeutic duplication)
  - Example: Milk of Magnesia 30 mL PO bid prn constipation; bisacodyl 10 mg PO daily prn constipation refractory to Milk of Magnesia
  - For "as needed" pain medications, clearly state which medication is used prn mild pain, which med is prn moderate pain, and which medication is prn severe pain
- Certain medications must state over what duration the infusion is administered
  - Potassium riders, magnesium riders, packed red blood cell transfusions
- List an indication when writing an order for radiology tests, antibiotic orders, and nuclear medicine tests (e.g., portable chest X-ray now, indication cough)

APPENDIX A19

DOCUMENTATION OF LABS AND NORMAL DRUG LEVELS

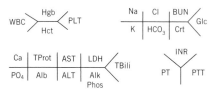

FIGURE A19.1. Standard Documentation Template for Lab Values

TABLE A19.1. Therapeutic Drug Levels

Drug	Therapeutic Levels	Drug	Therapeutic Levels
Carbamazepine	4–12 mcg/mL	Phenytoin	10–20 mcg/mL
Digoxin	0.5–2 ng/mL	Procainamide	4–10 mcg/mL
Gentamicin	4–10 mcg/mL (peak) 0.5–2 mcg/mL (trough)	Theophylline	10–20 mcg/mL
Lithium	0.5–1.3 mEq/L	Valproic acid	40–100 mcg/mL
Phenobarbital	10–40 mcg/mL	Vancomycin	10–20 mcg/mL

Source: Information available at www.globalrph.com/levels.htm.

MISCELLANEOUS TABLES AND FIGURES

TABLE A20.1. Triads of Diseases

Name	Triads
Alport's	Sensorineural deafness, progressive renal failure, and ocular anomalies
Beck's	Hypotension, JVD, and muffled heart tones in pericardial tamponade (a very insensitive triad)
Behcet's	Recurrent oral ulcers, genital ulcers, and iridocyclitis
Charcot's	Fever, jaundice, and RUQ pain in cholangitis (add AMS + shock = Reynold's pentad)
Cushing's	Bradycardia, hypertension, and irregular respirations in increased intracranial pressure
Gradenigo's	6th cranial nerve palsy, ear discharge, and retro-orbital pain in mastoiditis
Horner's	Ptosis, miosis, and anhydrosis in carotid or apical pleural disease
Hutchinson's	Interstitial keratitis, labyrinthine disease, and Hutchinson's teeth in congenital syphilis
Kartagener's	Bronchiectasis, recurrent sinusitis, and situs inversus
O'Donoghue's	Medial collateral and anterior cruciate knee ligament tears plus medial meniscus injury
Pregerson's	Lost prescription, sunglasses, and Toradol allergy in narcotic seeking
Reiter's	Arthritis, urethritis, and conjunctivitis in reactive arthritis (Reiter's disease)
Saint's	Hiatus hernia, colonic diverticula, and cholelithiasis
Sampter's	Asthma, nasal polyposis, and aspirin sensitivity
Virchow's	Trauma, hypercoagulable state, and/or immobility causing venous thromboembolic disease
Wernicke's	AMS, ataxia, and ophthalmoplegia in thiamin-deficiency encephalopathy
Whipple's	Symptoms of hypoglycemia, glucose is under 40, and prompt relief on glucose administration

Note: Many triads, though "classical," are not necessarily common

Source: Adapted from Pregerson DB *Tarascon Emergency Department Quick Reference Guide.* Sudbury, MA: Jones & Bartlett Publishing; 2011.

FIGURE A20.1. Temperature and Other Conversions

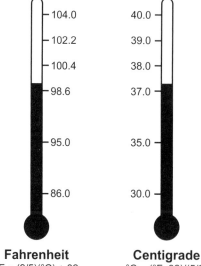

Fahrenheit
$°F = (9/5)(°C) + 32$

Centigrade
$°C = (°F-32)/(5/9)$

Source: Adapted from Pregerson DB. *Tarascon Emergency Department QuickReference Guide.*
Sudbury, MA: Jones & Bartlett Learning; 2011.

TABLE A20.2.   Eponymous Exam Signs

Eponym	Exam Finding	Disease
Adson's	Decreased radial pulse with neck turn and breath-hold	Thoracic outlet syndrome
Brudzinski's	Forced neck flexion produces hip + knee flexion	Meningitis
Cheyne-Stokes	Breathing alternates between fast and slow	CNS disease
Chvostek's	Facial spasm elicited by tapping facial nerve	Hypocalcemia
Dance's	Emptiness to palpation in RLQ	Intussusception
de Musset's	Head bobbing with each systole	Aortic insufficiency
Ewart's	Dull to percussion at L scapula	Pericardial effusion
Fathergill's	Abdomen more tender with abdomen tight/sit-up	Muscle strain
Grey Turner's	Flank ecchymosis	Retroperitoneal bleed
Hamman's	Crunching sound with each heartbeat	Pneumomediastinum
Hoffman's	Flicking tip of 3rd finger causes thumb flexion	Upper motor neuron disease
Homan's	Forced dorsiflexion of foot causes calf pain	DVT
Horner's	Ptosis, miosis, anhydrosis	Sympathetic lesion
Ishihara's	Color blindness cards	Color blindness
Janeway's	Painless red embolic hand lesions	Endocarditis
Kussmaul's	JVD increases with inspiration	Pericardial tamponade
Levine's	Clenched fist over chest	MI
Murphy's	Inspiratory splint with RUQ pressure	Cholecystitis
Nikolsky's	Lateral pressure on blister causes extension	Pemphigus, TEN, SSSS
Osler's nodes	Tender nodules on palms	Endocarditis
Phalen's	Prolonged wrist flexion causes median nerve paresthesia	Carpal tunnel syndrome
Pregerson's	Subpatella bulge with knee flexed	Knee effusion
Prehn's	Testicle pain relieved by support	Epididymitis
Psoas	Hip flexion versus resistance increases abdominal pain	Appendicitis
Quincke's	Nail bed pulsations with pressure	Aortic insufficiency
Romberg's	Falls with eyes closed	Decreased proprioception
Rovsing's	LLQ percussion causes RLQ pain	Appendicitis
Rumpel Leede	Petechiae from capillary leak after tourniquet or BP cuff	Dengue, RMSF, scarlatina
Steinberg	Thumb IP joint can project past ulnar edge of pinky	Marfan's
Thompson's	Calf squeeze does not cause plantar flexion	Achilles tendon rupture
Tinel's	Percussion of median nerve at wrist provokes parasthesia	Carpal tunnel syndrome
Traube's	Pistol shot sound at femoral artery	Aortic insufficiency
Trousseau's	Carpal spasm occurs when BP cuff inflated greater than systolic blood pressure for longer than 3 minutes	Hypocalcemia
Uhthoff's	Increased body temp causes worsening neuro sx/sn	Multiple sclerosis
Verneuil's	Distal press/percuss causes proximal pain	Fracture
Vircow's	Palpable left supraclavicular lymph node	Pancreatic or GI cancer
Von Graefe's	Lid lag with visual tracking from high to low	Grave's disease
Walker	1st and 5th digit encircling other wrist overlap proximal to DIP	Marfan's
Weber	Tuning fork to mid forehead heard asymmetrically	Hearing deficit
Yerganson's	Pain and weakness with resisted supination	Biceps tendonitis

Source: Reproduced from Pregerson DB. *Tarascon Emergency Department Quick Reference Guide*. Sudbury, MA: Jones & Bartlett Learning; 2011.

APPENDIX A21

TOP TEN LIST FOR BEING A GREAT MEDICAL STUDENT

1. Know your patients and take ownership of their care. Become the expert on your patients.
2. Come early and stay late. Never be late for rounds.
3. Be respectful and friendly to the entire medical team: attendings, residents, nurses, and ancillary staff
4. Dress professionally.
5. Be excited and enthusiastic about learning and contributing.
6. Be prepared for rounds. Always see your patients prior to rounds and formulate a plan on them (even if it is wrong).
7. Be an advocate for your patients and show genuine care for your patients as people, not just medical cases.
8. Read about your patients' medical problems daily.
9. Listen carefully to your patients. They will lead you to the answer if you let them talk. Also, do not dismiss your patients' complaints as "supratentorial" until every other possibility is excluded.
10. Take initiative. Ask your resident or attending if you can help with various tasks.

MISCELLANEOUS NEUROLOGIC TABLES AND FIGURES

TABLE A22.1.   Glasgow Coma Scale

Score	Eye Opening	Verbal Response	Motor Response
6	–	–	Follows commands
5	–	Normal conversation	Localizes pain
4	Spontaneous	Disoriented/inappropriate	Withdraws to pain
3	To voice	Incoherent	Decorticate posturing
2	To pain	Moans	Decerebrate posturing
1	None	None	No movement

Reflexes	Description
0	Absent
1+	Hypoactive
2+	Normal
3+	Hyperactive without clonus
4+	Hyperactive with clonus

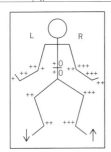

Note: large arrows at the feet represent the Babinski
reflexes of the toes and the reflexes on the trunk
represent the superficial abdominal reflexes

FIGURE A22.1.   Documentation of Deep Tendon Reflexes

TABLE A22.2.   Documentation of the Motor Exam

Grade 0/5	No muscle contraction
Grade 1/5	Muscle flicker, but no muscle movement
Grade 2/5	Muscle movement but can not lift against gravity
Grade 3/5	Can lift muscle against gravity, but not against resistance
Grade 4/5	Can move muscle against some resistance, but not full resistance
Grade 5/5	Full muscle strength

Conditions	Normal Eyes	Adie's Pupil	Argyl-Robertson	Horner's Syndrome	Mydriatic Medicine	Third Nerve Palsy
Normal light	● ●	● ●	• •	• ●	● ●	● ●
Dim light	● ●	● ●	• •	• ●	● ●	● ●
Bright light	• •	● ●	• •	• •	● •	● •
Accommodation	• •	• •	● ●	• •	● •	● ●
Pilocarpine	• •	• ●	• •	• •	● •	• •

FIGURE A22.2.   Pupillary Findings in Normal and Diseased Patients

Source: Reproduced from *Tarascon Emergency Department Quick Reference Guide* by D. Brady Pregerson.

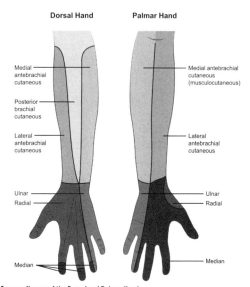

Dorsal Hand   **Palmar Hand**

Medial antebrachial cutaneous

Posterior brachial cutaneous

Lateral antebrachial cutaneous

Ulnar
Radial

Median

Medial antebrachial cutaneous (musculocutaneous)

Lateral antebrachial cutaneous

Ulnar
Radial

Median

FIGURE A22.3.   Sensory Nerves of the Dorsal and Palmar Hand

Source: Adapted from *Tarascon Emergency Department Quick Reference Guide* by D. Brady Pregerson.

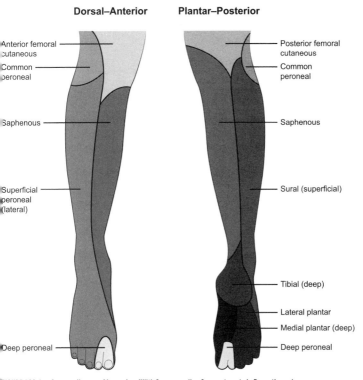

FIGURE A22.4.   Sensory Nerves of Lower Leg (With Corresponding Compartments in Parentheses)

Source: Adapted from *Tarascon Emergency Department Quick Reference Guide* by D. Brady Pregerson.

Feature A22.1   Folstein Mini-Mental Status Exam

Cognitive Screening Test

Part I: Direct Patient Testing

1. **Information for Delayed Recall Test**
    A. Give the patient a name and address to remember and recite it. Tell them to remember this information because you will ask about it again in a few minutes.
    B. Patient may have 4 attempts to correctly recite the information
    C. Example: Joe Smith, 54 Circle Drive, Dallas
    D. No points given for immediate recall

2. **Time Orientation Test**
    A. Ask the patient, "What is the date?"
    B. Patient must give the month, day, and year
    C. 1 point for an exact answer

3. **Clock Drawing Test**
    A. Give the patient a blank piece of paper
    B. Ask them to draw a clock face including all the numbers to indicate the hours of a clock
    C. Then, draw the hands of the clock to show a time of eleven fifteen (11:15)
    D. Two points possible: one point for part B and one point for part C

4. **Recent Events Test**
    A. Have the patient tell you something that has happened in the news recently (either national or local news item is acceptable)
    B. Patient must give a specific answer
    C. 1 point for a specific correct answer

5. **Delayed Recall Test**
    A. Ask the patient to recite the name and address they were asked to remember
    B. 5 points possible: 1 point each for first name, last name, street number, street name, and city

Scoring
A. A score of 9 signifies no significant impairment in cognition
B. Score of 5–8 if indeterminate; further testing is required
C. Score of 4 or below signifies cognitive impairment; further detailed testing is required to assess the degree of cognitive impairment

Part II: Family/Acquaintance Interview

Ask the friend or family member of the patient the following questions:

1. Does (name of patient) have more trouble remembering recent events now compared with before?
2. Does (name of patient) have more trouble remembering recent conversations a few days after they have happened*?
3. Has (name of patient) had more trouble recently finding the right word to say or use wrong words while speaking?
4. Is (name of patient) less capable of managing his/her finances recently†?
5. Is (name of patient) less capable of managing his/her medications recently†?
6. Does (name of patient) need more help with transportation to and from places†?

* Trouble remembering is due to cognitive impairment and not hearing impairment
† Trouble is due to cognitive impairment and not visual impairment
‡ Trouble is due to cognitive impairment and not physical impairment requiring assistance

Scoring
A. Each question can be answered "yes," "no," "don't know," or "not applicable"
B. Give 1 point to all answers that are either "no," "don't know," or "not applicable"
C. A total score of 0–3 indicates that cognitive impairment is present and that further detailed testing is indicated

Source: Adapted from *J Amer Geriatric Society*, 2002; Vol 50 (Issue 3): 530–34.

SNELLEN EYE CHART

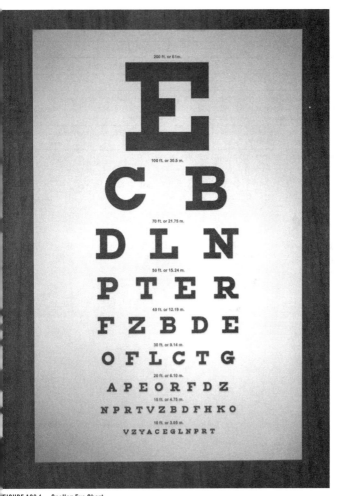

FIGURE A23.1.   Snellen Eye Chart
Source: © iStockphoto/Thinkstock

APPENDIX A24

PROPHYLAXIS FOR HOSPITALIZED ADULTS

TABLE A24.1. Risk Factors for Venous Thromboembolic Events in Hospitalized Patients

Advanced age older than 50 yo	Recent prolonged travel
Prolonged immobility	Major surgery in last 4 weeks
Recent trauma	Inflammatory bowel disease
Previous VTE	Central venous catheter

Medical conditions: severe burns, active cancer, stroke with paresis, inherited thrombophilia, polycythemia, myeloproliferative disorder, obesity, CHF, nephrotic syndrome, inflammatory bowel disease, acute MI, acute respiratory failure, sickle cell disease, paroxysmal nocturnal hemoglobinuria, and pregnancy

Medications: tamoxifen, raloxifene, thalidomide, lenalidomide, darbepoetin, epoetin α, bevacizumab, hormone replacement therapy, or systemic chemotherapy

Source: Information from *Arch Intern Med*, 2002; 162(11): 1245–8 and *NEJM*, 2001; 344(16): 1222–31.

TABLE A24.2.   Regimens for DVT Prophylaxis in Medical and Surgical Patients

Category	Options for DVT Prophylaxis
Low-risk patients • Age younger than 40, minor surgery*, no risk factors (RFs)†	• Early ambulation • Leg exercises
Moderate-risk patients • Minor surgery and RFs† • Surgery in pts 40–60 yo • Major surgery‡ and no RFs†	• Heparin§ 5000 U SQ q 8 h started 2 h preop • LMWH‖ (see dosing below) • Fondaparinux¶ 2.5 mg SQ daily • GCS or IPC
High-risk patients • Surgery, 40–60 yo and RFs† • Surgery older than 60 yo • Major surgery‡ younger than 40 yo and RFs† • High-risk medical patient†	• Heparin§ 5000 U SQ q 8 h started 2 h preop • LMWH‖ (see dosing below) • Fondaparinux¶ 2.5 mg SQ daily • GCS or IPC
Highest-risk patients • Major surgery‡ older than 40 yo and RFs† • THA, TKA, or HFS • Major trauma# • Spinal cord injury# • Critically ill medical patient	• Heparin§ 5000 U SQ q 8 h started 2 h preop • LMWH‖ (see dosing below) • Fondaparinux¶ 2.5 mg SQ daily • (Warfarin titrated to INR 2–3 option for THA or TKA) PLUS IPC
Moderate–high risk patients at high risk for bleeding	• GCS or IPC until bleeding risk is low • Initiate thromboprophylaxis when bleeding risk low

GCS = graduated compression stockings, IPC = intermittent pneumatic compression devices, THA = total hip arthroplasty, TKA = total knee arthroplasty, HFS = hip fracture surgery

* Eye, ear, dermatologic, laparoscopic, or arthroscopic operations

† Severe burns, immobility, prior VTE, active cancer, stroke with paresis, inherited thrombophilia, polycythemia, myeloproliferative disorder, obesity, CHF, nephrotic syndrome, inflammatory bowel disease, acute MI, acute respiratory failure, sickle cell disease, paroxysmal nocturnal hemoglobinuria, pregnancy, recent trauma, central venous catheter, mechanical ventilation, severe sepsis, shock, and use of the following meds: tamoxifen, raloxifene, thalidomide, lenalidomide, darbepoetin, epoetin α, bevacizumab, hormone replacement therapy, or systemic chemotherapy

‡ Thoracic, intraperitoneal, bariatric, open urologic, and gynecologic, cardiac, neurosurgical, and cancer operations

§ Caution starting heparin if initial PLT less than 50K and discontinue if PLT count falls 50% or more or to less than 100K

‖ LMWH = low molecular weight heparins: enoxaparin 40 mg SQ daily starting 1–2 h preop or 30 mg SQ q 12 h starting 12–24 h postop; dalteparin 2500 units SQ starting 1–2 h preop and 6–8 h postop, then 5000 units SQ daily (not approved for TKR); tinzaparin 75 units/kg SQ daily starting 10–12 h before THR/TKR; dosage adjustment required for CrCl 15–30 mL/min and adjust dose based on anti-FactorXa levels if weight exceeds 155 kg; avoid if CrCl is less than 15 mL/min; caution if initial platelet is less than 50K and discontinue if platelets fall by 50% or more or to a level less than 100K

¶ Give 6–8 h postop; avoid if CrCl is less than 30 mL/min, weight under 50 kg, thrombocytopenia with positive antiplatelet antibodies, epidural infusions, or endocarditis; no antidote if active bleeding develops; $T_{1/2}$ ~18 h

Thromboprophylaxis can generally be started within 36 h of major trauma or spinal cord injury unless intracranial bleeding, active internal bleeding, perispinal hematoma, or uncorrected coagulopathy present

Source: Adapted from *Chest.* 2012;141(Suppl 2):e227S–77S.

TABLE A24.3.   Staging and Treatment of Pressure Ulcers

Stage	Description	Treatment
I	Nonblanchable erythema of intact skin	Turn pt side-to-side at an oblique angle q 2 h, keep head of bed within 30°
II	Skin loss involving epidermis with or without dermis	Above, nonocclusive moist dressing, pressure-reducing devices*
III	Full thickness skin loss to subcutaneous tissue up to the level of the fascia	Above; debridement; hydrogel, alginate, hydrocolloid, or moistened gauze dressings
IV	Full thickness skin loss through fascia	Above, debridement, and surgical repair

* Static devices: foam, air mattress or mattress overlays; benefit of dynamic devices is unclear

Source: Adapted from *AFP*, 2008; 78(10): 1186–94.

1. <u>**RISK FACTORS FOR DECUBITUS ULCERS**</u>

- Malnutrition, immobility, dry skin, low body weight, multiple medical comorbidities, immunosuppression, coma, excessive local moisture, and lymphopenia

EQUATIONS

TABLE A25.1. Statistical Equations

		Disease Condition		
		Present	Absent	
Test	Positive	True positive (TP)	False positive (FP)	**Positive predictive value (PPV)**
	Negative	False negative (FN)	True negative (TN)	**Negative predictive value (PPV)**
		Sensitivity	Specificity	

SENSITIVITY

- Sensitivity $= TP/(TP + FN)$
- Sensitivity relates to the test's ability to identify positive results
- It refers to the proportion of people who have a disease and who test positive for the test
- Mnemonic is **"SNOUT"**: **SEN**sitive tests rule **OUT** disease
  - Negative result in sensitive test "rules out" disease

SPECIFICITY

- Specificity $= TN/(TN + FP)$
- Specificity relates to the test's ability to identify negative results
- It refers to the proportion of people who do **not** have a disease and who test negative for the test
- Mnemonic is **"SPIN"**: **SP**ecific tests rule **IN** disease
  - Positive result for a very specific test "rules in" the disease

POSITIVE PREDICTIVE VALUE (PPV)

- Positive predictive value $= TP/(TP + FP)$
- PPV is the proportion of people who test positive for a test who have a disease

NEGATIVE PREDICTIVE VALUE

- Negative predictive value $= TN/(TN + FN)$
- NPV is the proportion of people who test negative for a test who do **not** have a disease

APPENDIX A26

URINALYSIS INTERPRETATION

TABLE A26.1. Interpretation of Urine Dipstick

Category	Causes of Positive or Elevated Result
pH	Stones, RTA, infection
Protein	Detects albuminuria
RBC	Detects hematuria or myoglobinuria
Leukocyte esterase	Detects inflammation or infection
Ketones	Detects acetoacetate but not β-hydroxybutyrate
Nitrite	Detects presence of Gram-negative bacilli
Bilirubin	Elevated in hepatobiliary disease
Glucose	Elevated in hyperglycemia, pregnancy, and Fanconi syndrome

TABLE A26.2. Interpretation of Urinary Sediment

Category	Causes of Positive Result
RBC	Stones, infection, CA, trauma, renal infarct, glomerulonephritis (dysmorphic)
WBC	Infection, AIN, chronic cystitis
Epithelial cells	Skin contamination from clean catch specimen
Transitional cells	Bladder or ureteral dysplasia or cancer
RBC casts	Glomerulonephritis
WBC casts	AIN or pyelonephritis
Granular casts	ATN
Hyaline casts	Prerenal azotemia
Waxy casts	Prerenal azotemia
Crystals	Calcium oxalate, uric acid, cystine, or struvite crystals

Source: Adapted from *Am J Kidney Dis*, 2008; 51(6): 1052–67.

PERIPHERAL BLOOD SMEAR

INTERPRETATION OF WHITE BLOOD COUNT DIFFERENTIAL

- Dohle bodies, toxic granulations, or cytoplasmic vacuoles
  - 80% sensitivity for chronic inflammatory or infectious process
- Basophilia: chronic basophilic leukemia or myeloproliferative disorders
- Blasts: leukemia or lymphoma
- Auer rods: acute myelogenous leukemia
- Hypersegmented neutrophils: Vitamin B_{12} or folate deficiency
- Lymphocytosis
  - Reactive from viral infection or acute or chronic lymphocytic leukemia
  - If peripheral blood smear equivocal, differentiate by flow cytometry of blood
- Polycythemia suggests polycythemia vera especially with eosinophilia, thrombocytosis, microcytic indices, low erythropoietin levels, and Janus Kinase 2 (JAK2) mutation-positive
- Thrombocytosis
  - Infection, chronic inflammation, solid organ malignancy, myeloproliferative disorder, asplenia, iron-deficiency anemia, hemolysis, or acute bleeds
- Monocytosis: steroid use, pregnancy, asplenia, granulomatous disease, metastatic CA, chronic myelo-monocytic leukemia, lymphoma, radiation therapy, or post-MI
- Hypereosinophilic syndromes: absolute eosinophil count greater than 1500/mm³ for more than 6 months and end-organ dysfunction
  - Etiologies include hypereosinophilic syndrome, clonal eosinophilia, eosinophilic leukemia, Churg-Strauss syndrome, eosinophilic gastroenteritis or pneumonia, or helminthic infections (ascariasis, hookworms, strongyloides, trichinosis, visceral larva migrans, loiasis, onchocerciasis, schistosomiasis, clonorchiasis, paragonimiasis, fascioliasis, and fasciolopsiasis)

INTERPRETATION OF RED BLOOD CELL ABNORMALITIES

- Anisocytosis
- Poikilocytosis
- Spur cells: liver disease
- Bite cells: G6PD deficiency
- Pencil cells: advanced iron-deficiency disease
- Rouleaux formation: myeloma
- Schistocytes: microangiopathic hemolytic anemia
- Spherocytes: autoimmune hemolytic anemia
- Sickle cells: sickle cell anemia
- Stomatocytes: liver disease, alcohol abuse
- Target cells: liver disease, prior splenectomy, hemoglobinopathies
- Tear drop cells: myelofibrosis, myelophthisic anemia, thalassemia
- Basophilic stippling: sideroblastic anemia, megaloblastic anemia
- Heinz bodies: G6PD deficiency, thalassemia
- Howell-Jolly bodies: prior splenectomy or functional asplenia
- Nucleated RBC: hemolysis, extramedullary hematopoiesis

REFERENCES

Mayo Clin Proc, 2005;80(7):923–36.

INDEX

A

Abdominal pain, acute, 95–97
Abdominal x-ray interpretation, 391
Acetaminophen overdose, 401–402
Acid-base disorder, 313–314
Acidosis, 313–314
ACLS (advanced cardiovascular life
    support), 363–369
Acute abdominal pain, 95–97
Acute arterial insufficiency, 54
Acute back pain, 332–335
Acute cholangitis, 131, 133–134
Acute cholecystitis, 131–133
Acute diarrhea, 104–105
Acute hemorrhagic stroke, 230–233
Acute hepatitis, 110–113
Acute ischemic stroke, 225–229
Acute kidney injury, 319–322
Acute monoarticular arthritis, 331
Acute pain control, 406–410
Acute pancreatitis, 120–122
Acute pericarditis, 36–38
Admission order, format for, 370
Adrenal insufficiency, 79–81
Advanced cardiovascular life support
    (ACLS), 363
AIHA (autoimmune hemolytic
    anemia), 140
Alcohol
    intoxication, 402
    withdrawal syndrome, 357–358
Alkalosis, 313–314
Allergic/hypersensitivity reaction, 253
Alopecia, 253
Altered mental status in cancer
    patient, 277
Alzheimer's dementia, 234–235
Amphetamine withdrawal, 360
Analgesia. See Pain management
Anemia, 137–143
Angina, 3–7, 12–15
Antibiotics, 392–398. See also Infectious
    disease
Anticholinergic toxidrome, 400
Anticoagulation, perioperative, 157–159
Antidepressant toxicity, tricyclic, 403
Antiepileptic, 240
Antirheumatic drug,
    disease-modifying, 346
Antithrombotic, 25, 157–159
Aortic balloon valvotomy, 41
Aortic insufficiency, 39, 40, 42
Aortic stenosis, 39, 40
Aortic valve replacement, 41, 42
Arm sign, 5
Arrhythmia
    atrial fibrillation, 23–29
    bradyarrhythmia, 30–35, 366
    narrow-complex tachycardia, 367–369
    supraventricular tachycardia, 368
    ventricular fibrillation, 365
    ventricular tachycardia, 365
    wide-complex tachycardia, 369
Arthritis
    monoarticular, acute, 331
    polyarticular, 336–340
    rheumatoid, 341–348
    septic, 215–216

Ascites, 116–118
Aspergillus infection, 185, 204–210
Asthma, 298–302
Atrial fibrillation, 23–29
Autoimmune hemolytic anemia
    (AIHA), 140

B

Back pain, acute, 332–335
Bacterial respiratory disease, 178
Barrett's esophagus, 125–126
Bartonella infection, 180
Basic life support (BSL), 363
BBRACES criteria for syncope risk
    stratification, 63
Benzodiazepine overdose, 400
Biliary tract disorder, 131–134
Bleeding disorders, 144–145
Bone infection, 211–216
Boston criteria for heart failure, 17
Bowel
    disease, ischemic, 123–124
    obstruction, 129–130
Bradyarrhythmia, 30–35, 366
Brain metastasis, 281–282
Breast cancer, 257–259
BSL (basic life support), 363

C

Calcium
    disorder, 82–84
    repletion, 404
Calcium channel blocker
    toxicity, 402
Calcium stone, 329
Campylobacteriosis, 179
Cancer
    breast, 257–259
    chemotherapy, adverse effects of,
        253–256, 283–284
    colorectal, 260–262
    emergencies, 277–284
    leukemia, chronic, 263–265
    lung, 272–274
    lymphoma, 266–269
    multiple myeloma, 270–271
    prostate, 275–276
Candidiasis, 171–172, 181–183,
    204–210
Cardiac apex, displaced, 17
Cardiac device for heart failure, 20
Cardiomyopathy, 253
Cardiovascular disease. See also
    Arrhythmia
    cardiomyopathy, 253
    chest pain (angina), 3–7, 12–15
    congestive heart failure, 16–22
    evaluation, perioperative, 46–48
    heart failure, 9
    hypertension, 49–53
    myocardial infarction, 8–15
    non-st elevation acute coronary
        syndrome (NSTEMI), 12–15
    pericarditis, acute, 36–38
    peripheral arterial disease, 54–56
    shock, 57–60

    st elevation myocardial infarction
        (STEMI), 8–11
    syncope, 61–64
    valvular heart disease, 39–45
Cardioversion, 28
Catheter insertion, 377–379
Catheter-related bloodstream infection
    (CRABSI), 217–218
Cellulitis, 212
Central nervous system
    mass lesion, 169
    neurotoxicity, 195
Chagas disease, 195
Channelopathy, 242
Chemotherapy, adverse effects of,
    253–256, 283–284
Chest pain, 3–7
Chest x-ray, interpretation of, 389–390
Cholangitis, acute, 131, 133–134
Cholecystitis, acute, 131–133
Choledocholithiasis, 131, 133
Cholinergic toxidrome, 400
Chronic arterial insufficiency, 54–55
Chronic cough, 287–289
Chronic diarrhea, 105–107
Chronic kidney disease, 323–327
Chronic leukemia, 263–265
Chronic obstructive pulmonary disease
    (COPD) exacerbation, 303–305
Cirrhosis, 114–119
Clotting cascade, bleeding disorder, 144
CMV (cytomegalovirus) disease, 186–187
Coagulation, 144–145
Cocaine withdrawal, 360
Coccidioidomycosis, 185, 204–210
Cognitive screening test, 420
Colitis
    ischemic, 123–124
    ulcerative, 107–109
Colorectal cancer, 260–262
Complex partial seizure, 239
Congestive heart failure, 16–22
Constipation, 253
COPD (chronic obstructive pulmonary
    disease) exacerbation, 303–305
Coronary angiography, 6–7
Corticosteroid, 108, 405
Cough, chronic, 287–289
CRABSI (catheter-related bloodstream
    infection), 217–218
Crohn's disease, 107–109
Cryptococcal meningitis, HIV-positive
    patients, 183
Cryptosporidiosis, 174
Cvostek's sign, 83
Cystine stone, 329
Cystitis, 222–223
Cytomegalovirus (CMV) disease,
    186–187

D

Decubitus ulcer, 424
Deep tendon reflex, documentation
    of, 417
Deep vein thrombosis, 153–156, 423
Delirium, 236–237
Dementia, 234–235

Dermatomal map, 247
Diabetes mellitus, 67–71, 313–314
Diarrhea, 104–109
Diarrhea, chemotherapy, 253
Diffuse interstitial lung disease,
    308–309
Diffuse large b-cell lymphoma
    (DLBCL), 268
Discharge summary, format for, 374
Disease-modifying antirheumatic
    drugs, 346
Disease triad, 413
Diverticulitis, 127–128
DLBCL (diffuse large b-cell
    lymphoma), 268
Documentation, 412
Dressler syndrome, 11
Drug levels, normal, 412
Ductal carcinoma in situ, 257–259
Dysphagia, 125
Dyspnea, 290–291

E
Echocardiogram interpretation, 386–388
Electrocardiogram interpretation,
    386–388
Electrolyte repletion, 404
Empiric antibiotic, 392–394
Endocarditis, infective, 163–166
Endocrine disease
    adrenal insufficiency, 79–81
    calcium disorder, 82–84
    diabetes mellitus, 67–71
    panhypopituitarism, 91–92
    potassium disorder, 88–90
    SIADH, 254
    sodium disorder, 85–87
    thyroid disorder, 72–75, 76–78
Epidural analgesia, 410
Epileptic seizure, 238–241
Erysipelas, 212
Esophageal disorder, 125–126
Exam sign, eponymous, 415
Examination. See Physical exam
Extravasation reaction, 253
Eye chart, 421
Eye infection, 172

F
Fever, 161, 282
Fibrillation
    atrial, 23–29
    ventricular, 365
5-aminosalicylic acid derivative, 108
Folate dyscrasia, 125–126
Follicular lymphoma, 268
Folstein mini-mental status exam, 420
Frontotemporal dementia, 234–235
Fungal infection, invasive, 204–210

G
Gastroenterological disease
    abdominal pain, acute, 95–97
    biliary tract disorder, 131–134
    bowel obstruction, 129–130
    cirrhosis, 114–119
    diarrhea, 104–109
    diverticulitis, 127–128
    esophageal disorder, 125–126
    gastrointestinal bleeding, 98–100,
        101–103
    hepatitis, acute, 110–113
    HIV-positive patients, 171–172
    infection, 171–172

    ischemic bowel disease, 123–124
    pancreatitis, acute, 120–122
Gastroesophageal reflux disease (GERD),
    5, 125
Gastrointestinal bleeding
    lower, 101–103
    upper, 98–100
Gastrointestinal infection, 171–172
GBS (Guillain-Barre syndrome),
    247–248, 251
GERD (gastroesophageal reflux
    disease), 125
Glasgow coma scale, 417
Grand mal seizure, 239
Gram-stain interpretation, 399
Guillain-Barre syndrome (GBS),
    247–248, 251
Gynecomastia, 253

H
Hand innervation, 418
HBV (hepatitis B virus) infection, 191
HCV (hepatitis C virus) infection, 192
Healthcare-associated pneumonia,
    202–203
Heart disease. See Cardiovascular disease
Heart failure, 5, 16–22
Hematological disease
    anemia, 137–143
    anticoagulation, 157–159
    bleeding disorder, 144–145
    pancytopenia, 146
    sickle cell anemia, 142–143
    thrombocytopenia, 147–150
    venous thromboembolism, 151–156
Hematuria, 315–316
Hemolytic anemia, 137, 140–141
Hemoptysis, 292–294
Hemorrhagic cystitis, 253
Hemorrhagic stroke, acute, 230–233
Heparin-induced thrombocytopenia,
    148–149
Hepatic encephalopathy, 117
Hepatic hydrothorax, 118
Hepatitis
    acute, 110, 112–113
    B virus (HBV), 191
    C virus (HCV), 192
Hepatojugular reflux, 17
Hepatopulmonary syndrome, 117–118
Hepatorenal syndrome, 117
Hepatotoxicity, 253
Herpes simplex virus (HSV) infection,
    187–188
HHV (human herpesvirus) infection,
    188, 190
HIV-positive patient, infection in
    aspergillosis, invasive, 185
    bacterial respiratory disease, 178
    Bartonella, 180
    Campylobacteriosis, 179
    candidiasis, 181–183
    central nervous system mass
        lesion, 169
    Chagas disease, 195
    coccidioidomycosis, 185
    cryptosporidiosis, 174
    cytomegalovirus disease, 186–187
    gastrointestinal, 171–172
    hepatitis, 191, 192
    herpes simplex virus, 187–188
    histoplasmosis, 184
    human herpesvirus, 188, 190

    human papillomavirus, 190
    Isospora belli, 195
    leishmaniasis, 194–195
    malaria, 193–194
    meningitis, cryptococcal, 183
    meningoencephalitis, 168–169
    microsporidiosis, 175
    mycobacterium avium complex
        disease, 177
    ocular, 172
    pathophysiology, 167
    penicilliosis, 194
    pneumonia, 170–171, 173
    progressive multifocal
        leukoencephalopathy, 192
    pulmonary infection, 170–171
    Salmonellosis, 179
    Shigellosis, 179
    syphilis, 180–181
    Toxoplasma gondii encephalitis, 174
    tuberculosis, 176
    Varicella zoster virus, 189
Hodgkin's lymphoma, 266–269
Hospital-acquired pneumonia, 202–203
Hospital admission order, format for, 370
HPV (human papillomavirus)
    infection, 190
HSV (herpes simplex virus) infection,
    187–188
Human herpesvirus (HHV) infection,
    188, 190
Human papillomavirus (HPV) infection, 190
Hypercalcemia, 82–83, 281
Hypercalcemic crisis, 83, 281
Hyperglycemia, 67
Hyperkalemia, 89–90
Hypernatremia, 86–87
Hyperparathyroidism, 83, 313–314
Hypertension
    coronary, 49–53
    pulmonary, 310–311
Hypertensive emergency, 53
Hypertensive urgency, 52
Hyperthyroidism, 72–74
Hyperviscosity syndrome, 277–278
Hypocalcemia, 83–84
Hypogonadism, 253
Hypokalemia, 88
Hyponatremia, 85–86
Hypopituitarism, 91–92
Hypothyroidism, 76–78

I
Immunomodulating drugs, 108–109
Infectious disease. See also Antibiotic;
    HIV-positive patient, infection in
    antibiotic coverage by class, 395–398
    bone, 211–216
    catheter-related bloodstream
        infection, 217–218
    cystitis, 222–223
    empiric antibiotics for common
        infections, 392–394
    endocarditis, infective, 163–166
    fever, 161
    fungal infection, invasive, 204–210
    infective endocarditis, 163–166
    joints, 211–216
    meningitis, 196–199
    pneumonia, 200–203
    pyelonephritis, 222–223
    skin, 211–216
    soft tissue, 211–216
    tuberculosis, 219–221
    urinary tract infection, 222–223

Infective endocarditis, 163–166
Inflammatory bowel disease, 107–109
Inflammatory breast cancer, 259
Inflammatory pain syndrome, 410
Interstitial lung disease, diffuse, 308–309
Interventricular septum rupture, 10
Invasive breast cancer, 259
Ischemic bowel disease, 123–124
Ischemic colitis, 123–124
Ischemic stroke, acute, 225–229
Isospora belli infection, 195

J
Jaundice, painless, 131, 132
Joint infection, 211–216
Jugular venous distention, 17

K
Kidney disease. *See* Renal disease

L
Laboratory values, documentation of, 412
LACI (lacunar infarct), 226
Lacunar infarct (LACI), 226
Large vessel vasculitis, 352–355
Left ventricular aneurysm, 11
Left ventricular mural thrombus, 11
Left ventricular wall rupture, 10
Leg innervation, 419
Leishmaniasis, 194–195
Leukemia, chronic, 263–265
Levine sign, 5
LGIB (lower gastrointestinal bleeding), 101–103
Lower gastrointestinal bleeding (LGIB), 101–103
Lower leg innervation, 419
Lung cancer, 272–274
Lung disease, diffuse interstitial, 308–309
Lupus erythematous, systemic, 349–351
Lymphoma, 266–269

M
MAC (mycobacterium avium complex) disease, 177
Macrocytic anemia, 137
Magnesium repletion, 404
Malaria, 193–194
Malignant spinal cord compression, 278
Medical student, advice for, 416
Medium vessel vasculitis, 352–355
Meningitis, 183, 198–199
Meningoencephalitis, 168–169
Mental status, altered, 277
Mesenteric ischemia, 123–124
Metastatic breast cancer, 259
MGC (myasthenia gravis crisis), 248–249, 251
Microcytic anemia, 137
Microsporidiosis, 175
Mitral regurgitation, 10, 39–40, 44
Mitral stenosis, 39, 40, 43
Mitral valve repair/replacement, 44
Monoarticular arthritis, acute, 331
Motor exam documentation, 418
Mucositis, 253
Multiple myeloma, 270–271
Multiple sclerosis, 249–250, 251
Murmur, heart, 39–40
Myasthenia gravis crisis (MGC), 248–249, 251

Mycobacterium avium complex (MAC) disease, 177
Myelosuppression, 253
Myocardial infarction, 5, 8–15
Myopathy, 242, 245, 250–251
Myxedema coma, 76, 78

N
Narrow-complex tachycardia, 367
Necrotizing soft tissue infection (NSTI), 213–214
Negative predictive value (NPV), 425
Neisseria meningitidis, 196
Nephrolithiasis, 328–329
Nephrotic syndrome, 317–318
Nephrotoxicity, 253
Nerve, sensory, 418, 419
Neurological disorder
  delirium, 236–237
  dementia, 234–235
  seizures, 238–241
  stroke, 225–233
  weakness, 242–251
Neutropenic fever, 282
Non-Hodgkin's lymphoma, 266–269
Non-small cell lung cancer (NSCLC), 272–274
Non ST-elevation acute coronary syndrome (NSTEMI), 12–15
Nonimmune-mediated hemolytic anemia, 141
Normocytic anemia, 137, 139–141
NPV (negative predictive value), 425
NSCLC (non-small cell lung cancer), 272–274
NSTEMI (non st-elevation acute coronary syndrome), 12–15
NSTI (necrotizing soft tissue infection), 213–214

O
Obstructed bowel, 129–130
Ocular infection, 172
Oncological disease. *See* Cancer
Opiate withdrawal syndrome, 359
Opioid
  overdose, 400
  side effect management, 409
Order writing, 411
Osteomyelitis, 214–215
Ototoxicity, 253
Overdose, 400–403
Oxfordshire Ischemic Stroke Subtypes, 225–226

P
PACI (partial anterior circulation infarct), 225
Pain management, acute, 406–410
Pain syndrome, inflammatory, 410
Painless jaundice, 131, 132
Palm sign, 5
Palmar-plantar dysesthesia, 253
Pancreatitis, acute, 120–122
Pancytopenia, 146
Panhypopituitarism, 91–92
Paraneoplastic syndrome, 282–283
Parkinson's disease, 234–235
Partial anterior circulation infarct (PACI), 225
Patient-controlled analgesia (PCA), 409
Patient history, format for, 371
PCA (patient-controlled analgesia), 409

Penicilliosis, 194
Peptic ulcer disease, 99–100
Percutaneous mitral balloon valvotomy, 43
Pericarditis, 11
Pericarditis, acute, 36–38
Perioperative cardiovascular evaluation, 48
Peripheral arterial disease, 54–56
Peripheral blood smear interpretation, 425
Peripheral neuropathy
  chemotherapeutic agents, adverse effect of, 253
  weakness, 242, 244–245, 246, 250
Phosphorus repletion, 404
Physical exam
  eponymous signs, 415
  format for, 371
  motor, 418
Pleural effusion, 295–297
Plexopathy, 242, 251
Pneumonia, 5, 170–171, 173, 200–203
POCI (posterior circulation infarct), 226
Pointing sign, 5
Poisonings, 400–403
Polyarticular arthritis, 336–340
Portopulmonary hypertension, 118
Positive predictive value (PPV), 425
Posterior circulation infarct (POCI), 226
Potassium
  disorder, 88–90
  repletion, 404
PPV (positive predictive value), 425
Pregnancy in sickle cell anemia, 143
Prescription writing, 411
Pressure ulcer, 424
Procedure note template
  central venous catheter
    femoral, 379
    internal jugular, 378
    subclavian, 377
  endotracheal intubation, 384
  general requirements, 375
  lumbar puncture, 382
  paracentesis, 381
  radial arterial line insertion, 376
  Swan-Ganz catheter, 385
  thoracentesis, 380
  tube thoracostomy, 383
Progressive multifocal leukoencephalopathy, 192
Prophylaxis, 422–424
Prostate cancer, 275–276
Prosthesis-associated osteomyelitis, 215
Pulmonary disease
  asthma, 298–302
  chronic cough, 287–289
  COPD, 303–305
  diffuse interstitial lung disease, 308–309
  dyspnea, 290–291
  hemoptysis, 292–294
  pleural effusion, 295–297
  pulmonary embolism, 5, 153–156
  pulmonary evaluation and management, 306–307
  pulmonary hypertension, 310–311
Pulmonary embolism, 5, 153–156
Pulmonary evaluation and management, perioperative, 306–307
Pulmonary hypertension, 310–311
Pulmonary infection, 170–171
Pulmonary toxicity, 253
Pulseless arrest algorithm, 364
Pupillary finding, 418
Pyelonephritis, 222–223

R
Radiation therapy, adverse effects of, 283–284
Radiculopathy, 242, 251
Red blood cell abnormality, 427
Reflex, deep tendon, 417
Renal disease
    acid-base disorder, 313–314
    acute kidney injury, 319–322
    chronic kidney disease, 323–327
    hematuria, 315–316
    nephrolithiasis, 328–329
    nephrotic syndrome, 317–318
Reset osmostat, 86
Respiratory disease. *See* Pulmonary disease
Rheumatoid arthritis, 341–348
Rheumatological disease
    arthritis, 215–216, 331, 336–348
    back pain, acute, 332–335
    lupus erythematous, systemic, 349–351
    septic arthritis, 215–216
    vasculitis, systemic, 352–355

S
Salicylate toxicity, 402
Salmonellosis, 179
SBP (spontaneous bacterial peritonitis), 116–117
SCLC (small cell lung cancer), 272–274
Secondary generalized partial seizure, 239
Seizures, 238–241
Sensitivity, 425
Sensory nerve, 418, 419
Septic arthritis, 215–216
Shigellosis, 179
Shock, 57–60
SIADH (syndrome of inappropriate antidiuretic hormone secretion), 86, 254, 282
Sick cell syndrome, 86
Sickle cell anemia, 142–143
Simple partial seizure, 239
Skin
    infection, 211–216
    rash and discoloration, 253
Small cell lung cancer (SCLC), 272–274
Small vessel vasculitis, 352–355
Snellen eye chart, 421
SOAP progress note, format for, 372

Sodium disorder, 85–87
Soft tissue infection, 211–216
Specificity, 425
Spinal cord compression, malignant, 278
Spinal root lesion, 246
Spontaneous bacterial peritonitis (SBP), 116–117
ST-elevation myocardial infarction (STEMI), 8–11
Staghorn calculi, 329
Staphylococcal infection, 211–212
Statistical equation, 425
Status epilepticus, 238
STEMI (st-elevation myocardial infarction), 8–11
Stomatitis, 253
Streptococcal infection, 196, 211–212
Stroke, 225–229, 230–233
Struvite calculi, 329
Substance abuse abstinence disorder
    alcohol, 357–358
    opiate withdrawal syndrome, 359
    sympathomimetic withdrawal syndrome, 360
Superior vena cava syndrome, 278–279
Supraventricular tachycardia, 368
Surgical site infection, 213
Swan-ganz catheter insertion, 385
Sympathomimetic toxidrome, 400
Sympathomimetic withdrawal syndrome, 360
Syncope, 61–64
Syndrome of inappropriate antidiuretic hormone secretion (SIADH), 86, 254, 282
Syphilis, 180–181
Systemic lupus erythematous, 349–351
Systemic vasculitis, 352–355

T
Tachycardia
    narrow-complex, 367–369
    supraventricular, 368
    ventricular, 365
    wide-complex, 369
TACI (total anterior circulation infarct), 225
TE (*Toxoplasma gondii* encephalitis), 174
Temperature conversion chart, 414
Thrombocytopenia, 147–150
Thyroid disorder, 76–78
Thyroid storm, 72, 74

Total anterior circulation infarct (TACI), 225
Toxidromes, 400–403
    antidotes, 401
Toxoplasma gondii encephalitis (TE), 174
Transfer summary, format for, 373
Treadmill testing, 7
Triad of disease, 413
Tricyclic antidepressant toxicity, 403
Trousseau's sign, 83
Tuberculosis, 176, 219–221
Tumor lysis syndrome (TLS), 279–280

U
UGIB (upper gastrointestinal bleeding), 98–100
Ulcer, pressure, 424
Ulcerative colitis, 107–109
Unstable angina, 12–15
Upper gastrointestinal bleeding (UGIB), 98–100
Urate stone, 329
Urinalysis interpretation, 426
Urinary tract infection, 222–223

V
Valvular heart disease, 39–45
Varicella zoster virus (VZV) infection, 189
Vascular dementia, 234–235
Vascular disease. *See* Cardiovascular disease
Vasculitis, systemic, 352–355
Venous thromboembolism, 151–156, 422
Ventricular fibrillation, 365
Ventricular tachycardia, 365
Vertebral osteomyelitis, 215
Vision chart, 421
Vomiting from chemotherapy, 254
VZV (varicella zoster virus) infection, 189

W
Weakness, 242–251
White blood cell count differential, 427
Wide-complex tachycardia, 369
Withdrawal syndrome, 357–360

X
X-ray interpretation, 389–391